Teach Yourself
VISUAL
Weight Training

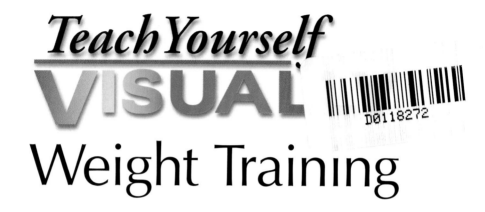

Visual

From
maranGraphics®

&

Wiley Publishing, Inc.

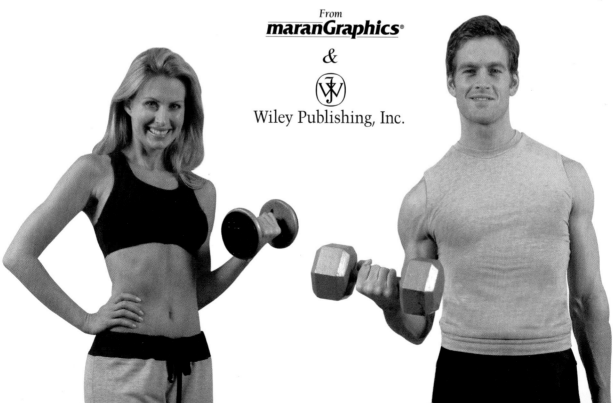

Teach Yourself VISUALLY™ Weight Training

Published by
Wiley Publishing, Inc.
909 Third Avenue
New York, NY 10022

Published simultaneously in Canada

Library of Congress Control Number:

ISBN: 0-7645-2582-4

Manufactured in the United States of America

10 9 8 7 6 5 4

1K/QR/QV/QT/MG

Trademark Acknowledgments

Important Numbers

For U.S. corporate orders, please call maranGraphics at 800-469-6616 or fax 905-890-9434.

For general information on our products and services, please contact our Customer Care Department within the U.S. at 800-762-2974, outside the U.S. at 317-572-3993 or fax 317-572-4002.

Permissions

Food Guide Pyramid

U.S. Department of Agriculture (USDA) and the U.S. Department of Health and Human Services (DHHS).

Wiley Publishing, Inc.   is a trademark of Wiley Publishing, Inc.

U.S. Corporate Sales

Contact maranGraphics at (800) 469-6616 or fax (905) 890-9434.

U.S. Trade Sales

Contact Wiley at (800) 762-2974 or fax (317) 572-4002.

VISUAL TESTIMONIALS

"I write to extend my
thanks and appreciation
for your books.
They are clear, easy to follow,
and straight to the point.
Keep up the good work!
I bought several of your books
and they are just right!
No regrets! I will always
buy your books because
they are the best."

Seward Kollie
Dakar, Senegal

"I just had to let you and
your company know how
great I think your books are.
I just purchased my third
Visual book (my first two
are dog-eared now!) and,
once again, your product has
surpassed my expectations.
The expertise, thought, and
effort that go into each book
are obvious, and I sincerely
appreciate your efforts.
Keep up the wonderful work!"

Tracey Moore
Memphis, TN

"I am an avid fan of
your Visual books.
If I need to learn anything,
I just buy one of your books and
learn the topic in no time.
Wonders! I have even trained
my friends to give me
Visual books as gifts."

Illona Bergstrom
Aventura, FL

"I have quite a few of your
Visual books and have been
very pleased with all of them.
I love the way the
lessons are presented!"

Mary Jane Newman
Yorba Linda, CA

"Like a lot of other people,
I understand things best
when I see them visually.
Your books really make
learning easy and
life more fun."

John T. Frey
Cadillac, MI

maranGraphics is a family-run business
located near Toronto, Canada.

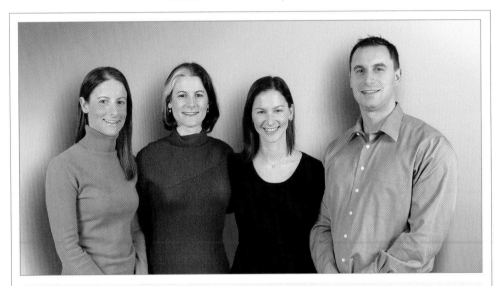

At maranGraphics, we believe in producing great consumer books–one book at a time.

Each maranGraphics book uses the award-winning communication process that we have been developing over the last 28 years. Using this process, we organize photographs and text in a way that makes it easy for you to learn new concepts and tasks.

We spend hours deciding the best way to perform each task, so you don't have to! Our clear, easy-to-follow photographs and instructions walk you through each task from beginning to end.

We want to thank you for purchasing what we feel are the best books money can buy. We hope you enjoy using this book as much as we enjoyed creating it!

Sincerely,

The Maran Family

Please visit us on the Web at:
www.maran.com

CREDITS

Author:
maranGraphics
Development Group

Content Architect:
Ruth Maran

Technical Consultant:
Mindy Parmar, BA Kin.,
CAT(C), CSCS

Nutritional Consultant:
Abby Langer, BA, DPD, RD

Project Manager:
Judy Maran

Copy Development and Editing:
Raquel Scott
Roderick Anatalio
Wanda Lawrie

Editing:
Roxanne Van Damme
Megan Robinson

Layout Designer:
Sarah Jang

**Front Cover, Gym Backgrounds
and Overviews:**
Designed by Russ Marini

Photographic Retouching:
Russ Marini
Steven Schaerer

Front Cover Consultant:
Domo Kovacevic,
A.C.E., C.F.C.

**Wiley Vice President and
Executive Publisher:**
Kathy Nebenhaus

Wiley Staff:
Dawn Barnes
Roxane Cerda
Cindy Kitchel
Lisa Murphy
Susan Olinsky

Models:
Ryan Hamilton
Judy Maran
Keith Mclean
Chantal Nadeau
John Tarnowski

**Photography and
Post Production:**
Robert Maran

ACKNOWLEDGMENTS

Thanks to the dedicated staff of maranGraphics, including Roderick Anatalio,
Sarah Jang, Kelleigh Johnson, Wanda Lawrie, Jill Maran, Judy Maran,
Robert Maran, Ruth Maran, Russ Marini, Megan Robinson,
Steven Schaerer, Raquel Scott and Roxanne Van Damme.

Finally, to Richard Maran who originated the easy-to-use graphic format
of this guide. Thank you for your inspiration and guidance.

SPECIAL THANKS TO

Canadian BodyWorks Fitness

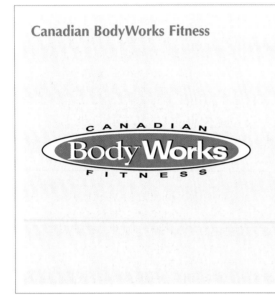

Special thanks to *Canadian BodyWorks Fitness* for allowing us to take photographs in their gym.

Canadian BodyWorks Fitness is a 24-hour health and fitness club. BodyWorks Fitness is founded on the principles of providing a high level of cleanliness, caring, personal support, comfort and fun. The staff at BodyWorks Fitness strive to consistently meet members' ultimate expectations, as well as provide them with a memorable experience and most importantly, exceptional value.

www.canadianbodyworks.com

Life Fitness

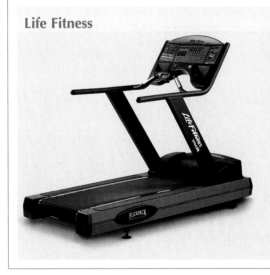

Special thanks to *Life Fitness* for allowing us to show photos of their equipment in parts of our book.

Life Fitness is a popular brand of fitness equipment found in health clubs worldwide. Their home equipment is also widely recommended by fitness experts in the U.S. and around the world. Life Fitness products are user-friendly, well-designed, incorporate advanced technology and help you practice personalized and effective workouts.

www.lifefitness.com

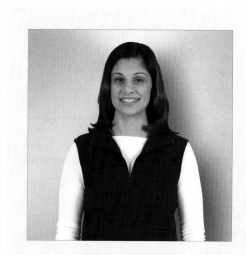

Mindy Parmar is a Certified Athletic Therapist CAT(C) and Personal Trainer (PTS and ACE). Her education includes an Honors Degree in Kinesiology and Health Science (B.A. Hons., Kin.). Mindy has received certification as a personal trainer from the American Council on Exercise (ACE) and is certified as a Strength Conditioning Specialist (CSCS) by the National Strength Conditioning Association (NSCA).

Mindy teaches First Aid and CPR through the Red Cross. She also instructs and certifies fitness professionals to achieve their personal trainer certifications. In addition, Mindy teaches the Prevention and Treatment of Sports Injuries at Seneca College for the Fitness Certificate Program. Mindy's future goals include completing her Doctorate in Acupuncture, becoming certified as a Registered Holistic Nutritional Consultant and attending Osteopathy school.

A few words from Mindy Parmar...

I would like to thank maranGraphics for this opportunity to create a useful tool that promotes a healthy and fit lifestyle. I would also like to thank my loving husband, Sanjay, for all his support throughout the process. I have truly enjoyed the process of putting this book together. I am certain this book will be an excellent resource for people of all fitness levels.

ENJOY!!

And pursue your dreams of achieving a healthy and fit body.

Table of Contents

Table of Contents

Table of Contents

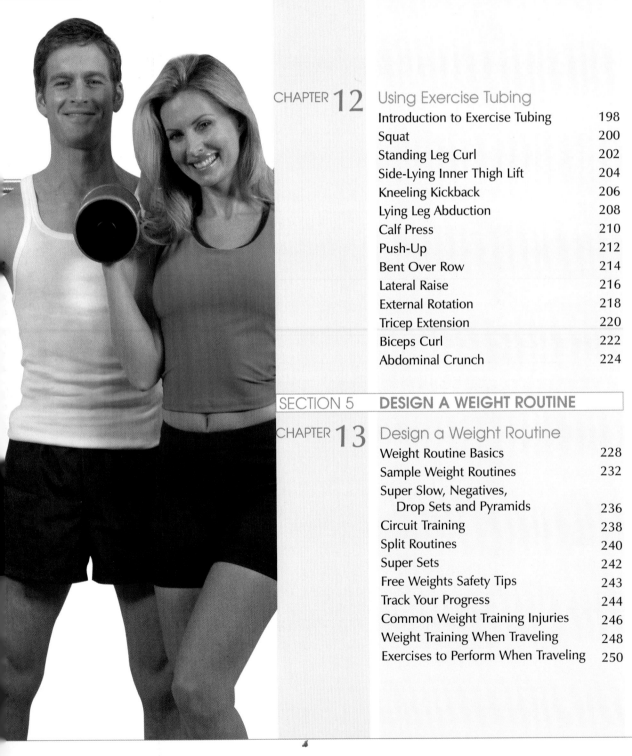

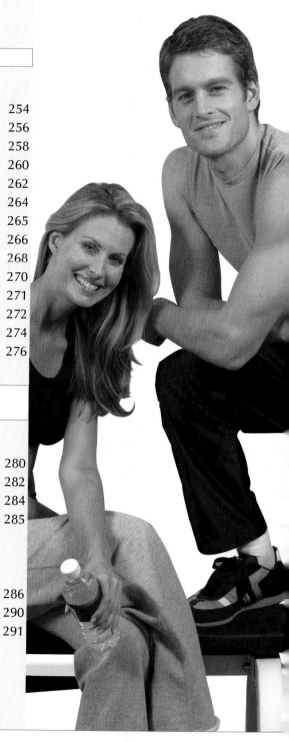

Section 1

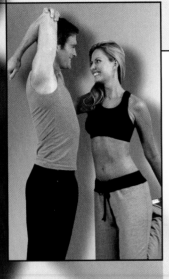

If you are new to weight training, you probably have a lot of questions you need answered before you begin. What are the names of the muscles I will be working? Should I weight train at home or at a gym? Are there certain things I should consider when choosing a gym or a personal trainer? What should I wear when weight training? Section 1 provides the answers to all these questions and more.

Weight Training Basics

In this Section...

Weight Training Basics

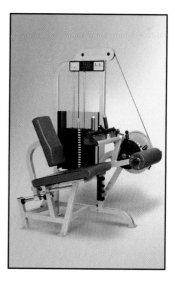

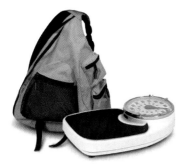

the benefits of
weight training

Weight training has a number of benefits, which include reducing stress and improving your energy level. You may want to consult with your doctor before starting a weight training program, especially if you have medical problems, past injuries or have not been physically active for over a year. If you have concerns, you can also hire a personal trainer to design a safe training program for you.

Increases Strength

Weight training increases your muscle strength. Your muscles become more efficient and stronger as a result of the stress placed on them when lifting weight. Weight training also helps prevent muscle atrophy as you become older.

Prevents Injuries

When you have strong muscles, you have better control, balance and coordination to perform everyday activities. Strong muscles protect your joints from injury.

Helps Control Your Weight

Weight training helps control your weight by raising your resting metabolic rate, which means you burn more calories throughout the day. The more muscle you have, the higher your resting metabolic rate.

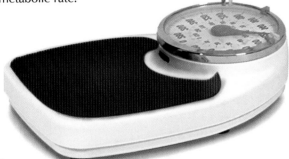

Improves Sports Performance

Stronger muscles allow you to move better and can improve your performance in sports, such as swimming, tennis and basketball.

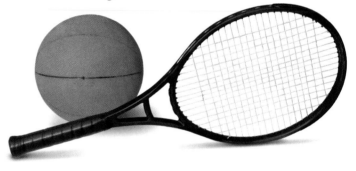

Improves Appearance

By enhancing the tone and shape of your muscles, weight training can help you look better as well as improve your posture.

Strengthens Bones

Weight training is a weight bearing exercise that places stress on your bones, and when bones are stressed, they become stronger. Building strong bones helps prevent osteoporosis, which is a disease where bones become brittle.

weight training
misconceptions

There are many weight training misconceptions that can discourage people from joining a gym and working out. Here is some information that can help clear up these misconceptions.

"Weight training will make me too big."

This is a common misconception, especially among women. In reality, you need to lift very heavy weight for many years before you would gain a significant amount of muscle mass. Women do not have as much testosterone in their bodies as men, which is one of the main hormones that allows you to gain muscle mass.

"Weight training takes a long time."

To get a good workout, you do not need to spend a few hours every day in the gym. You can achieve results by exercising 30 to 45 minutes a day, 3 to 4 times a week. If you are training for more than 2 hours, you are either working out inefficiently or talking too much while resting between sets.

"One weight training routine can work for everyone."

A single weight training program that works for everyone does not exist. Your weight training routine should be specifically designed to meet your needs and goals. Be careful not to be persuaded into following a program that your friend swears by or that you read about in a magazine. After developing your weight training routine, you can make modifications to adjust the program to meet your changing needs and schedule.

"Weight training can reduce fat in a specific area of my body."

This misconception is referred to as spot reducing. In reality, weight training cannot reduce fat in a specific area of your body, but it can reduce the fat throughout your entire body. When you work specific muscle groups, you are simply toning the muscles underneath the fat. The best way to lose fat is through a combination of proper diet, exercise and weight training.

"Weight training will not help me lose weight."

Weight training increases your metabolism which in turn helps you burn more calories. You will find that weight training is an important element of many weight loss programs. People who try to lose weight by diet alone are actually losing muscle in addition to fat. Weight training helps you lose weight while keeping your muscles strong and well-toned.

"Stretching is a great way to warm up before weight training."

Stretching does not provide a proper warm-up before weight training. To properly warm up, you should perform at least 5 minutes of cardiovascular exercise to help slowly increase your heart rate and blood flow. You can stretch after your warm-up or at the end of your workout.

major muscles in your body

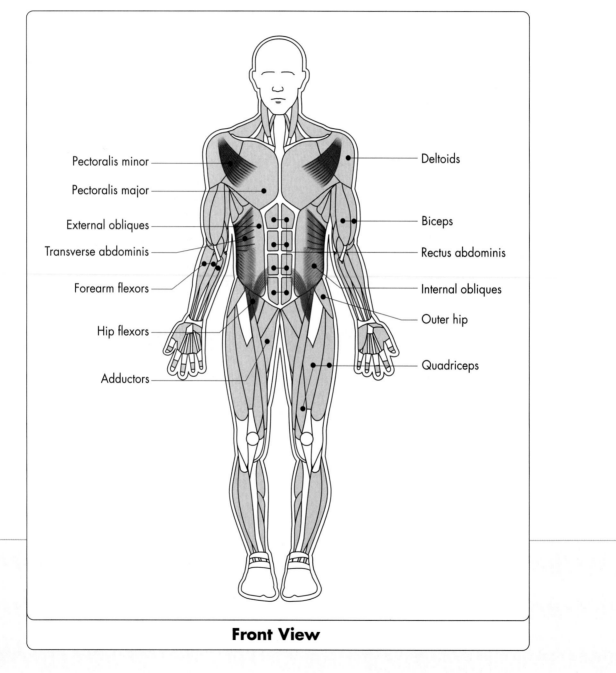

Pectoralis minor

Pectoralis major

External obliques

Transverse abdominis

Forearm flexors

Hip flexors

Adductors

Deltoids

Biceps

Rectus abdominis

Internal obliques

Outer hip

Quadriceps

Front View

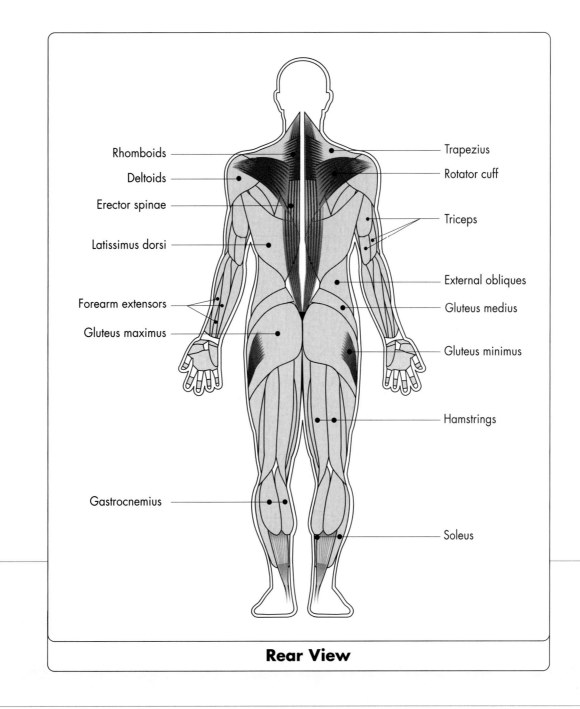

Rhomboids

Deltoids

Erector spinae

Latissimus dorsi

Forearm extensors

Gluteus maximus

Gastrocnemius

Trapezius

Rotator cuff

Triceps

External obliques

Gluteus medius

Gluteus minimus

Hamstrings

Soleus

Rear View

weight training at home or at a gym

After you decide to start a weight training program, the next step is to determine whether to work out at home or join a gym. There are several factors to consider before deciding which option is best for you.

WEIGHT TRAINING **AT HOME**

Privacy

If you are self-conscious or shy about exercising in public, you may find weight training in the privacy of your own home appealing. Some personal trainers may be willing to train you in your home, but if hiring a personal trainer is beyond your budget, there is a wide selection of exercise videos and books that you can use for instruction and motivation.

Cost

Although the initial cost of setting up a home gym can be quite large, investing in a home gym can be cheaper in the long run than maintaining a long-term gym membership. However, a drawback of owning your own equipment is that you may not be able to replace or update your equipment as often as a gym.

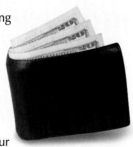

No Waiting

Working out at home means you do not have to wait to use a machine or rush to finish your workout so someone else can use the equipment. Having your own machines can allow you to exercise more efficiently, without interrupting your rhythm or having to wait between sets.

Convenience

Convenience is one of the most important reasons people choose to weight train at home. If your schedule is unpredictable, you may find it difficult to fit in your workouts with a gym's hours. Working out at home allows you 24-hour access to the equipment and also saves you travel time if you do not live or work close to a gym.

Personalized Environment

Designing your personal workout space can make exercising interesting and fun. You can paint your walls bright colors or hang motivational posters on the walls. You can place the equipment where you like, whether facing a window or in front of the television and listen to your own music without having to wear earphones.

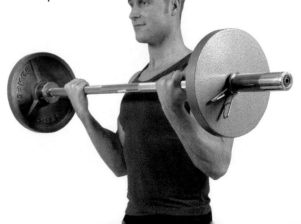

WEIGHT TRAINING **AT A GYM**

Safety

Working with heavy weights can be dangerous if you do not have a spotter standing by to assist you. In a gym, there is always someone around to help and staff members may alert you if you are doing something that can result in injury.

Motivation

If you live in a busy household, it might be difficult to stick to a workout routine amid distractions of family life that constantly demand your time and attention. Getting away to a gym eliminates many of those distractions and being in an environment where everyone is exercising can help motivate you.

Meet New People

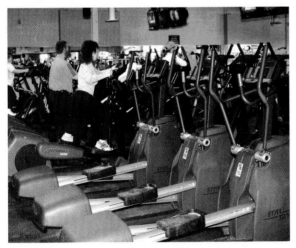

A public gym is a great place to meet and interact with new people. If your social life needs a boost, joining a gym will provide an opportunity to make new friends while getting in shape.

Equipment Choices and Facilities

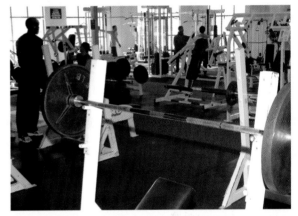

Public gyms have a wider selection of machines than you would usually be able to afford or accommodate at home. If you are easily bored, varying your exercises will help keep you interested and motivated to continue your fitness program. Also, public gyms often have additional facilities, such as a swimming pool, sauna or steam room.

Advice

Some gyms offer introductory programs to help you start with a basic weight training program to get familiar with the equipment. While you are working out, you should also be able to get advice from staff on how to adjust or use a machine.

No Loss of Living Space

Weight training equipment can be bulky, consuming a large amount of space. If you cannot spare enough room at home to safely set up or store equipment, working out at a gym may be your best option.

set up a home gym

If you decide to weight train at home, there are several factors to consider before setting up a home gym.

When choosing the area to set up the gym, consider traffic flow, safety, the equipment you want to include and whether you will want to expand the gym in the future. You should also determine the amount of space available in the area, since this will determine what you can fit in the room.

Your home gym should include components for weight training as well as aerobic and flexibility training. Make sure the equipment you purchase is appropriate to your interests and current fitness level but will also be able to adjust as your fitness level increases.

Dumbbells

Dumbbells are more versatile than barbells, which makes dumbbells a more practical purchase for your home gym. For best results, start with 5 pairs of dumbbells of varying weight instead of buying only one pair and using them for every exercise.

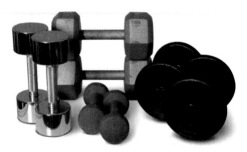

DUMBBELL RACK

Using a rack to store your dumbbells can help save space, keep your workout area tidy and make it easier for you to retrieve dumbbells. If space is limited, consider a vertical rather than a horizontal rack, since the vertical rack requires less space.

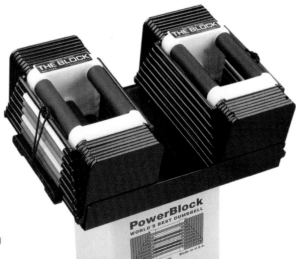

ADJUSTABLE DUMBBELLS

You may want to consider an adjustable dumbbell kit, which consists of two short bars and several weight plates that you can clamp on to the bars. While adjustable dumbbells can save space and money, constantly adding and removing weight plates can become time consuming. You can also purchase adjustable dumbbells, such as a PowerBlock, that allow you to easily add and remove weight. To select the amount of weight you want to lift, you insert a pin into a hole that corresponds to the weight. When you remove the dumbbell from the block, the dumbbell will contain only the amount of weight you selected.

Barbells

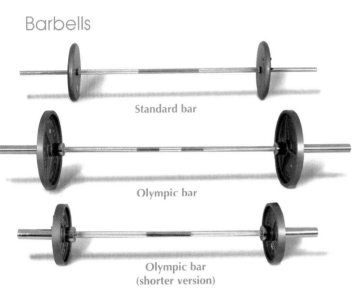

Standard bar

Olympic bar

Olympic bar
(shorter version)

Adding a barbell to your home gym allows you to lift heavier weights and vary your workout. You can get barbells with fixed weights, but barbells that consist of a bar that you can add weight plates to are more practical. There are different types of bars available, such as a standard bar or Olympic bar. A standard bar can vary in length from 5 to 7 feet, weighs around 20 lbs and is ideal for home use. An Olympic bar, which is about 7 feet and weighs 45-pounds, is usually used when working large muscle groups, such as your legs, back and chest. The Olympic bar is also available in shorter versions which range from 5 to 6 feet long and weigh approximately 35 pounds. The shorter Olympic bar is usually used when working smaller muscle groups, such as shoulders, biceps and triceps. The bar you use depends on the amount of weight you want to lift.

Plates for barbells are available in weights of 2.5 to 45 pounds and can be stored on a weight tree that you can purchase separately. You should also obtain collars you can place at the ends of the bar to prevent the weights from slipping off.

Mirror

Placing a mirror in your weight training area allows you to watch your form, which is especially important when lifting free weights. You should use a full-length mirror large enough to show your entire body. If the mirror stands on the floor, be careful about placing dumbbells or barbells where they can roll into the mirror.

Bench

You should choose a sturdy bench that can be adjusted from a flat to vertical position with different degrees of incline. The decline feature is not as important as the incline feature, since it is not often used. Before making your decision, inspect the bench carefully and test it in as many ways as you can by sitting or lying on the bench and adjusting the incline to make sure the mechanism works properly and is easy to use.

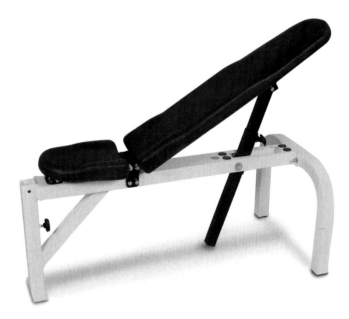

set up a home gym

Exercise Tubing

Exercise tubing is an inexpensive, lightweight and portable tool you can use to vary your normal strength training routine. Tubing is especially useful if you do not have a lot of space to store your equipment. While exercise tubing will not give you the same results as intense strength training with weights, tubing is good for toning and defining your muscles. For more information on exercise tubing, see page 198.

Exercise Ball

Exercise balls are large, inflatable vinyl balls that can be used in a variety of exercises, including strength training and stretching. You can use an exercise ball instead of a bench to add variety and increase the difficulty of many exercises. Using an exercise ball helps improve your stability and balance by strengthening your core muscles, which include your lower back and abdominal muscles. For more information on exercise balls, see page 168.

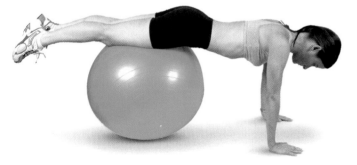

Cardiovascular Equipment

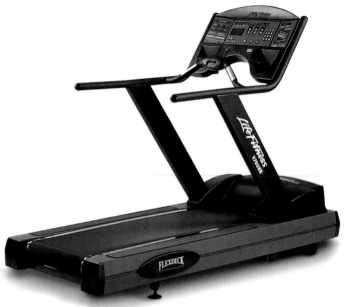

The type of cardiovascular equipment you buy for your home gym will depend largely on the amount of space and money you have available. You can purchase many of the cardiovascular machines used in public gyms to use at home. Some popular cardiovascular machines for home use include treadmills, stationary bikes, stair climbers, elliptical crosstrainers and rowing machines. If you do not have room for a machine, you can get a good cardiovascular workout by jumping rope, walking or running.

Exercise Mat

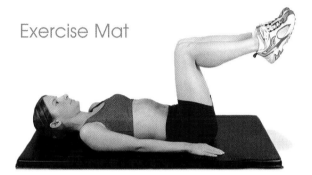

An exercise mat provides a cushion between your body and the floor to make floor exercises, such as abdominal crunches and stretching, more comfortable to perform. Unlike a towel or blanket, an exercise mat will not bunch up and most mats can be folded and stored in a corner. Mats are available in different thicknesses. When choosing a mat, select one that is thick enough to protect your knees from digging into the floor when performing kneeling exercises and long enough to fit your body from the top of your head to your tailbone.

Equipment Mat

Equipment mats are usually placed under exercise equipment to keep the equipment in place and protect your carpet and floors from the impact of heavy equipment. Mats are especially useful for cardiovascular equipment, such as treadmills. Mats help reduce noisy vibrations that can wear down equipment and prevents dust and fibers from the floor or carpet from getting into the mechanical parts of the equipment. You can also place a mat in the area where you lift free weights to protect your floor from accidents, such as a dropped dumbbell.

Multigym

Since most people do not have room at home to accommodate different weight machines, the multigym, which combines several weight lifting stations into one machine, provides a practical solution. A multigym can give you a good overall weight workout, but the machine is not as smooth as the ones you will find in health clubs. Some multigyms have two weight stacks, so two people can work out at the same time. You should choose a multigym that is space-efficient and includes good safety features. Make sure the frame and seats are sturdy and the pads are thick and durable. Try out the machine to ensure that moving parts, such as the weight stack, move smoothly, the machine adjusts easily to fit your body and is comfortable and easy to use.

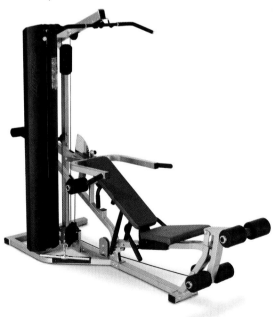

weight training equipment

Initially, the weight training equipment you see in a gym might seem complicated and intimidating, but once you try them, you will find that they are easy to use. This section provides an overview of the basic strength training equipment available at gyms.

Barbells

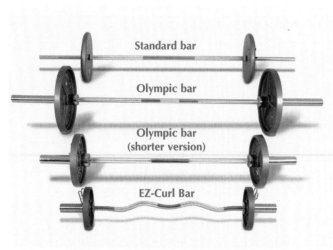

Standard bar

Olympic bar

Olympic bar
(shorter version)

EZ-Curl Bar

Barbells come in a variety of designs, but mainly consist of a bar to which you can add weight plates. Gyms normally carry four main types of barbells: standard bars, Olympic bars, EZ-Curl bars and fixed barbells.

STANDARD BAR
This bar can be 5 to 7 feet in length, weighs about 20 pounds and is used when working smaller muscle groups, such as shoulders, biceps and triceps.

OLYMPIC BAR
This straight bar is about 7 feet long, weighs 45 pounds and is usually used when working large muscle groups, such as legs, back and chest. The Olympic bar is also available in shorter versions, which range from 5 to 6 feet long and weigh approximately 35 pounds.

EZ-CURL BAR
This is a W-shaped bar about 4 feet long, which is used to work smaller muscle groups, such as biceps and triceps.

FIXED BARBELLS
These barbells have weights permanently fastened to the ends so you do not need to add or remove weight plates. Fixed barbells come in a variety of weights, ranging from 20 to 150 pounds.

WEIGHT PLATES
Weight plates are usually stored on vertical racks, called weight trees, next to barbells. These plates are available in weights of 2.5, 5, 10, 25, 35 and 45 pounds and each has a hole in the center that allows you to slide it onto the bar. Some plates may also have additional holes you can use to lift or carry them.

COLLARS
To secure the weights to the bars, you should use collars, which are devices like screws or clips that you can place on the bar to prevent the weight plates from rattling or falling off.

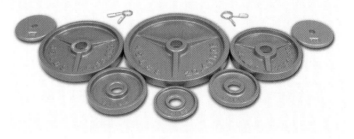

Dumbbells

Dumbbells come in different shapes, sizes, weights and materials. They can be made from chrome or steel, or coated with rubber to help lessen the impact on surfaces, such as floors, when dropped. Depending on the design, some dumbbells can have a

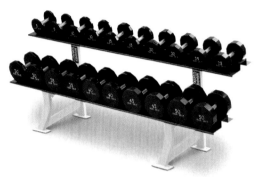

better grip than others. You can usually find dumbbells arranged on a rack in order of weight—from lightest to heaviest—in a mirrored area of the gym. Keep in mind that the weight indicated on a dumbbell may not be accurate, since the weight of the handle may not be included in the total weight.

Bench

A bench is useful for performing many weight training exercises. Benches come in different designs. Some benches can be adjusted to a flat, vertical, incline or decline position for different exercises.

FLAT: Flat benches come in various lengths, heights and widths.

VERTICAL: Vertical benches provide back support to protect your lower back muscles during sitting exercises.

INCLINE: Incline benches have adjustable backs that can be positioned flat, straight up or at different angles of incline. Changing the angle of the bench for an exercise emphasizes different muscles. Some incline benches cannot be positioned flat or may be positioned at a fixed incline.

DECLINE: Decline benches slope downward to allow you to lie with your head lower than your feet, which is useful for exercises that strengthen the lower portion of your chest.

Weight Stack Machines

Weight stack machines, which are the most popular type of machines available, are ideal for beginners because they are simple to use. These machines contain a stack of rectangular weight plates with notches where you can insert a metal rod, called a pin, to select the amount of weight you want to lift.

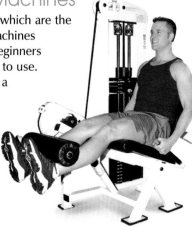

Plate Loaded Machines

Plate loaded machines combine the flexibility and feel of free weights with most of the safety features of traditional weight machines. These machines have bars where you can place the weight plates you want to lift. Some plate loaded machines have free-floating levers that allow you to move in a variety of ways, rather than a fixed path. Plate loaded machines may also allow you to work one side of your body at a time, which is useful for strengthening your muscles equally.

weight training equipment

Exercise Ball

Many gyms have large, inflatable vinyl balls, called exercise balls, which can be used in a variety of strength training exercises. Using an exercise ball helps improve your stability and balance by strengthening your core muscles, which include your lower back and abdominal muscles. For more information on exercise balls, see page 168.

Roman Chair

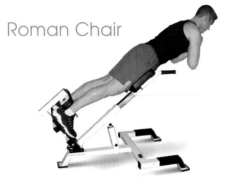

Roman Chairs are used for lower back and abdominal exercises, such as back extensions and side crunches. You can perform only a limited number of exercises on this piece of equipment. The design of the Roman Chair, such as the angle of the pad or how your feet are supported, may vary.

Preacher Curl Bench

This bench is designed for specific exercises that isolate your bicep muscles, such as preacher curl. The preacher curl bench usually has a rack where you can rest your barbell.

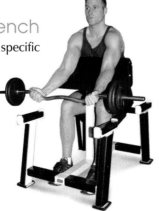

Smith Machine

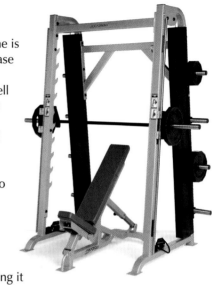

The Smith machine is designed to increase the safety and efficiency of barbell exercises, such as bench presses, overhead lifts and squats. The machine has a barbell confined to a vertical track so the bar can travel only straight up or down. This helps guide your movements, making it easier to maintain proper form. Many Smith machines also have adjustable safety stops that prevent the weight from being lowered below a certain point. If you accidentally drop the bar, the safety stops will catch the weight to save you from injury.

Power Cage

If you are lifting heavy weight without a spotter, a power cage can make the task easier. A power cage is generally a large metal frame with a series of hooks attached. You can place the barbell on the hooks at the desired height so you do not need to hold the barbell while getting into position for the exercise. Unlike the Smith machine, there are no tracks to guide your movement once you lift the weight.

Cable Machines

Cable machines consist of one or two vertical towers to which cable pulleys are attached. Cable machines offer more exercise options than other machines, since you can adjust the height of the pulley to various positions, such as above your head or close to the floor. You can also fasten a number of different attachments to the pulley to perform a wide variety of exercises.

SHORT, STRAIGHT BAR
This attachment is commonly used for upper body exercises using both arms.

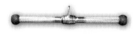

V-SHAPE BAR
This is commonly used for upper body exercises using both arms.

EZ-CURL BAR
This attachment is used for upper body exercises using both arms.

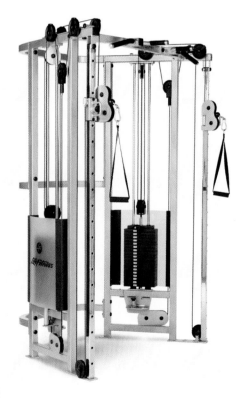

HORSESHOE HANDLE
This handle is useful for single-arm exercises that allow you to work each side separately.

ROPE
This attachment is great for arm exercises, such as biceps and triceps.

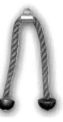

ANKLE STRAP
You wrap this strap around your ankle to perform lower body exercises. Most new straps use Velcro to secure the strap, while older models use a buckle.

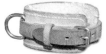

free weights versus
weight machines

While free weights and weight machines are both effective for developing strength, each has its own set of advantages and disadvantages. In general, machines are better for beginners, while free weights, which include barbells and dumbbells, work well for intermediate to advanced users. For best results, you can incorporate both free weights and machines into your weight training program.

FREE WEIGHTS

Advantages

VERSATILE Free weights allow you to perform hundreds of exercises to work all the muscle groups in your body.

WORK SEVERAL MUSCLE GROUPS AT ONCE Free weights often employ additional muscle groups to stabilize your body as you work the targeted muscles.

IMPROVE COORDINATION AND BALANCE Using free weights helps sharpen your coordination and balance, since you need to keep your body stable and maintain proper form during the exercises.

AFFORDABLE Free weights cost less and consume less space than machines.

Disadvantages

GREATER RISK OF INJURY Lifting heavy weights without a spotter or without maintaining proper form increases your chances of getting injured.

MORE TIME Using free weights can increase your workout time if you frequently need to add or remove plates from a barbell or locate dumbbells between exercises.

MORE CONCENTRATION AND FOCUS Using free weights requires more concentration and focus than using machines, since you need to control the weight on your own.

INTIMIDATING Barbells and heavy dumbbells can seem intimidating, especially to beginners.

Dumbbells versus Barbells

While barbells allow you to lift more weight with both hands simultaneously, dumbbells can help correct strength imbalances, since each side is required to lift its own weight. Dumbbells also allow you to perform more exercise variations than barbells.

WEIGHT MACHINES

Advantages

SAFE Weight machines are generally safer than free weights. Since you are not holding the actual weights, there is no chance of injury from dropping weights. This allows you to lift heavier weights without a spotter.

EASY TO USE Most machines simply require you to insert a pin into the weight stack to select the amount of weight you want to lift.

ISOLATE MUSCLES Weight machines allow you to target a specific muscle group without using other muscles too much.

MAINTAIN FORM Weight machines help guide and control your movements, making it easier to maintain proper form.

LESS TIME You can usually complete your workout in a shorter time, since you do not need to transfer weight plates to a barbell or locate dumbbells between exercises.

Disadvantages

IMPERFECT FIT If you are much bigger or much smaller than the average person, you may have trouble positioning your body properly when using some machines. Most machines are not designed for people under 5'5".

PROMOTE MUSCLE IMBALANCES Exercises using machines usually involve working the muscles on both sides of your body at once. If you have muscle imbalances, your stronger side can end up lifting more of the weight, which often results in your weaker side getting weaker and your stronger side getting stronger.

LIMITED OPTIONS You are usually restricted to a specific movement when using a machine so you are able to perform only one type of exercise on a machine.

COSTLY Machines can be expensive and bulky, which can make them impractical for home use if you have a tight budget or limited space.

choosing a gym

Once you decide to exercise at a gym, there are several factors to consider before signing up.

If you do not know of any gyms in your area, you can drive around your neighborhood, ask friends or check the local yellow pages. When you find a gym that interests you, try to obtain a day pass or trial membership, which will allow you to try the gym before committing to a membership. You should visit a gym at the time you plan to normally exercise to get a better idea of how crowded the gym will be at that time.

If you find gyms intimidating or overwhelming, keep in mind that once you become familiar with the surroundings, you will overcome your initial discomfort.

Cost

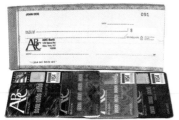

Joining a gym can be costly, so carefully consider what is included when you sign up and how you may be able to save on membership fees. For example, if the fee does not include an item you want, such as towel service, you can ask whether they will include the item at no cost to make the deal. Often gyms offer discounts when you join with a friend or at certain times of the year, such as after Christmas or during the summer. Restricted memberships may also be available at a reduced rate if you do not want to use all the facilities or you are willing to exercise during off-peak hours. The type of membership you choose will also determine the cost, as a month-to-month membership is usually more expensive in the long run than an annual membership. Also, keep in mind that some gyms charge an initiation fee.

Hours of Operation

The gym's hours of operation should correspond with your schedule. For example, if you prefer to exercise at 8 p.m. on weekends, you should make sure the gym is open at that time.

Location

You should choose a gym that is close to your home or work. You will have a better chance of maintaining your fitness program if your gym is easy to access and provides basic conveniences, such as adequate parking.

Contract

Before signing a contract, take the time to read the document carefully, consider your decision and do not feel pressured to sign on the spot. You should consider the gym's reputation and the length of time it has been operating. Also, take into account the flexibility of the contract. Some gyms allow you to put your membership on hold if you cannot use the gym for long periods, such as when you take a long vacation. Keep in mind that a gym may require 30 to 60 days written notice before canceling your contract. Depending on where you live, you may have the legal right to cancel your membership within a few days of signing without incurring a penalty.

Cleanliness

You should make sure all facilities, such as the gym area, bathrooms, locker rooms, sauna and steam room, are clean and fit for use. Also, ensure there is adequate water pressure in the showers and toilet paper in the bathrooms.

Ambience

It is important that you feel comfortable and welcome at the gym. Take note of the atmosphere of the place on your first visit. Factors such as the type of music played and the demeanor of the other members can affect your level of motivation and enjoyment when exercising. If you feel intimidated or uncomfortable when you enter a gym, it may not be the right gym for you.

Staff

A good gym should always have staff available to answer your questions about an exercise or a piece of equipment. Make sure staff members are approachable and helpful, as well as professional and well-informed.

Affiliation with Other Gyms

If you travel frequently, you may want to join a gym that is part of a chain or is affiliated with gyms in other cities. An affiliated gym in another city may allow you to use their facilities free or for a discounted rate, which will help make it easier to maintain your fitness program while you are traveling.

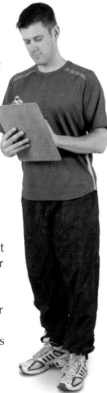

Extra Conveniences and Facilities

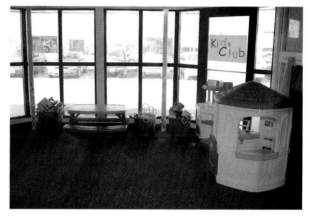

Some gyms offer only the bare essentials, while others provide additional conveniences, such as childcare, massages, saunas or fitness classes. Some gyms might also have televisions you can watch while exercising or audio outputs on the cardio machines that allow you to listen to your CDs without using your own CD player. Some gyms allow you to rent lockers. This allows you to leave your personal items, such as shampoo, deodorant and CDs, at the gym.

Equipment

When you visit the gym, observe the quality, selection and types of equipment available and whether there is a time limit on some machines, such as treadmills, to ensure everyone gets a fair chance to use the machines. It is also important to ensure the gym has the machines you regularly use. Make note of the condition of the equipment, such as whether all the machines run smoothly, the weight plates are rust-free and the upholstery on the equipment is in good condition.

choosing a personal trainer

A personal trainer can provide the motivation and instruction you need to start and maintain a weight training program. Since a standard qualification for personal trainers does not exist, it is important that you consider your options carefully before hiring a trainer.

Once you find a personal trainer you like, you should arrange a trial session to get to know the trainer better before committing to a long-term program.

Try to avoid basing your decision on the trainer's appearance, as this is not a good indicator of how well the trainer can teach or motivate you.

In addition to motivating and instructing you, a trainer should be able to provide a customized program that includes the five components of good health: strength training, weight management, cardiovascular exercise, basic nutrition and flexibility training.

Find a Personal Trainer

When you join a gym, you may automatically receive a free introductory session with a personal trainer. You can also find a personal trainer by asking friends, checking fitness clubs in your area or contacting professional organizations, such as some of the associations listed below.

Qualifications

You should make sure your personal trainer's certifications are current and are from recognized professional associations. Trainers need to upgrade their skills about once a year to maintain certification.

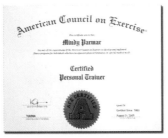

Accredited professional associations include:

Aerobics and Fitness Association of America (AFAA)

The National Academy of Sports Medicine (NASM)

American Council on Exercise (ACE)

International Sports Sciences Association (ISSA)

American College of Sports Medicine (ACSM)

National Strength and Conditioning Association (NSCA)

Cost and Availability

Hiring a personal trainer can be costly, but you may be able to save if you shop around. Generally, more experienced trainers will have higher rates than newly certified trainers. Trainers usually charge a fee per session, but you may be able to negotiate a reduced rate for a package or for semi-private sessions if you sign up with a friend. To avoid future problems, make sure all fees, cancellation and billing policies are clearly set out in writing. Also ensure the trainer will be available at the times you want to exercise.

Certified in CPR and First Aid

Though rare, accidents can happen while exercising with a trainer, so you need to make sure your trainer is certified in CPR (cardiopulmonary resuscitation) and first aid and can handle emergencies.

Check References

One of the best ways to learn about a trainer is to talk to his or her clients. You can ask questions about the trainer's strengths and weaknesses and find out if the trainer is dependable, knowledgeable and professional.

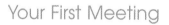

Your First Meeting

Most trainers will set up a first meeting to get acquainted with you. During this meeting, the trainer should discuss your exercise and health history, your present fitness level and your goals. You may need to perform several fitness tests to give the trainer a better idea of your fitness level so he or she can customize a program for you.

Experience

You should consider the type and amount of experience a trainer has and whether the trainer's experience is relevant to your needs. If you have previous injuries or special needs, you should choose a trainer whose experience and style of training best suit you.

Liability Insurance

You should make sure the trainer has liability insurance, which will cover the trainer if you get injured while exercising with the trainer and decide to take legal action.

Track Progress

Before starting a training program, a trainer should help you determine your short-term and long-term goals and establish a way to keep track of your progress.

Warning Signs

There are several warning signs that a trainer may not be a good choice. A trainer who is unwilling to supply references, proof of qualifications or liability insurance probably has something to hide. Be wary of a trainer who is unaware of current developments in the field of exercise or who acknowledges only his or her own style of training. You should stay away from a trainer who makes unrealistic promises, tries to push you beyond your capacity or offers to sell you dietary supplements.

Personality

A trainer's personality can affect your level of motivation and enjoyment when exercising. You should choose a trainer who is easy to talk to, is interested in your goals and who will motivate you through positive reinforcement. A trainer should never make you feel uncomfortable or incompetent. You may also want to consider whether you feel more comfortable with a male or female trainer.

clothing and accessories

Wearing suitable clothing and using the proper accessories can make your workouts comfortable and safe.

Shoes

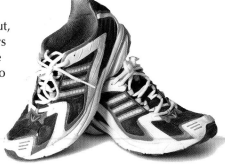

When working out, you should always wear comfortable shoes. It is best to wear shoes with rubber soles for better grip and balance. For safety reasons, most gyms will not allow you to wear sandals or loafers while lifting weights. If you were to accidentally drop a weight on your feet while wearing sandals, your toes would not be protected.

Weight Training Belts

Weight training belts are made of thick, dense leather or synthetic material and are about six inches in width. The belt is typically worn around your waist, just above your hips, to help protect your back when lifting heavy weight. It is a misconception that using a weight training belt is necessary to keep your back supported. It is actually best not to wear weight training belts since they hinder the development of your back and abdominal muscles. These muscles are strengthened when you perform exercises that require you to keep your back supported. Wearing a weight training belt is similar to using a crutch and gives you a false sense of security when trying to lift heavier weight.

Weight Training Gloves

You can wear weight training gloves that fit snugly on your hands without restricting movement. Weight training gloves typically have padded palms and cut-off finger tips for ventilation. The gloves can give you a more secure grip and prevent your hands from slipping off barbells, dumbbells and handles. They also protect your hands from blisters and calluses when lifting weight.

Chalk

You can use gym chalk to reduce the moisture on your hands and improve your grip. This is especially useful when you plan to lift very heavy weight.

Wraps

Wraps are typically made of tensor type material and are fastened around wrists, knees and elbows using Velcro. People like to wear wraps for extra support. However, similar to weight training belts, it is best not to wear wraps at all especially if you have an injury or joint pain. Wearing wraps gives you a false sense of security. If you have problems with any of your joints, it is safer to avoid using wraps and skip the exercise instead.

Wrist Straps

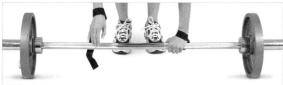

Wrist straps are made of sturdy, non-stretch material and are commonly used when performing lat pulldowns and barbell deadlifts. The material is wrapped around your wrists and then wrapped around the bar you will be lifting to make it easier to grip the bar. However, similar to weight training belts and wraps, you do not need to use wrist straps while lifting weight. Wearing wrist straps gives you a false sense of security that your wrists are stronger than they actually are. Wrist straps prevent your hand and forearm muscles from becoming stronger. If you find that you need wrist straps, you are probably lifting more weight than you can handle.

Weight Lifting Pads

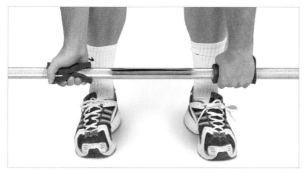

Weight lifting pads are placed in the palms of your hands when lifting weight to improve your grip and to prevent blisters and calluses. They are made of spongy, rubber material and are typically square or circular in shape. Weight lifting pads are not as convenient to use as weight training gloves.

Clothing

You should wear comfortable clothing that allows you to move freely and perform exercises properly. Try to dress modestly and avoid wearing heavy clothing that can restrict your movements or conceal mistakes in your posture. If you are working on a specific area of your body, you may find it easier if you wear clothing that allows you to see the muscles being worked. For example, you can wear shorts when working your lower body or wear a tank top when working your arms. When you perform exercises that require you to spread your legs, make sure to wear tights or long shorts.

weight training etiquette

When working out at a gym, it is important that you follow particular rules of etiquette. As with everyday social situations, you should always be polite and courteous. Although there may be rituals and customs unique to each gym, there are some general rules you should follow to avoid being frowned upon by other gym members.

Return Weights After Use

Failing to return weights back to the rack after finishing an exercise is one of the most common mistakes people make at a gym. People can end up tripping on weights that are left unattended on the floor. When you finish using a pair of dumbbells or when you remove a weight plate from a barbell, you should make sure you return the weights back to their proper place on the rack.

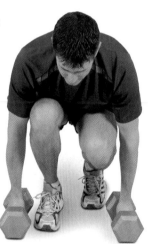

Share Equipment

Sharing equipment is very important when working out at a gym. If people are waiting to use a machine, you should avoid sitting on the machine while resting between sets. If you are waiting to use a machine, do not hover over the person currently using the machine. If the gym is very busy, you may want to ask another member to "work in" with you. Working in means taking turns using the exercise machine so one person is using the machine while the other is resting.

Cardiovascular Equipment

To make it fair to everyone exercising, your gym may require people to sign up before using popular cardiovascular equipment, such as treadmills and bikes. Make sure you check the sign-up sheet before hopping on to an available machine, especially when your gym is very busy. Some gyms limit the time each person can use a machine. When a lot of people are waiting, you should avoid staying on a machine for more than 20 minutes.

Wear Appropriate Clothing

Make sure you wear clothing that is comfortable and breathable. You should also make sure you wear clean clothing and avoid using strong perfume, cologne or aftershave when working out. For safety reasons, you should wear the proper footwear, such as a good pair of running shoes.

Do Not Carry Around Your Gym Bag

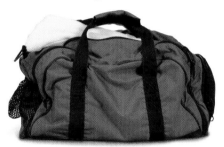

You should use a locker to store your gym bag. Do not bring your gym bag to the exercise area. Since most gyms have limited space between machines, placing your gym bag on the floor can take up valuable floor space and present a potential hazard to other people exercising.

Do Not Monopolize the Drinking Fountain

Be considerate of other gym members when using the drinking fountain. When people are lined up to use the drinking fountain, do not stand at the fountain while trying to catch your breath or choose this time to fill up your water bottle. You should first let everyone in line get a drink before filling up your water bottle.

Keep Noise to a Minimum

When working out at a gym, you should avoid making loud noises. Loud groaning or music may distract other gym members from their exercise. Try to limit your noise to heaving breathing. You should also avoid hooting and hollering in the gym. If you are working out with friends, try to keep the volume of your conversation to a minimum to avoid annoying other gym members.

Locker Room Etiquette

You should do your part to keep all areas of the locker room clean. When you are finished using a towel, make sure you place it in a laundry basket instead of simply leaving the towel on a bench or on the floor. Also, avoid cluttering an entire counter with your grooming products or dumping the contents of your bag on a bench. When using the shower, do not take extra long showers especially when people are waiting to use the facilities. After taking a shower, make sure you take all your belongings with you, such your shampoo bottle, soap and razor.

Do Not Drop or Slam Weights

As part of an effort to exercise safely, you should gently lower the weight down after each exercise. Dropping or slamming the weight down is not only noisy and bad for the equipment, but it is also a potentially dangerous behavior.

Wipe Down Equipment

As common courtesy, you should always wipe your sweat off all equipment, including machines and exercise mats, once you are finished using them. Most gyms provide towels and disinfectant spray for this purpose. If not, you could bring your own towel for wiping down the equipment.

Section 2

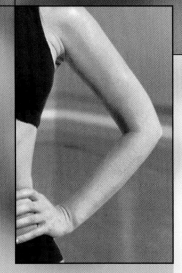

Toning and strengthening your upper body involves working your chest, back, shoulders, triceps, biceps, wrists and abdominals. Working your upper body is beneficial for improving your posture and enhancing your ability to play sports that require upper body strength. Of course, there are also aesthetic benefits to making your upper body look strong and toned. Section 2 takes you through the exercises you can perform to work your upper body.

Work Your Upper Body

In this Section...

Work Your Chest
Dumbbell Bench Press
Barbell Bench Press
Dumbbell Fly
Push-Up
Assisted Dip
Chest Press Machine
Pec Fly Machine
Cable Crossover

Work Your Shoulders
Dumbbell Shoulder Press
Lateral Raise
Bent Over Lateral Raise
Front Raise
Reverse Fly
Shoulder Press Machine
Dumbbell External Rotation
Dumbbell Internal Rotation

Work Your Back
Lat Pulldown
One-Arm Dumbbell Row
Bent Over Barbell Row
Dumbbell Shrug
Assisted Chin-Up
Upright Row
Back Extension on a Roman Chair
Seated Cable Row

Work Your Triceps
Bench Dip
Tricep Kickback
Triceps Pushdown
Barbell Triceps Press
Dumbbell Overhead Triceps Extension
Lying Barbell Triceps Extension
Triceps Extension Machine

Work Your Biceps and Wrists
Seated Dumbbell Curl
Barbell Curl
Concentration Curl
Preacher Curl
Hammer Curl
Cable Biceps Curl
Arm Curl Machine
Wrist Curl and Reverse Wrist Curl

Work Your Abdominals
Abdominal Crunch
Twist Crunch
Reverse Crunch
Abdominal Machine
Leg Raise
Plank
Side Plank
Bridge

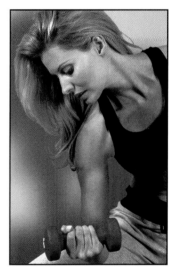

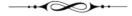

dumbbell bench press

The dumbbell bench press is a great exercise for working your chest. In addition, this exercise strengthens your triceps and the front of your shoulders.

The dumbbell bench press is similar to the barbell bench press shown on page 32, but the use of dumbbells instead of a barbell works your chest more and helps develop equal strength in your arms since each arm is lifting its own weight.

As you perform this exercise, do not arch your back in an effort to lift the weights. As with any exercise, you should use only as much weight as you can lift while maintaining proper form. If you are lifting heavier weights, you should work with a spotter.

You can place your feet flat on the floor for better balance and stability or on the bench to help flatten your back. If you cannot place your feet flat on the floor, place them on the bench.

You should be careful when performing this exercise if you have shoulder, elbow or wrist problems.

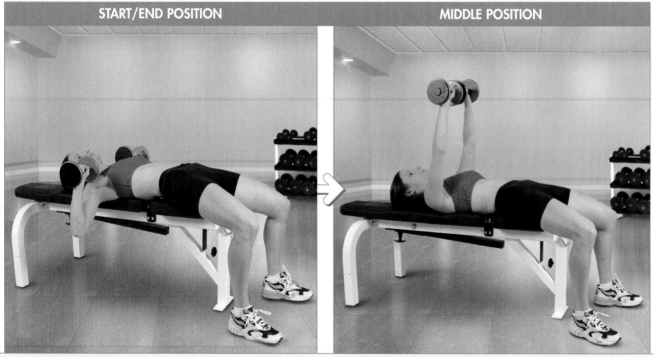

| START/END POSITION | MIDDLE POSITION |

1 Hold a dumbbell in each hand.

2 Lie on your back on a bench and position your feet flat on the floor or on the bench. Tighten your abdominal muscles to help protect your back.

3 Hold the dumbbells at your sides, with your elbows bent and positioned slightly below your shoulders. Your palms should face forward and your elbows should point down to the floor. You should feel a slight stretch in your outer chest.

4 Slowly push the dumbbells up above the middle of your chest. The dumbbells should almost touch.

• Make sure you keep your hips and shoulders on the bench and your legs and feet stationary for better support.

5 Slowly lower the dumbbells back to the starting position.

How can I work my upper or lower chest more?

To work the upper part of your chest more, you can perform the dumbbell bench press while lying on an incline bench. This variation also works the front of your shoulders more. To work the lower part of your chest more, you can perform this exercise while lying on a decline bench.

Can I perform a similar exercise using a cable machine?

Yes. Position a cable on a tower of a cable machine at roughly shoulder height and attach a handle to the cable. Stand with your back to the tower and your left foot in front of your right foot. Your feet should be shoulder width apart. Hold the handle with your right hand and position your elbow to the side at shoulder height, with your forearm parallel to the floor and your palm facing down. Place your left hand on your hip and extend your right arm as if you are performing a punch. After completing a set, repeat the exercise with your left arm. For more information on cable machines, see page 17.

DON'T

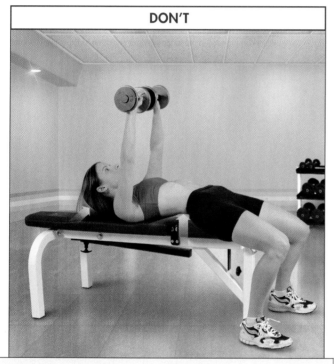

- Do not arch your back or wiggle your body to help lift the weights.
- Do not lift your head off the bench.
- Do not lock your elbows when you straighten your arms.
- Do not allow the dumbbells to sway toward your head.

MUSCLES TARGETED

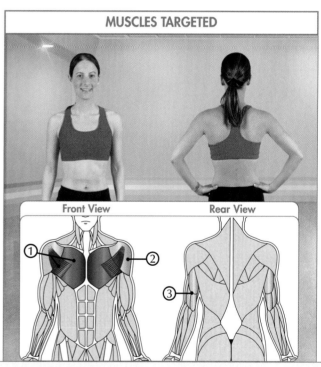

Front View   Rear View

Targeted muscles:
① chest (*pectoralis major and minor*)

Additional muscles:
② front shoulders (*anterior deltoids*)
③ triceps

barbell bench press

Bodybuilders consider the barbell bench press to be the king of all chest exercises. In addition to building strength and mass in your chest area, the barbell bench press strengthens your shoulders and triceps. This exercise is also good for developing overall upper body strength.

When performing this exercise, you should focus on maintaining proper form. Keep your abdominal muscles tight and your back flat on the bench. Do not arch your back or raise your hips off the bench to help lift the weight. When you straighten your arms, do not raise the barbell too high or lock your elbows.

You can choose to place your feet on the floor or on the bench. Placing your feet on the floor gives you better stability, while placing your feet on the bench helps reduce the stress on your back.

Use extra caution performing the barbell bench press if you have problems with your shoulders, elbows or wrists.

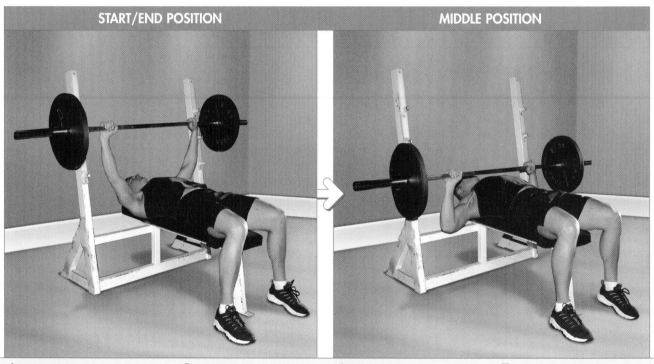

START/END POSITION **MIDDLE POSITION**

1 Lie on your back on a bench and position your feet flat on the floor or on the bench. Tighten your abdominal muscles to help protect your back.

2 Hold the bar slightly wider than shoulder width apart.

3 Lift the bar over the middle of your chest. Keep your elbows slightly bent.

4 Slowly lower the bar to about an inch from the middle of your chest. Your elbows should end up slightly below your shoulders.

5 Pause for a moment and then slowly raise the bar back to the starting position. Push your shoulder blades into the bench while raising the bar.

How can I put more emphasis on my upper or lower chest?

To put more emphasis on your upper chest, you can perform the barbell bench press while lying on an incline bench. The use of an incline bench also works the front of your shoulders a bit more. To put more emphasis on your lower chest, you can perform the barbell bench press while lying on a decline bench.

Is there a safer way to perform the barbell bench press?

You can use the Smith machine to safely perform the bench press. The machine features adjustable bar stops that prevent the weight from being lowered below a certain point. If you lose control of the bar, the Smith machine will catch the weight to save you from injury. The Smith machine also helps guide your movement and allows you to feel more stable and balanced. For more information on the Smith machine, see page 16.

DON'T

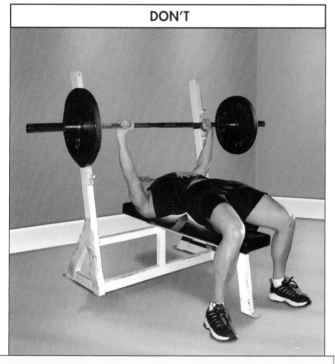

- Do not arch your back or wiggle your body to help you lift the weight. Keep your back on the bench and your legs and feet stationary for better support.

- Do not press the bar up too high. Your shoulders should not lift off the bench.

- Do not lift your head off the bench or lock your elbows.

MUSCLES TARGETED

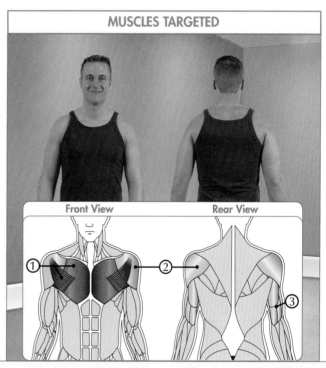

Targeted muscles:
① chest *(pectoralis major and minor)*

Additional muscles:
② shoulders *(deltoids)*
③ triceps

dumbbell fly

The dumbbell fly shapes and defines your chest. The exercise also strengthens the front of your shoulders.

To perform the dumbbell fly, you lie on a bench with the dumbbells raised above your chest and then you lower the dumbbells in an arc out to your sides. You then raise the dumbbells in an arc back to the starting position. When raising the dumbbells, visualize your arms wrapping around someone you are giving a hug. You should perform the dumbbell fly in a smooth, continuous motion and avoid using too much weight.

Any erratic movements or the use of too much weight may result in injury to the rotator cuff muscles in your shoulders.

It is important to maintain the proper form when performing this exercise. You should keep your elbows bent as you lift and lower the weights. Straightening your arms can put excessive pressure on your elbows and shoulder joints. You should also remember not to lower your elbows below the level of your shoulders as this will strain your shoulder muscles.

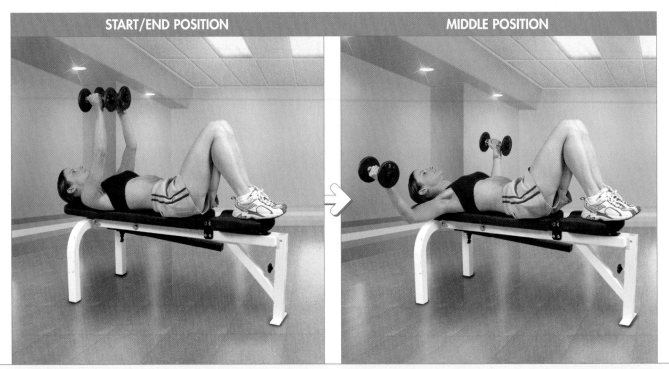

START/END POSITION   **MIDDLE POSITION**

1 Hold a dumbbell in each hand.

2 Lie on your back on a bench and position your feet flat on the floor or on the bench. Keep the dumbbells close to your chest.

3 With your palms facing each other, raise the dumbbells directly above your chest until your arms are almost straight. The dumbbells should almost touch. Make sure your back is flat against the bench.

4 With your elbows slightly bent, slowly lower the dumbbells out to your sides in a semicircular motion until your elbows are level with your shoulders. You should feel a slight stretch in your outer chest.

5 Pause for a moment and then slowly raise the dumbbells back to the starting position.

When performing the dumbbell fly, how can I work my upper or lower chest more?

To work your upper chest more, you can perform the dumbbell fly while lying on an incline bench. To work your lower chest more, you can perform this exercise while lying on a decline bench. When performing the dumbbell fly on a decline bench, you should have someone assist you with picking up and releasing the weights.

Can I perform a similar exercise using a cable machine?

Yes. You can perform the cable fly using a cable machine. Position the cables on each tower of the cable machine at the lowest setting and then attach handles to the cables. Place a flat bench between the towers. Grasp one handle at a time and then lie on your back on the bench. You can now perform the exercise in the same manner described below. For more information on cable machines, see page 17.

DON'T

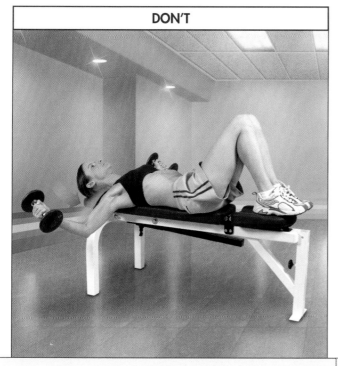

MUSCLES TARGETED

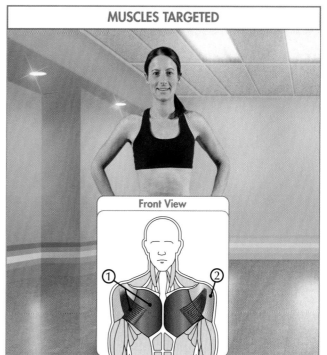

Front View

- Do not lower your arms below your shoulders as this will strain your shoulder muscles.
- Do not arch your back to help raise the dumbbells.
- Do not bend your wrists during the exercise. Keep your wrists straight and in line with your arms.

Targeted muscles:
① chest *(pectoralis major and minor)*

Additional muscles:
② front shoulders *(anterior deltoids)*

push-up

Push-ups are an excellent exercise for building upper-body strength and endurance and should be an important element of your strength training program. Push-ups work your chest, as well as your shoulders and triceps. Performing push-ups can help improve your ability to throw, which is useful in sports such as baseball or football.

One of the best features of push-ups is that it requires no weights or special equipment. All you need is an area large enough to accommodate your body length.

As you do push-ups, remember to keep your abdominal muscles tight to support your lower back. Also keep your face pointing toward the floor and your head in line with your back. Allowing your head to bob up and down as you move can result in neck strain. When you push yourself up, extend your arms as straight as you can without locking your elbows. If you have shoulder, elbow, wrist or lower back problems, consider modifying this exercise.

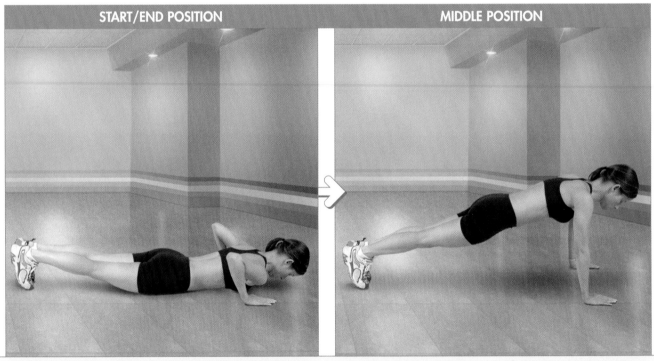

START/END POSITION **MIDDLE POSITION**

1 Lie on your stomach on the floor with your legs together and straight and the balls of your feet touching the floor. Tighten your abdominal muscles to help protect your back.

2 Bend your elbows and place your palms on the floor beside your shoulders, fingers pointing forward.

3 Slowly straighten your arms to raise your body off the floor. Make sure you keep your back and legs straight.

4 Slowly lower your body until your chest is a few inches off the floor.

Is there an easier way to do push-ups?

Yes. You can try performing modified push-ups or wall push-ups. To do modified push-ups, lay on the floor as you would for regular push-ups, except put your knees on the floor to help support your weight. You can keep your lower legs on the floor or raise them slightly, but do not cross your legs at the ankles. To do wall push-ups, stand about two feet away from a wall with your weight on the balls of your feet. Place your palms flat on the wall, a bit wider than shoulder width apart. Bending your elbows, lean into the wall and then push yourself back up.

I don't find regular push-ups challenging enough. How can I make them harder?

You can do push-ups with your feet elevated to make the push-ups more challenging. Get into the push-up position as you would for regular push-ups, except put your feet on a bench or step and place your hands on the floor.

DON'T

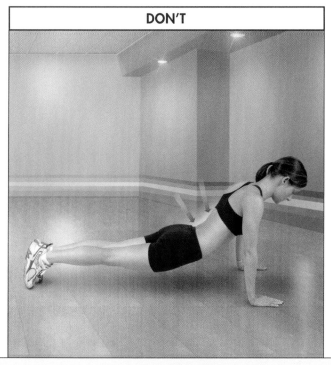

- Do not allow your back to slouch when you lift your body off the floor.

- Do not lock your elbows.

- Do not allow your head to tilt forward. Keep your head and neck aligned with your back.

MUSCLES TARGETED

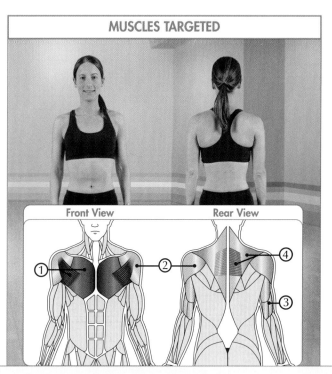

Targeted muscles:
① chest *(pectoralis major and minor)*

Additional muscles:
② shoulders *(deltoids)*
③ triceps
④ upper back *(rhomboids and trapezius)*

assisted dip

The assisted dip primarily works your chest and triceps, but also works the front of your shoulders. Using the assisted dip machine is one of the best ways to gain strength in your upper body.

The assisted dip machine allows you to practice dips without having to lift your entire body weight. When you do not have to lift your entire body weight, you can focus on using proper form. Even though the dips are assisted, you should take care when performing this exercise if you have

shoulder, elbow or wrist problems.

Choosing the amount of weight to use on the assisted dip machine may be confusing, since you need to select the opposite of what would apply to other exercises. The assisted dip machine counterbalances your body weight, so you need to choose a heavier weight to make the exercise easier or a lighter weight to make the exercise more difficult. Beginners may find that setting the weight between 60 and 70 percent of their body weight is most effective.

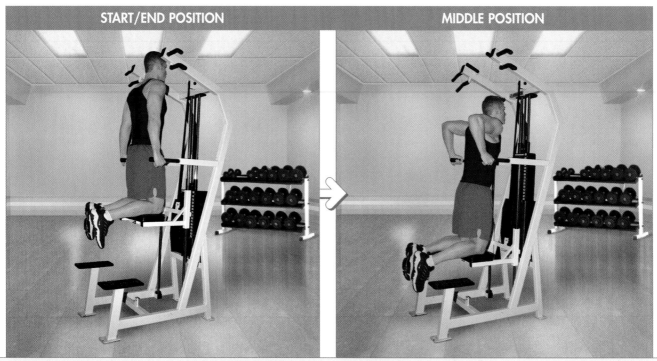

START/END POSITION　　　**MIDDLE POSITION**

1 Position your knees on the knee pad of an assisted dip machine.

2 Grip the lower bars with your palms facing in. Straighten your arms. Make sure your back is straight and you tighten your abdominal muscles to help protect your back.

3 Slowly lower your body until your upper arms are parallel to the floor. Keep your elbows close to your sides.

4 Slowly straighten your arms to lift your body back to the starting position.

Can I change the grip on an assisted dip machine?

On some assisted dip machines, you can adjust the handles to make the grip wider or narrower. The grip you select depends on which muscles you want to concentrate on. A wider grip allows you to focus on working your chest. A narrower grip allows you to focus on working your triceps.

How can I perform more advanced dips?

You can use a dip station to perform non-assisted dips that require you to lift and lower your entire body weight. A dip station is similar to an assisted dip machine but does not have a knee pad or weight stack. Grip the handles of the dip station with your palms facing in. Lift yourself onto the dip station bars, straighten your arms and then bend your knees and cross your ankles. Lower and lift your body using the same arm movement as you would on an assisted dip machine. You should take care when performing non-assisted dips if you have lower back problems.

DON'T

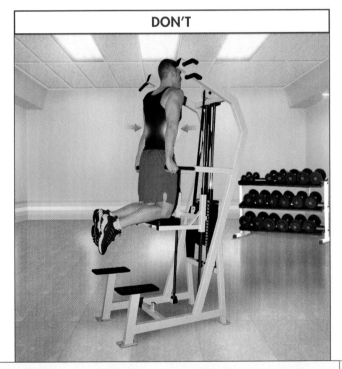

- Do not lock your elbows. Keep your elbows slightly bent at all times.
- Do not arch your back or shrug your shoulders.
- Do not push your head forward. Keep your head and neck in line with your body.
- Do not lower your body below the position at which your upper arms are parallel to the floor.

MUSCLES TARGETED

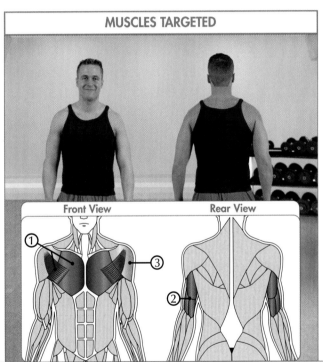

Targeted muscles:
① chest *(pectoralis major and minor)*
② triceps

Additional muscles:
③ front shoulders *(anterior deltoids)*

chest press machine

The chest press machine focuses on your chest, but also strengthens the front of your shoulders and your triceps. This machine allows you to perform an exercise similar to the bench press. For information on the bench press, see pages 30 and 32. Since the chest press machine does not require you to work with free weights, you have more stability than when performing the bench press. This added stability will help you isolate your chest muscles. When using the chest press machine, you should take extra care if you have shoulder, elbow or wrist problems.

It is important to maintain correct form when using the chest press machine. As you push the handles forward, make sure you do not push too quickly and end up locking your elbows. Your elbows should always be slightly bent. You should also not lift your shoulders, head or buttocks off the pad to help you push the weight forward. Remember to keep your abdominal muscles tight and make sure you do not arch your back.

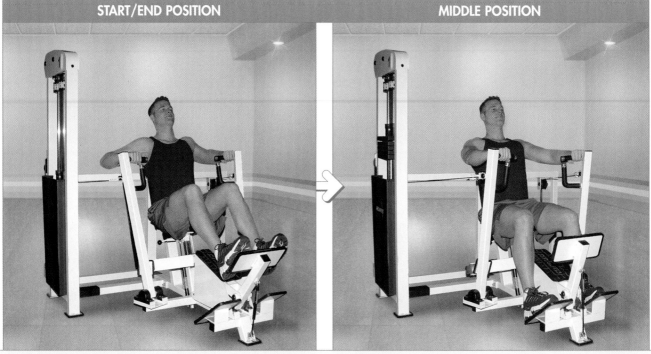

START/END POSITION **MIDDLE POSITION**

1 Sit on a chest press machine. Tighten your abdominal muscles to help protect your back.

2 If the machine has a foot lever to move the handles forward, press down on the lever.

3 Grasp the horizontal handles, both palms facing down, elbows out to your sides. Your hands should line up with the center of your chest.

• You can adjust the seat height to obtain the desired position.

4 Remove your feet from the foot lever to transfer the weight to your hands. Position your feet on the floor or footrest.

5 Slowly push the handles forward until your arms are straight, elbows slightly bent.

6 Slowly bend your arms until your hands are in front of your chest.

7 When you have completed your set, press down on the foot lever, release the handles and then slowly release the foot lever to lower the weight.

Is there a way to make the exercise more difficult?

Some chest press machines have vertical handles you can use to make the exercise more difficult. The vertical handles make the exercise more challenging because you no longer have as much help from your shoulders to push the weight forward. Using vertical handles will work the middle of your chest more to emphasize the separation between your chest muscles. When you use vertical handles, your palms face each other and your elbows are beside your body.

How can I emphasize my upper chest and the front of my shoulders more?

You can use an incline chest press machine to emphasize your upper chest and the front of your shoulders more. An incline chest press machine is similar to the regular chest press machine except you lie back on an incline and push the weight up instead of forward. When performing this exercise, grasp the handles with your palms facing forward, point your elbows out to the sides and avoid locking your elbows as you push the handles up.

DON'T

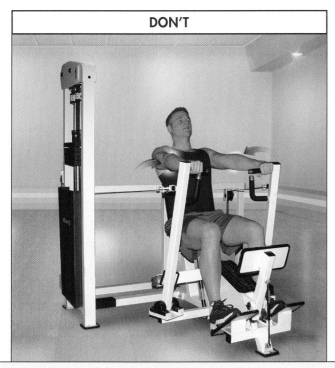

- Do not lock your elbows when you straighten your arms.
- Do not lift your shoulders, head or buttocks off the pad.
- Do not arch your back.
- Do not bend your wrists.
- Do not bring your arms too far back. Your elbows should not pass shoulder level.

MUSCLES TARGETED

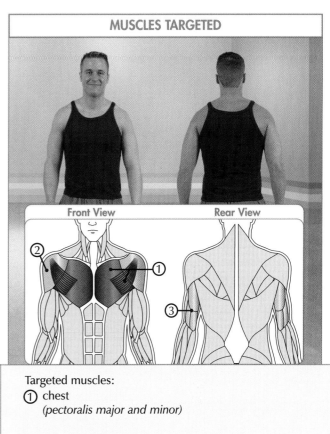

Targeted muscles:
① chest
(pectoralis major and minor)

Additional muscles:
② front shoulders
(anterior deltoids)
③ triceps

pec fly machine

The pec fly machine helps give your chest better definition by working the outer and upper edges of your chest. In addition to strengthening your chest, the machine also strengthens the front of your shoulders and your biceps.

The pec fly machine works the same muscles as the dumbbell fly. For information on the dumbbell fly, see page 34. The pec fly machine gives you more stability, making the exercise easier to perform than the dumbbell fly. As a result, you can try using slightly heavier weights on the pec fly machine. Despite the added stability, you should be careful performing this exercise if you have shoulder, elbow or neck problems.

If you find you are slamming the weights down onto the stack between repetitions, you are going too quickly. Keep the exercise slow and steady as you concentrate on your form. Do not allow your arms to go too far back when you return to the starting position. Also, make sure you keep your upper body and head on the back pad.

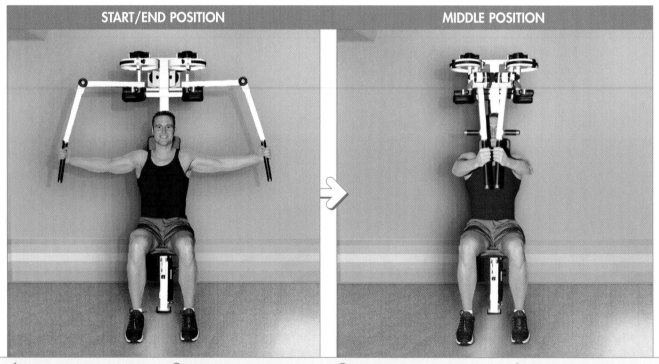

START/END POSITION **MIDDLE POSITION**

1 Sit on a pec fly machine with your feet flat on the floor or on the footrest, roughly shoulder width apart. Keep your back straight and tighten your abdominal muscles to help protect your back.

2 Grasp the handles with both palms facing forward. Your hands should be at shoulder height.

• You should be able to adjust the seat height to obtain the desired position.

3 Slowly push the handles toward the center of your body until both hands almost touch.

4 Slowly move your arms out to your sides to return to the starting position.

How can I ensure I do not injure my shoulders in this exercise?

To avoid shoulder injury, you should ensure that your elbows are in line with your shoulders at the start and end of each repetition. Some pec fly machines have handles you can adjust to make sure you do not bring your arms too far back. If the machine you are using does not have adjustable handles, you should begin the exercise by turning your body to one side at a time to bring each handle to the proper starting position.

Can I make this exercise easier?

You can use the pec deck machine to make this exercise easier by bringing your arms closer to your body. This machine is similar to the pec fly machine, except your forearms rest against pads and your elbows are bent at 90-degree angles. Be sure to watch your form carefully because it is very easy to cheat when using the pec deck machine.

DON'T

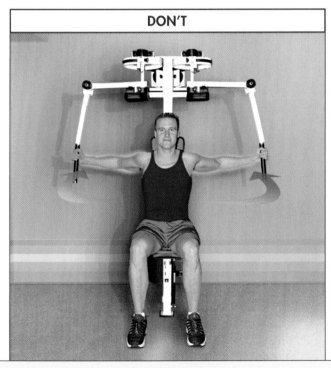

- Do not bring your arms too far back since this can injure your shoulders.

- Do not arch your back or lift your upper body or head off the back pad.

- Do not bend your wrists or shrug your shoulders.

MUSCLES TARGETED

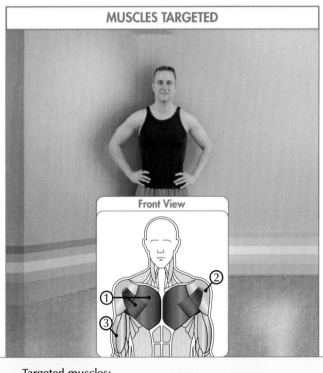

Front View

Targeted muscles:
① chest (*pectoralis major and minor*)

Additional muscles:
② front shoulders (*anterior deltoids*)
③ biceps

cable crossover

The cable crossover primarily strengthens and defines your chest, but also builds strength in the front of your shoulders. This exercise can help improve your performance in sports that require a strong upper body, such as baseball, tennis, hockey and golf. You should be careful performing this exercise if you have shoulder, elbow, wrist or lower back problems.

It is important to concentrate on maintaining proper form when performing the cable crossover. Make sure you use your chest to pull the handles of the cable

machine down to your sides and in front of your body. To help isolate your chest, keep your wrists straight, your elbows slightly bent and your shoulders back throughout the exercise. Also, remember to keep your knees slightly bent and your upper body erect. Your head, neck and back should be in a straight line.

As you perform the cable crossover, make sure you exhale as you pull the handles of the cable machine down.

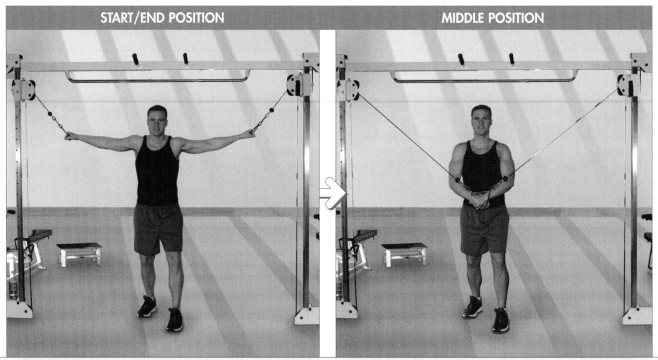

| START/END POSITION | MIDDLE POSITION |

1 Position the cable on each tower of a cable machine at the highest setting. Attach a handle to each cable.

2 Grasp a handle in each hand, palms facing down.

3 Stand in the center of the machine with your feet roughly shoulder width apart and one foot slightly forward. Make sure your feet are flat on the floor and your knees are slightly bent. Tighten your abdominal muscles to help protect your back.

4 Keeping a slight bend in your elbows, slowly pull the handles down to your sides and slightly in front of you until one wrist is in front of the other wrist. As you pull the handles down, slowly rotate your wrists so your palms face your stomach.

5 Pause for a moment and then slowly raise your arms up and out to your sides until your hands are at shoulder height.

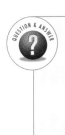

How can I work my lower chest more in this exercise?

To work your lower chest more, you can position the cable on each tower of a cable machine at the lowest setting. Grasp a handle in each hand with your palms facing your body and stand slightly in front of the center of the machine. Then pull the handles in front of you, just below chest height, so that your palms end up facing the ceiling. This modification also works your biceps.

Can I work each side of my body separately?

Yes. If you want to focus on one side of your body at a time, you can perform the cable crossover using only one arm at a time. Perform a full set with one arm and then switch arms and perform another set with your other arm. You can place the hand you are not using on your hip as you perform the exercise.

DON'T

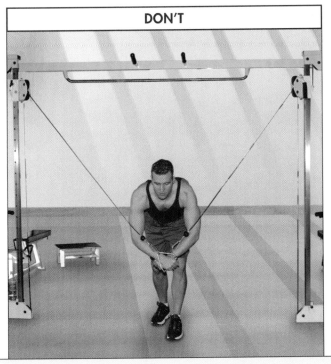

- Do not lean forward. Keep your head, neck and back in a straight line.

- Do not bend your wrists.

- Do not lock your elbows or knees. Keep your elbows and knees slightly bent.

MUSCLES TARGETED

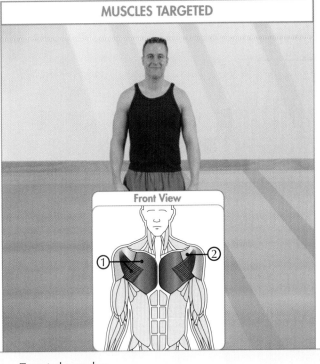

Front View

Targeted muscles:
① chest (*pectoralis major and minor*)

Additional muscles:
② front shoulders (*anterior deltoids*)

dumbbell shoulder press

The dumbbell shoulder press, also called the overhead press or military press, works your shoulders and upper back as well as your triceps. This is a good exercise for building strong, wide shoulders. Strengthening your shoulders helps make overhead pushing or lifting movements easier. If you have neck, shoulder, lower back or elbow problems, you should be careful when performing this exercise.

You can perform dumbbell shoulder presses while sitting or standing. If you choose to sit, use a bench with back support. Supporting your back helps you avoid using your lower back during the exercise so you must do most of the work with your shoulder muscles.

When you raise the dumbbells, press your arms straight up over your head, but do not lock your elbows. Keep your head and neck straight, your abdominal muscles tight and your back erect. If you find that you need to arch your back excessively to lift the dumbbells, consider using lighter weights.

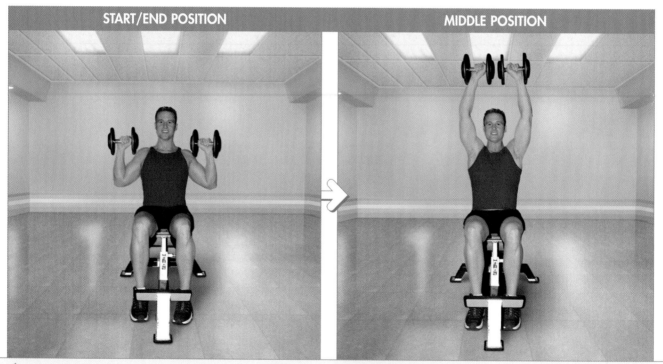

START/END POSITION MIDDLE POSITION

1 Hold a dumbbell in each hand.

2 Sit on a bench with back support and place your feet flat on the floor roughly shoulder width apart.

• Keep your back straight and head up. Tighten your abdominal muscles to help protect your back.

3 Position the dumbbells just above your shoulders with your elbows pointing down and palms facing forward.

4 Slowly raise the dumbbells above your head until they almost touch. Your arms should end up as straight as possible without locking your elbows.

• When your arms are straight, you should be able to see the weights without tilting your head back.

5 Slowly lower the dumbbells back to the starting position.

Is there a way to change how the exercise works my shoulders?

You can slightly change the emphasis of the exercise by holding the dumbbells in a different way. To work the front part of your shoulders more, perform the shoulder press as usual, but hold the dumbbells with your palms facing each other instead of forward.

Can I use a barbell to perform shoulder presses?

Yes. Sit on a bench just behind the bar of a barbell rack or a Smith machine. Make sure the bench or machine has a back support. Grip the bar with your hands a bit wider than shoulder width apart and palms facing forward. The height of the bar should allow your elbows to bend about 90 degrees. Lift the bar off the rack and hold it at about chin level. Slowly press the bar straight up above your head and then slowly lower the bar back to the starting position. For information on the Smith machine, see page 16.

DON'T

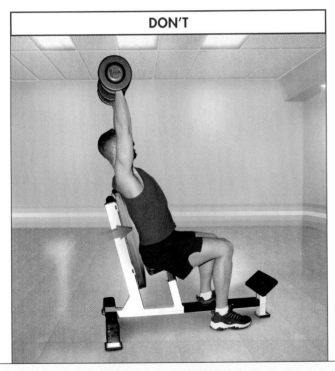

- Do not arch your back or wiggle your body to help you lift the dumbbells. Keep your back flat against the pad.
- Do not lock your elbows or allow the dumbbells to sway back and forth.
- Do not lower the dumbbells below the starting position.

MUSCLES TARGETED

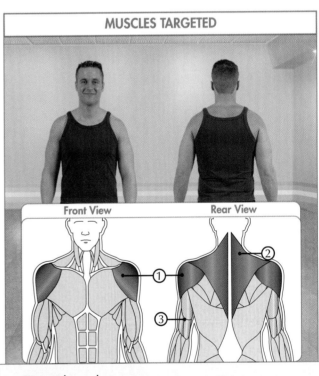

Front View Rear View

Targeted muscles:
① shoulders *(anterior and middle deltoids)*
② upper back *(upper trapezius)*

Additional muscles:
③ triceps

lateral raise

The lateral raise works the muscles of your shoulders and upper back. This is a good exercise for building strength and defining the shape of your shoulders, which can even out the overall look of your body.

As with any exercise, you should be careful to use proper form when performing the lateral raise, but you should be especially careful if you have neck or lower back problems. You should not perform this exercise if you have shoulder problems. Remember to keep your palms facing down as you lift the dumbbells to ensure your shoulders, rather than your biceps, are doing the work.

You should also make sure you keep your elbows slightly bent throughout the exercise to take the pressure off your elbows.

To prevent injuries, avoid raising your arms above your shoulders and moving your upper body forward or back as you lift the weights. Maintaining good posture and tight abdominal muscles throughout the exercise will help you avoid back strain. You can also perform the lateral raise while sitting on a chair or bench to provide better stability for your back while working your shoulders.

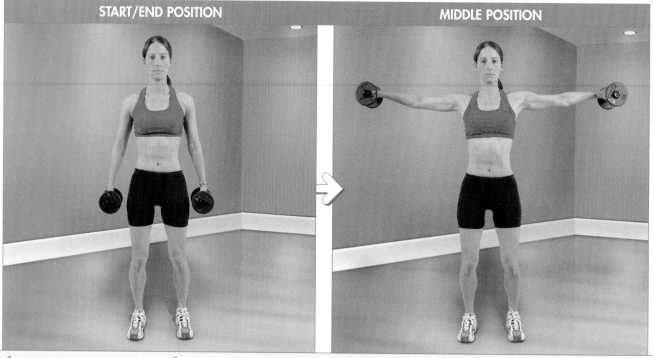

START/END POSITION   **MIDDLE POSITION**

1 Hold a dumbbell in each hand with your arms at your sides and both palms facing inward.

2 Stand straight with your feet roughly shoulder width apart. Tighten your abdominal muscles to help protect your back.

3 Slowly raise the dumbbells out to your sides until they are at shoulder height. Keep your arms straight, elbows slightly bent and palms facing down as you lift the dumbbells.

4 Pause for a moment and then slowly lower the dumbbells back to your sides.

I have weak shoulders. Is there an easier way to perform the lateral raise?

If you have problems with your shoulders, you can take some of the strain off your shoulders by performing the lateral raise with your elbows bent at 90-degree angles. Start the exercise with your elbows bent, palms facing inward and the dumbbells in front of your body. Keep your elbows bent throughout the exercise.

Can I modify the lateral raise to help work my rotator cuff muscles?

You can easily modify the lateral raise to work your rotator cuff muscles by performing the exercise with your palms facing forward instead of inward. Strengthening your rotator cuff muscles can help your performance in sports that require upper body strength. This variation also works the middle part of your shoulders.

DON'T

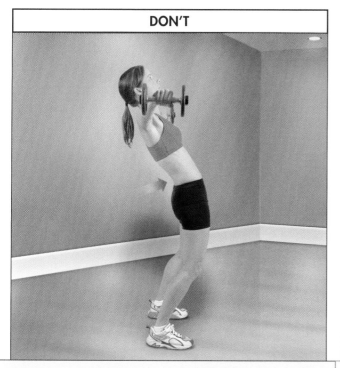

- Do not arch your back, lean forward, lean back or swing back and forth to help you lift the dumbbells. Keep your back straight at all times.
- Do not raise your arms above your shoulders.

MUSCLES TARGETED

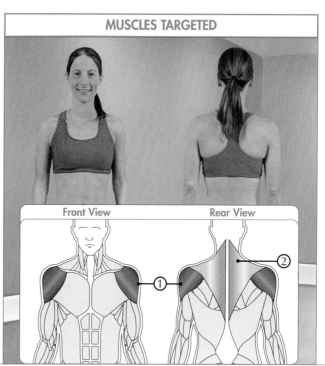

Front View   Rear View

Targeted muscles:
① middle shoulders (*middle deltoids*)

Additional muscles:
② upper back (*upper trapezius*)

bent over lateral raise

The bent over lateral raise focuses on the muscles in the back of your shoulders and your middle and upper back. This exercise can make activities that involve lifting easier and can help improve your posture.

Isolating the back of your shoulder muscles can help give your shoulders a more balanced appearance. Since this exercise works your shoulders, you should take care when performing this exercise if you have shoulder or neck problems.

When performing the bent over lateral raise, there are several things you should keep in mind to maintain proper form. Make sure you bend forward from your hips and keep your back straight so that your upper body is parallel to the floor. As you lift the weight, you should maintain a slow, controlled arm movement and keep the rest of your body still. You may have to make a conscious effort to not raise your upper body as you lift the weight.

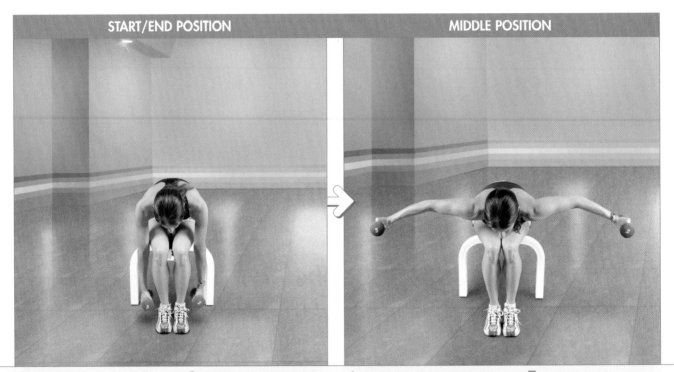

START/END POSITION | **MIDDLE POSITION**

1 Hold a dumbbell in each hand.

2 Sit on the edge of a bench with your legs together. Bend forward from your hips so your upper body is parallel to the floor. Tighten your abdominal muscles to help protect your back.

3 Allow your arms to hang straight down, elbows slightly bent, both palms facing in.

4 Slowly raise the dumbbells out to your sides until your elbows are at shoulder height. Keep your arms straight, elbows slightly bent and palms facing down. Squeeze your shoulder blades together as you lift the dumbbells.

5 Pause for a moment and then slowly lower the dumbbells back to your sides.

Is there a more advanced bent over lateral raise?

Yes. The standing bent over lateral raise is a more advanced exercise because it requires you to maintain your balance and stability while lifting the weight. With your feet shoulder width apart and your upper body at a 45-degree angle with the floor, perform the same arm movement as you would when seated.

How can I work each side separately?

You can use a cable machine to work each side separately. Position a cable on a tower of a cable machine at the lowest setting and then attach a handle to the cable. Stand with your feet shoulder width apart, with one side of your body facing the tower. Then grip the handle with the hand furthest away from the cable. With your upper body at a 45-degree angle with the floor, perform the same arm movement as you would when seated. Repeat for your other side. For more information on cable machines, see page 17.

DON'T

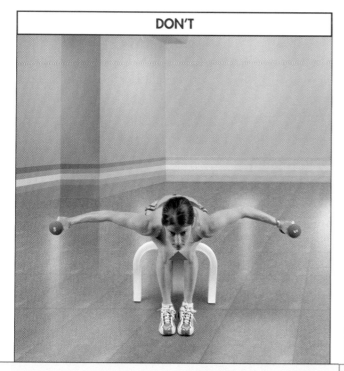

MUSCLES TARGETED

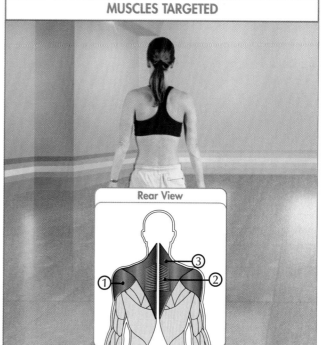

- Do not turn your head left or right or tilt your head up or down. Keep your head and neck in line with your body.

- Do not lock your elbows or raise them past your shoulders.

- Do not hunch your back or move your upper body as you raise and lower the dumbbells. Your back should be straight and your upper body should remain parallel to the floor.

Targeted muscles:
① rear shoulders (*posterior deltoids*)
② middle back (*rhomboids*)
③ upper back (*upper trapezius*)

front raise

The front raise can improve the overall shape of your shoulders by working the front of your shoulders. Strengthening the front of your shoulders can also help you perform everyday tasks, such as lifting objects and reaching up to take an object off a shelf.

While performing the front raise, make sure you do not lean back or forward or arch your back to help you lift the weight. You should also try not to lift the weight by rocking your body back and forth. Concentrate on using only your shoulders to lift the weight. As you raise your arms, keep your elbows slightly bent and make sure you do not raise your arms above shoulder height.

If you want to focus on strengthening one shoulder at a time, you can alternate between your left and right arm to lift the dumbbells. Keep alternating arms until you finish a set.

You should use caution when performing the front raise if you have shoulder or neck problems.

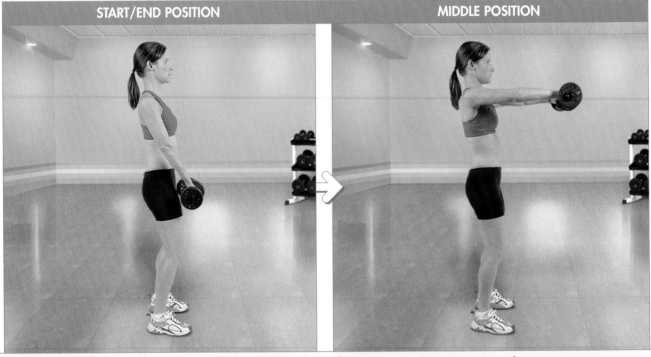

START/END POSITION　　　**MIDDLE POSITION**

1 Hold a dumbbell in each hand in front of your thighs, both palms facing your body.

2 Stand straight with your feet roughly shoulder width apart. Make sure your knees and elbows are slightly bent. Tighten your abdominal muscles to help protect your back.

3 Slowly raise your arms in front of you until your arms are parallel to the floor.

4 Slowly lower the dumbbells back to the starting position.

How can I protect my back more when performing the front raise?

To protect your back more, you can perform the front raise while sitting on a bench with a back support. Position your arms beside your body with your palms facing in and then rotate your wrists as you raise your arms so your palms end up facing the floor. This modification helps isolate the front of your shoulders more by making it more difficult to use other muscles to lift the weight.

Can I perform the front raise using a cable machine?

Yes. Position a cable on a tower of a cable machine at the lowest setting and then attach a handle to the cable. Stand to the side of the handle with your back facing the tower, your feet shoulder width apart and your knees slightly bent. Grasp the handle with your palm facing backward and then perform the same arm movement as described below. When you complete a set with one arm, repeat the exercise using your other arm. For more information on cable machines, see page 17.

DON'T

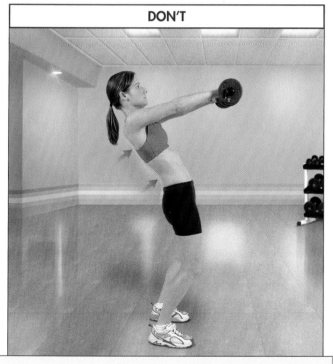

MUSCLES TARGETED

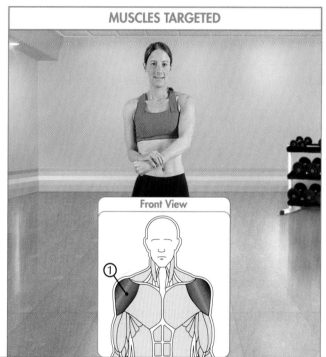

Front View

- Do not arch your back, lean forward or lean back to help lift the dumbbells. Keep your back straight at all times.

- Do not raise your arms above your shoulders.

- Do not lock your elbows. Keep your elbows slightly bent at all times.

- Do not tilt your head forward or back. Keep your head, neck and back in a straight line.

Targeted muscles:
① front shoulders *(anterior deltoids)*

reverse fly

The reverse fly works the back of your shoulders, as well as your upper back and triceps. You use a pec fly/rear deltoid machine or a rear deltoid fly machine to perform this exercise.

Since most shoulder exercises work the front of your shoulders, performing the reverse fly to work the back of your shoulders allows you to strengthen the muscles in your shoulders evenly. The reverse fly can also help improve your posture, which is a

benefit of developing strong shoulders.

You should be careful performing this exercise if you have shoulder or neck problems. To avoid injuring your shoulders, do not press your arms too far back when you push the handles outward. Also concentrate on performing the exercise in a slow, controlled manner, while keeping your back straight, your abdominal muscles tight and your head and neck in line with your back.

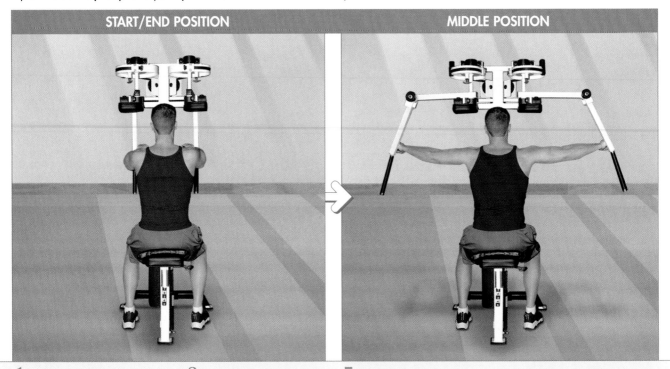

| START/END POSITION | MIDDLE POSITION |

1 If you are using a pec fly/rear deltoid machine, adjust the arms of the machine so the handles are as close to the weight stack as possible.

2 Sit on the machine with your chest firmly against the pad.

3 Position your feet flat on the floor or on the footrest.

4 Grasp the handles with both palms facing down. Your hands should be at shoulder height.

• You can adjust the seat height to obtain the desired position.

5 Keeping your elbows slightly bent, slowly push the handles out to your sides until your arms line up with your body.

• Make sure you keep your back straight and you tighten your abdominal muscles to help protect your back.

6 Slowly move your hands back toward the center of your body to return to the starting position.

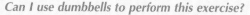

How can I work one arm at a time?

Working one arm at a time allows you to focus on strengthening each arm independently. This is useful when one of your arms is stronger than the other and you want to balance the strength in your arms. Perform the exercise as described below, except grasp the front of the chest pad for support with one arm while you work the other arm. After completing a set with one arm, repeat the exercise with your other arm.

Can I use dumbbells to perform this exercise?

Yes. Grasp a light dumbbell in each hand and sit on a bench with back support. Position your feet shoulder width apart. Extend your arms straight out in front of you at shoulder level with your palms facing down and your elbows slightly bent. Bring your arms out to the sides until the dumbbells are in line with your body and then slowly move your arms forward to return to the starting position. Using dumbbells helps strengthen your shoulders equally and makes the exercise harder since you have to balance the weight.

DON'T

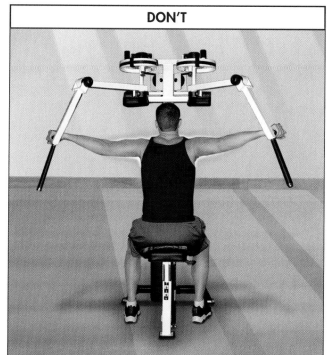

- Do not bring your arms too far back since this can injure your shoulders.

- Do not lean back or bend your neck.

- Do not lock your elbows or bend your wrists.

- Do not shrug your shoulders.

MUSCLES TARGETED

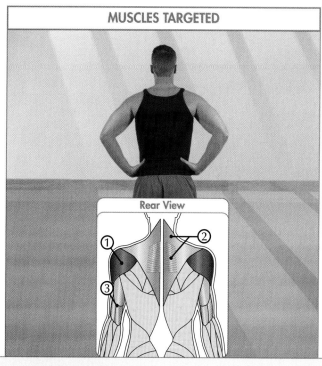

Rear View

Targeted muscles:
① rear shoulders
(posterior deltoids)

Additional muscles:
② upper back
(trapezius and rhomboids)
③ triceps

shoulder press machine

The shoulder press machine mainly works the middle and front of your shoulders, but also strengthens your triceps and upper back. This exercise helps develop stronger shoulder muscles, which makes lifting objects over your head easier. The shoulder press machine is safer and easier to use than free weights because you do not need to worry about balancing the weight or the weight falling on you.

As you use the shoulder press machine, keep your shoulders relaxed. You should also remember to maintain proper form. Avoid lifting your head off the bench as you press the handles up and tighten your abdominal muscles to help protect your back.

If you have problems with your shoulders, elbows or neck, you should be careful when using this machine. In particular, do not use too much force as you press the handles up to avoid putting excess stress on your elbows.

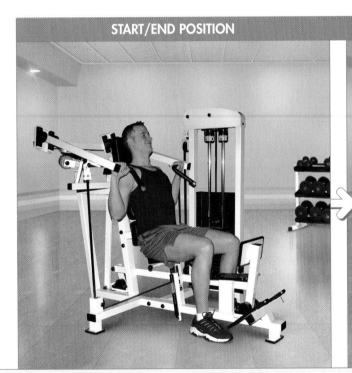

START/END POSITION

MIDDLE POSITION

1 Sit on a shoulder press machine with your feet flat on the floor, roughly shoulder width apart. Make sure your back is straight and tighten your abdominal muscles to help protect your back.

2 Grasp the horizontal handles with your palms facing forward. Your hands should be level with your shoulders and your elbows pointed toward the floor.

• You should be able to adjust the seat height to obtain the desired position.

3 Slowly press the handles up until your arms are straight, elbows slightly bent.

4 Slowly lower the handles until your arms are just above the starting position.

How can I focus on working the front of my shoulders more?

Most shoulder press machines have another set of handles that allow you to focus on the front of your shoulders more. Perform the same exercise described below, except hold the other set of handles with your palms facing each other instead of forward.

Can I use the shoulder press machine to balance the strength between my arms?

Some shoulder press machines allow you to work on one arm at a time to help balance the strength between your arms. This is useful for preventing your strong arm from getting stronger and your weak arm from getting weaker. When working on each arm separately, you should use less weight.

DON'T

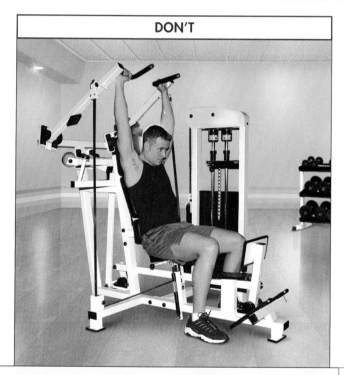

- Do not lift your head off the bench.
- Do not arch your back or wiggle your body to help you lift the weight. Keep your back flat against the pad.
- Do not shrug your shoulders while pressing the weight up.
- Do not lock your elbows. Keep your elbows slightly bent at all times.

MUSCLES TARGETED

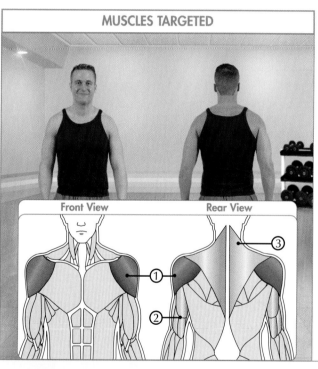

Targeted muscles:
① middle and front shoulders
  (middle and anterior deltoids)

Additional muscles:
② triceps
③ upper back *(upper trapezius)*

dumbbell external rotation

The dumbbell external rotation works the muscles deep in your shoulders, which are called the rotator cuff muscles. The rotator cuff muscles are responsible for rotating and stabilizing your arm in its socket. As a result, strengthening the rotator cuff muscles can help improve your performance in any throwing or racquet sports, such as baseball or tennis.

To maintain proper form when performing this exercise, you can visualize your shoulder acting as a hinge that opens when you raise your arm and

closes when you lower your arm. As you lift the weight, make sure you keep your body stationary and only move your arm as far back as is comfortable for you. If you have recently injured your rotator cuff muscles, use caution when performing this exercise.

You may feel strain in your neck while performing this exercise. To reduce the strain on your neck, lie on your outstretched arm. Placing a towel under your neck may help to make the exercise even more comfortable.

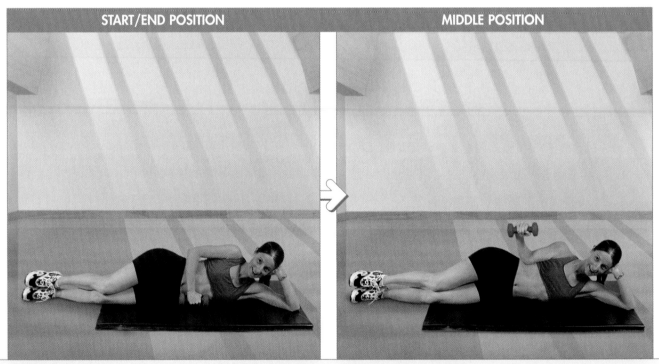

START/END POSITION · **MIDDLE POSITION**

1 Hold a dumbbell in your right hand.

2 Lie on your left side on the floor or on a bench with your legs together, knees slightly bent. Rest your head in your left hand or lie on your outstretched left arm.

3 Position your right elbow at your side, bend your elbow at a 90-degree angle and rest your right forearm on your stomach, palm facing your stomach.

4 Keeping your upper arm stationary, slowly raise your right hand as far as you can. Tighten your abdominal muscles to help protect your back.

5 Slowly lower your right hand back toward your stomach.

6 After completing a set with your right arm, switch sides and repeat the exercise with your left arm.

Is there a standing variation of this exercise?

Yes. To perform a standing variation of this exercise, stand with your feet shoulder width apart as you hold a dumbbell out to one side at shoulder height. With your palm facing the floor, bend your elbow to bring your forearm forward until your arm forms a 90-degree angle. Keeping your upper arm at shoulder height, raise your forearm so that your palm faces forward and then lower your forearm back to the starting position. Once you complete a set, repeat the exercise with your other arm.

What should I do if I find a heavy dumbbell awkward to lift?

You can use a cable machine to perform the exercise instead of using a dumbbell. Position a cable on a tower of a cable machine at hip height and attach a handle to the cable. Stand with your feet shoulder width apart with one side of your body facing the tower. Grip the handle with the hand furthest away from the cable. Then perform the same movement as you would when lying down. For more information on cable machines, see page 17.

DON'T

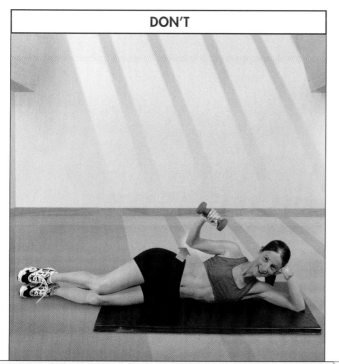

MUSCLES TARGETED

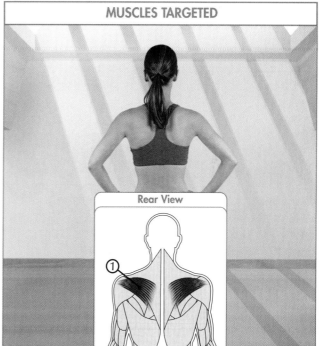

Rear View

- Do not lift your elbow off your side or bend your wrist when raising or lowering your arm.

- Do not rock your body back and forth. Keep your body stationary.

- Do not strain your neck. Rest your head in your free hand or lie on your outstretched arm.

Targeted muscles:
① deep shoulder muscles *(rotator cuff)*

dumbbell internal rotation

The dumbbell internal rotation focuses on the rotator cuff. The rotator cuff is located deep in your shoulders and is responsible for rotating and stabilizing your arm in its socket. For this reason, strengthening your rotator cuff can help improve your performance in any throwing or racquet sports, such as football or squash.

It may help you maintain proper form when performing this exercise if you visualize your shoulder acting as a hinge that closes when you raise your arm and opens when you lower your arm. As you lift and lower your arm, make sure you do not rock your body back and forth to help you lift the weight. Instead, you should keep your body stationary.

Be careful performing this exercise if you have recently injured your rotator cuff. You should also take care to not strain your neck when performing this exercise. To make sure you do not strain your neck, rest your head on the floor or on a rolled up towel.

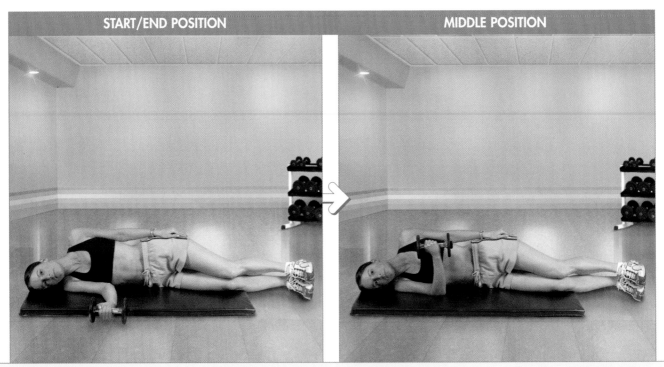

START/END POSITION | **MIDDLE POSITION**

1 Hold a dumbbell in your right hand.

2 Lie on your right side on the floor or on a bench with your legs together, knees slightly bent. Position your left arm at your side. Tighten your abdominal muscles to help protect your back.

3 Position your right elbow at your side, bend your elbow at a 90-degree angle and rest your arm on the floor.

4 Keeping your upper right arm stationary, slowly raise your right hand toward your body.

5 Slowly lower your right hand back to the starting position.

6 After completing a set with your right arm, switch sides and repeat the exercise with your left arm.

What should I do if I find a heavy dumbbell awkward to lift?

You can use a cable machine to perform the exercise instead. Position a cable on a tower of a cable machine at hip height and then attach a handle to the cable. Stand with your feet shoulder width apart with one side of your body facing the tower. Grip the handle with the hand closest to the cable and then perform the same movement as you would when lying down. For more information on cable machines, see page 17.

How can I make the exercise more difficult?

Position a cable on a tower of a cable machine at shoulder height and then attach a handle to the cable. Stand with your back facing the tower and your feet shoulder width apart with one foot in front of the other. Reach your right hand over your right shoulder to grip the handle with your palm facing forward. With your upper arm parallel to the floor, bring your forearm up until your arm forms a 90-degree angle. Keep your upper arm stationary as you pull the handle forward so your palm faces the floor and then return to the starting position. Once you complete a set, repeat the exercise with your other arm.

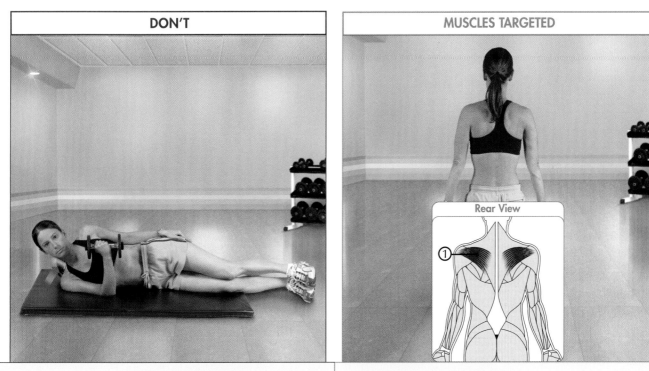

DON'T	MUSCLES TARGETED

Rear View

- Do not strain your neck. You can rest your head on the floor or on a rolled up towel.

- Do not rock your body back and forth. Keep your body stationary.

Targeted muscles:
① deep shoulder muscles
   (rotator cuff)

lat pulldown

The lat pulldown targets two of the major muscles of your back and is a great exercise for adding mass to your back and obtaining the desirable V-shape. This exercise also strengthens your shoulders and biceps.

The lat pulldown is a common exercise in many weightlifters' routines and is especially valuable for athletes, such as swimmers, rowers and rock climbers, who benefit from having a powerful upper body.

While performing this exercise, you should concentrate on maintaining proper form. Keep your back straight and your abdominal muscles tight to help protect your back. Do not swing your body back and forth or lean back too far to help you pull down the weight.

After you have completed a set, you should stand up and slowly lower the weight back down onto the stack. Do not just release the bar and let the weight come crashing down onto the stack.

You should be very careful when performing lat pulldowns if you have shoulder, elbow, lower back or neck problems.

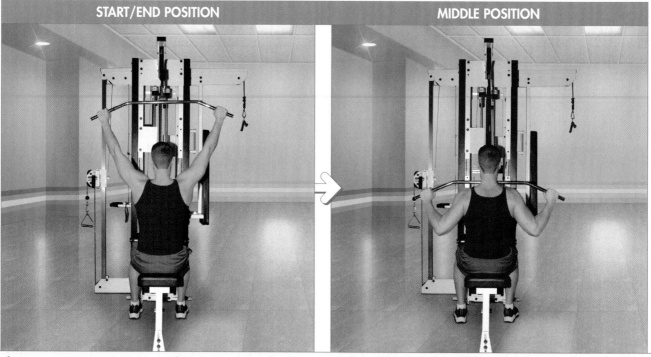

START/END POSITION → **MIDDLE POSITION**

1 Sit on a lat pulldown machine and position your upper thighs under the thigh pad and your feet flat on the floor.

• You can adjust the height of the seat or thigh pad to the desired position.

2 Stand up and grasp the bar with both palms facing forward and your hands slightly wider than shoulder width apart.

3 Still grasping the bar, sit down and lean back slightly from your hips.

4 Drop your shoulders and squeeze your shoulder blades together as you slowly pull the bar down to the top of your chest.

• Keep your back straight and your elbows pointing toward the floor.

5 Pause for a moment and then slowly straighten your arms to raise the bar back to the starting position.

6 When you have completed a set, stand up to slowly lower the weight.

How can I work my biceps and forearms more?

You can perform the reverse-grip lat pulldown to work your biceps and forearms more. To perform the reverse-grip lat pulldown, perform the steps below, except turn your palms to face your body and grasp the bar with your hands shoulder width apart. This lat pulldown variation also works the inner part of your back *(latissimus dorsi)* more.

How can I put more focus on the lower part of my back and the rear of my shoulders?

You can perform the straight arm lat pulldown to put more focus on the lower part of your back *(latissimus dorsi)* and the rear of your shoulders. Stand behind the seat of a lat pulldown machine, with your feet about shoulder width apart. Grasp the bar with your palms facing the floor and your hands shoulder width apart. Bend your elbows and knees slightly and tighten your abdominal muscles. Then slowly pull the bar down to your thighs, keeping your arms straight.

DON'T

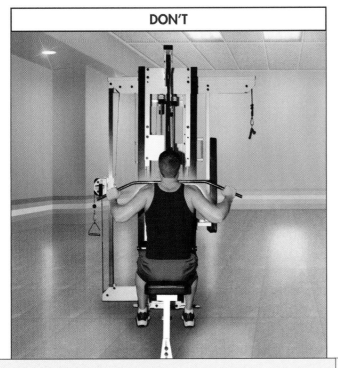

- Do not shrug your shoulders.
- Do not lean too far back, swing back and forth or arch your back to help pull the bar down.
- Do not lift your body off the seat when you raise the bar back to the starting position.
- Do not bend your wrists or lock your elbows.
- Keep your head, neck and back in a straight line.

MUSCLES TARGETED

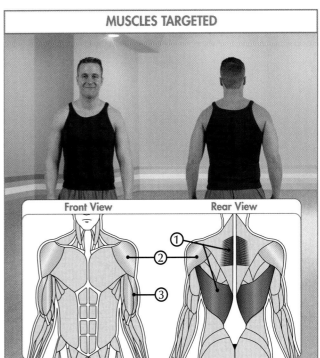

Front View   Rear View

Targeted muscles:
① back *(latissimus dorsi* and *rhomboids)*

Additional muscles:
② shoulders *(deltoids)*
③ biceps

one-arm dumbbell row

The one-arm dumbbell row works your back, with a secondary emphasis on the back of your shoulders and your biceps. This exercise is useful if you want to add mass and definition to the muscles in your back.

You may have a tendency to focus on the movement of your arm in this exercise. Remember, however, that this is primarily a back exercise, so you should concentrate on using your back muscles to lift the weight. With proper focus on your back, this exercise can strengthen each side of your back to correct any imbalances in your back muscles.

To maintain proper form, you should keep your abdominals tight and your back straight and parallel to the floor at all times. You will know that you are lifting the correct amount of weight if you can squeeze your shoulder blade when you pull your elbow back. You should not have to twist your body or jerk or swing the dumbbell forward to lift the weight.

Use caution performing this exercise if you have shoulder, neck or lower back problems.

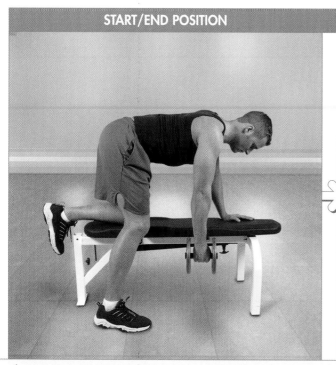

START/END POSITION   **MIDDLE POSITION**

1 Position your right foot flat on the floor beside a flat bench with your knee slightly bent. Position your left knee on the bench.

2 Lean forward and position your left hand on the bench to support your upper body.

• Make sure your back is straight and parallel with the floor.

3 Allow your right arm to hang straight down. Reach down and pick up a dumbbell off the floor, palm facing in.

4 Slowly raise the dumbbell by pulling your elbow as far back as you can. Squeeze your shoulder blade and keep your arm close to your side.

• Tighten your abdominal muscles to help protect your back.

5 Slowly lower the dumbbell back to the starting position.

6 After completing a set with your right arm, position your right hand and right knee on the bench and repeat with your left arm.

How can I make the exercise more intense?

You can rotate your wrist as you perform the exercise, which helps work your back muscles more. Start with your palm facing backward. As you raise the dumbbell, rotate your wrist so that your palm ends up facing your body. You may find it helpful to visualize yourself starting a lawn mower as you perform this exercise.

Can I perform a variation of the one-arm dumbbell row using the cable machine?

Yes. Position a cable on a tower of a cable machine at the lowest setting and attach a handle to the cable. Stand one foot in front and slightly to the side of the tower with your feet shoulder width apart and your knees slightly bent. Then bend from the hips to position your upper body at a 45-degree angle with the floor. Grip the handle so your arm is extended in front of you and your palm is facing the floor. As you perform the exercise, use the same arm movement as described in the steps below, except turn your wrist so your palm ends up facing your body. Perform a full set on one side and then repeat on your other side.

DON'T

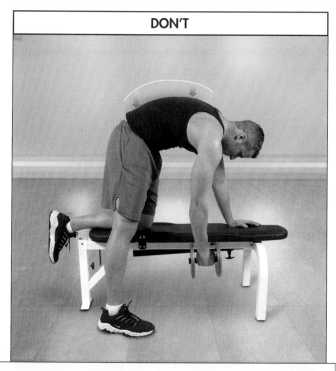

- Do not arch or hunch your back. Keep your back straight and parallel with the floor at all times.
- Do not twist your body or swing the dumbbell forward to help you lift the weight.
- Do not bend your neck. Keep your head, neck and back in a straight line.
- Do not lock the knee of the leg you are standing on or the elbow of the arm supporting your body.

MUSCLES TARGETED

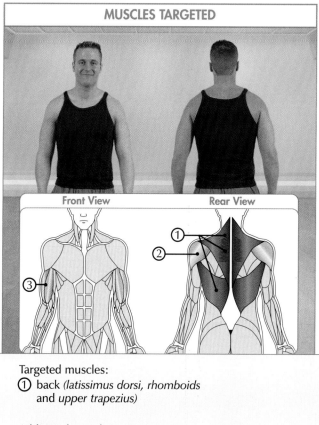

Front View　　Rear View

Targeted muscles:
① back (*latissimus dorsi, rhomboids* and *upper trapezius*)

Additional muscles:
② rear shoulders (*posterior deltoid*)
③ biceps

bent over barbell row

The bent over barbell row targets the major muscles of your back, but also works the back of your shoulders. Regular practice of this exercise can help you strengthen and add mass to your upper back.

When performing the bent over barbell row, remember to bend at your hips, not your waist. As you bend your arms to raise the barbell, do not hunch your back to help lift the weight. You should keep your back straight and your abdominal muscles tight throughout the exercise to help protect your back. You should also keep your elbows close to your sides as you lift and lower the weight. As with any exercise, you should perform all movements in a slow, controlled manner to benefit the most from the exercise.

To avoid injury, do not lock your elbows or knees during the exercise. You should also avoid bending your wrists or neck. You should be careful performing the bent over barbell row if you have lower back, shoulder or neck problems.

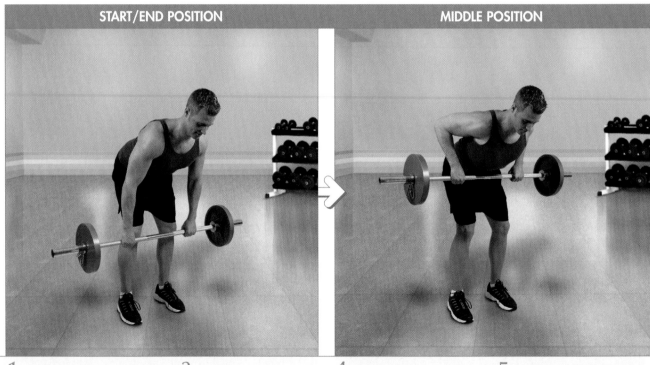

START/END POSITION   **MIDDLE POSITION**

1 Stand behind a barbell with your feet flat on the floor roughly shoulder width apart and your knees slightly bent.

2 Grasp the bar roughly shoulder width apart with your palms facing back and your elbows slightly bent.

3 Bend forward from your hips at a 45-degree angle. Keep your back straight and tighten your abdominal muscles to help protect your back.

4 Slowly bend your arms to raise the bar to your stomach.

5 Pause for a moment and then slowly straighten your arms to lower the bar.

Can I perform bent over rows using dumbbells?

Yes. You can perform bent over rows using dumbbells instead of a barbell. Perform the steps below, holding the dumbbells with your palms facing back. Since each arm is lifting its own weight, using dumbbells strengthens the left and right sides of your back independently to help correct any imbalances in your back muscles.

How can I work my biceps when performing bent over rows?

In addition to working your back and the back of your shoulders, you can work your biceps by grasping the barbell or dumbbells with your palms facing forward. Holding the barbell or dumbbells with your palms facing forward also gives you a greater range of motion. As a result, you can pull your elbows back further to work your back, the back of your shoulders and your biceps more.

DON'T

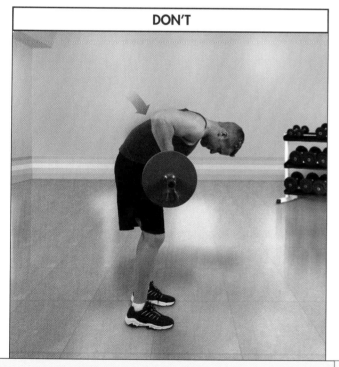

- Do not hunch your back to help you lift the weight.

- Do not allow your elbows to move away from your body. Keep your elbows close to your sides.

- Do not lock your knees or elbows.

- Do not bend your wrists or neck.

MUSCLES TARGETED

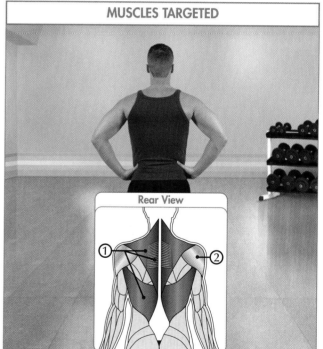

Rear View

Targeted muscles:
① back (*latissimus dorsi, rhomboids* and *trapezius*)

Additional muscles:
② rear shoulders (*posterior deltoids*)

dumbbell shrug

The dumbbell shrug is a simple but effective way to strengthen your upper back and shoulders. Shrugs help develop the muscles between your shoulders and neck, increasing the strength and stability of your neck. Greater neck stability is beneficial for people who participate in contact sports or activities that pose a high risk for neck and head injuries, such as football. Strengthening your upper back and shoulders can also help make it easier to perform some everyday tasks, such as carrying a heavy bag over your shoulder.

If you have neck or lower back problems, you should be careful when doing this exercise.

To prevent unnecessary strain on your shoulder joints, avoid rolling your shoulders in a circle as you shrug. Instead, concentrate on lifting your shoulders straight up and straight down for each movement. You may notice that your range of motion tends to decrease as your muscles get tired, but try to perform the full range of movement throughout the entire exercise.

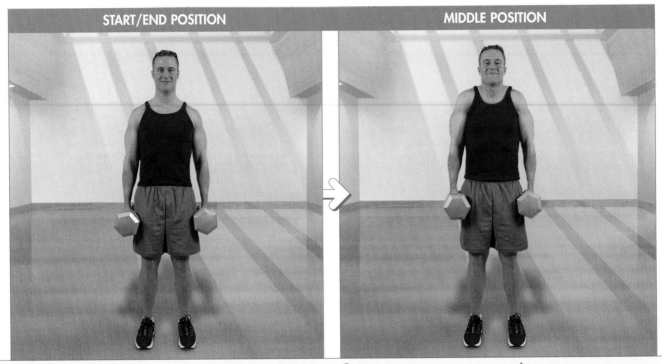

START/END POSITION | **MIDDLE POSITION**

1 Hold a dumbbell in each hand at your sides, with your elbows slightly bent and both palms facing in.

2 Stand straight with your feet roughly shoulder width apart, knees slightly bent and your head up. Tighten your abdominal muscles to help protect your back.

3 Slowly raise your shoulders as close to your ears as possible.

4 Pause for a moment and then slowly return your shoulders to the starting position.

QUESTION & ANSWER

How do I perform shrugs using a barbell?

Stand with your feet shoulder width apart and hold the barbell behind you with your hands at your sides, elbows slightly bent and your palms facing back. Raise your shoulders towards your ears, squeezing your shoulder blades together. Then return to the starting position. The barbell shrug works more of your upper middle back and is more effective than the dumbbell shrug since your arms are positioned further back. If you are not comfortable holding the barbell behind your back, you can hold it in front of your thighs instead.

Is there a machine I can use to do this exercise?

Yes. Some gyms have a shrug machine. Sit at the machine and grasp the handles at your sides with your palms facing in. If necessary, adjust the seat height to make sure your elbows are slightly bent when you grasp the handles. Lift the handles as you raise your shoulders and slowly lower the handles as you lower your shoulders. The shrug machine may help you lift more weight without losing your balance.

DON'T

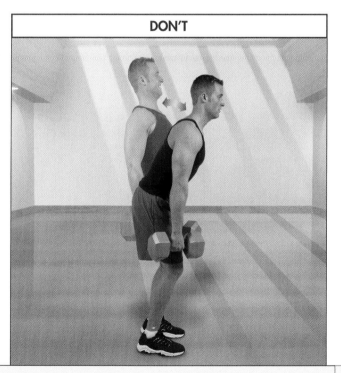

- Do not rock your body back and forth to help you lift the dumbbells.
- Do not roll your shoulders in a circle. Shrug your shoulders straight up and down.
- Do not lock your elbows. Keep your elbows slightly bent at all times.
- Do not tilt your head. Keep your head, neck and back in a straight line.

MUSCLES TARGETED

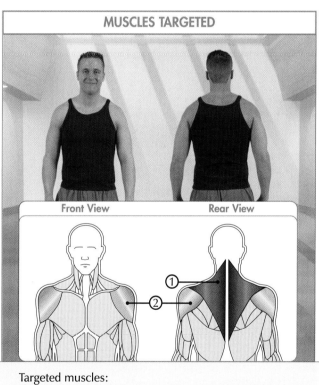

Front View   Rear View

Targeted muscles:
① upper back *(upper trapezius)*

Additional muscles:
② shoulders *(deltoids)*

assisted chin-up

Assisted chin-ups mainly work your back, but also strengthen your shoulders and biceps. This is an exercise that gives shape to your back and builds strength in your entire upper body. Greater upper body strength is beneficial for people who participate in activities that involve pulling their own body weight, such as swimming and rock climbing.

Using an assisted chin-up machine allows you to lift only a part of your body weight. The assisted chin-up machine counterbalances your body weight, so you need to choose a heavier weight to make the exercise

easier or a lighter weight to make the exercise more difficult. Depending on the type of assisted chin-up machine you are using, you may need to kneel or stand on a platform.

As you perform assisted chin-ups, you must keep your shoulders relaxed so they do not draw up towards your ears. You should also keep your abdominal muscles tight to help protect your back. You should be careful performing this exercise if you have problems with your neck, shoulders or elbows.

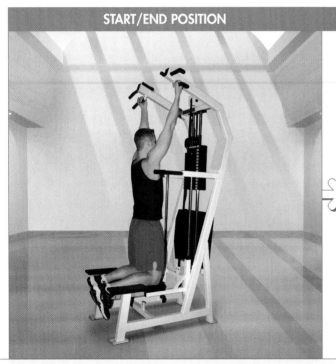

START/END POSITION

MIDDLE POSITION

1 Position your knees on the platform of an assisted chin-up machine.

2 Grasp the upper handlebars roughly shoulder width apart with both palms facing you. Straighten your arms.

• Make sure your back is straight and you tighten your abdominal muscles to help protect your back.

3 Slowly raise your body by bending your arms until your chin is at handle level.

4 Slowly straighten your arms to lower your body back to the starting position.

How can I put more focus on my biceps, forearms and the front of my shoulders?

Some assisted chin-up machines have another set of handles or a handle that extends to allow you a different grip so you can put more focus on your biceps, forearms and the front of your shoulders. Perform the same exercise described in the steps below, except hold the handles with your palms facing each other instead of towards you.

How can I perform more difficult chin-ups?

You can use a chin-up bar to perform non-assisted chin-ups that require you to lift and lower your entire body weight. When you are hanging from the chin-up bar, you need to bend your knees and cross your ankles. If you have lower back problems, you should be careful performing non-assisted chin-ups.

What is the difference between chin-ups and pull-ups?

The difference between chin-ups and pull-ups is the way you grasp the handlebars. When performing pull-ups, you grasp the handlebars one and a half shoulder width apart with your palms facing away from you. Pull-ups target your back muscles to give you more of a V shape.

DON'T	MUSCLES TARGETED
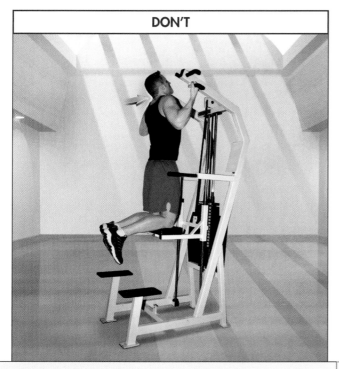	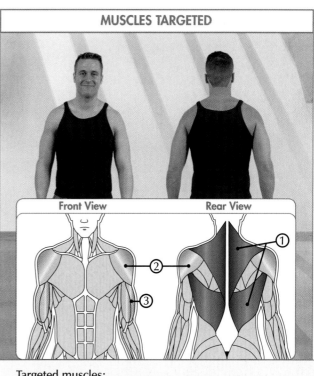

- Do not bend your neck backwards or shrug your shoulders.
- Do not lean back or arch your back to help you lift your body.
- Do not bend at the hips as you lift your body.
- Do not lock your elbows.

Targeted muscles:
① back (*latissimus dorsi* and *trapezius*)

Additional muscles:
② shoulders (*deltoids*)
③ biceps

upright row

The upright row can add definition and shape to your back and shoulders. This exercise works your upper and middle back, as well as the middle and front of your shoulders and your biceps. You should be careful performing upright rows if you have neck or shoulder problems.

If you find a barbell too heavy to use for this exercise, you can use an EZ curl bar, which weighs less. To use an EZ curl bar, hold the bar in the same way you would hold a barbell, except position your hands inside the curves, near the center of the bar.

Instead of pulling the bar up with your hands, focus on raising your elbows and the rest of your arm will follow naturally. To get the most out of this exercise, try to maintain a continuous flow of movement by slowly pulling the bar up right after lowering it, without resting at the bottom or allowing your back and shoulder muscles to relax between repetitions.

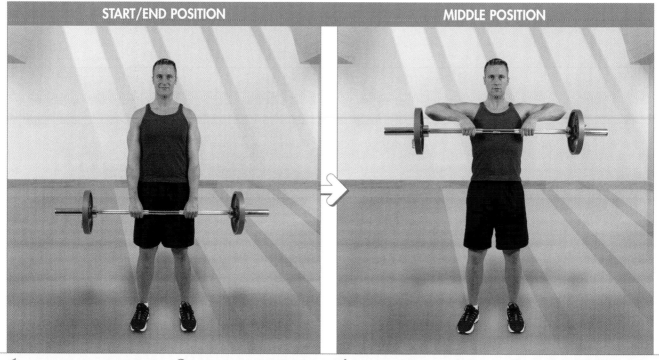

START/END POSITION　　**MIDDLE POSITION**

1 Grasp a barbell with your hands roughly shoulder width apart and both palms facing back.

2 Stand straight with your feet roughly shoulder width apart and your knees slightly bent.

3 Allow your arms to hang straight down so your palms face the front of your thighs. Make sure your elbows are slightly bent.

4 Slowly bend your arms to lift the bar straight up until your hands are level with your upper chest. Your elbows should not pass your shoulders.

• Make sure you keep your back straight and tighten your abdominal muscles to help protect your back.

5 Pause for a moment and then slowly straighten your arms to lower the bar back to the starting position.

How can I use dumbbells to perform this exercise?

To use dumbbells to perform upright rows, hold a dumbbell in each hand in front of your thighs, with your palms facing your body. Then lift and lower the dumbbells as you would a barbell. Using dumbbells, instead of a barbell, is useful when the muscles on one side of your body are stronger than the muscles on the other side and you want to correct the imbalance. Since each side works independently, the stronger side cannot compensate for the weaker side.

Can I use a cable machine to perform upright rows?

Yes. Position a cable on a tower of a cable machine at the lowest setting and then attach a straight bar to the cable. Grasp the bar with your hands shoulder width apart and your palms facing your body. Stand close to the tower with your feet shoulder width apart and then pull the bar up until your hands are level with your upper chest. Using a cable machine allows you to lift more weight and offers a different resistance than free weights.

DON'T

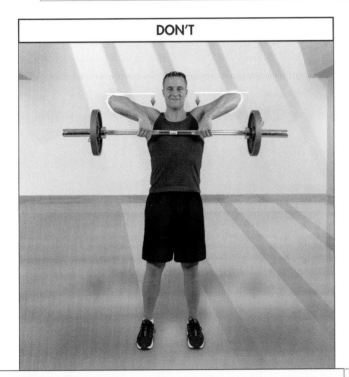

- Do not lift the bar too high. Your elbows should not pass your shoulders.

- Do not bend your wrists.

- Do not lean back or rock your body back and forth to help you lift the weight.

- Do not allow your hands to be higher than your elbows when lifting the bar.

MUSCLES TARGETED

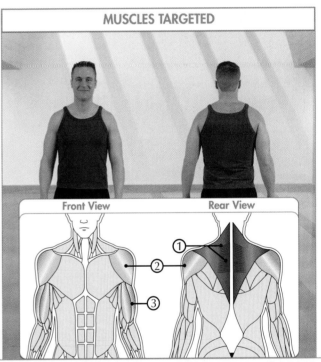

Front View   Rear View

Targeted muscles:
① upper and middle back
   (*trapezius* and *rhomboids*)

Additional muscles:
② middle and front shoulders
   (*medial and anterior deltoids*)
③ biceps

back extension on a roman chair

The back extension on a Roman chair is a great exercise for your lower back. Performing this exercise can help you with everyday activities that require lower back strength. In addition to strengthening your lower back, the back extension on a Roman chair also works your buttocks.

When performing the back extension on a Roman chair, make sure you keep your back straight at all times. You should also avoid bending your neck during the exercise. Keep your head, neck and back in a straight line as you lift and lower your upper body.

If you want to make this exercise more intense, you can try placing your hands lightly behind your head with your elbows out to your sides while making sure not to interlace your fingers. You can also try performing the exercise while holding a weight plate close to your chest.

You should not perform this exercise if you have lower back problems.

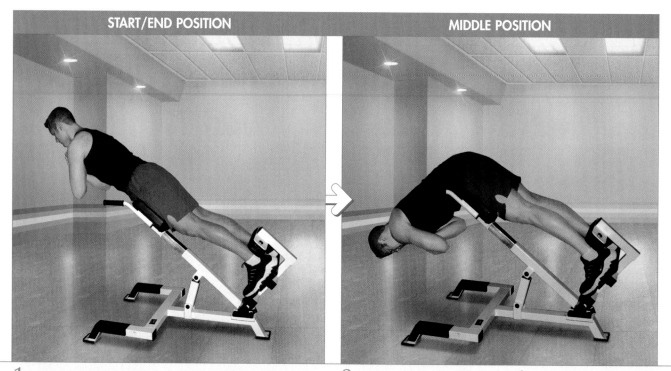

START/END POSITION

MIDDLE POSITION

1 Lie face down on a Roman chair with your ankles positioned securely under the ankle pads. Make sure your upper thighs are on the pad and your hips are positioned at the end of the pad.

• You may need to adjust the pad height to obtain the desired position.

2 Start with your entire body straight. Place your hands across your chest.

3 Slowly lower your body as far as you can by bending at the hips. Make sure your back remains straight at all times.

4 Slowly raise your body back to the starting position.

Can I perform back extensions without using a Roman chair?

Yes. Lie on your stomach on an exercise mat, with your arms stretched out in front of you and your legs straight out behind you. Raise your right arm and your left leg off the floor. Make sure you do not bend your knee while lifting your leg. Hold for 2 to 3 seconds before lowering, and then raise your left arm and right leg. Alternate between opposite arms and legs until you have completed a set. This variation is also good for people with back problems.

I find the back extension on a Roman chair too difficult because of my weak lower back. Is there a similar exercise I can perform?

Yes. You can use a back extension machine, which is ideal if you have a weak lower back or are recovering from a back injury. Sit on a back extension machine and attach the seat belt to secure yourself in place. Adjust the foot plate to make sure your knees are bent at 90-degree angles. Push the roller pad back using your lower back muscles. Pause for a moment and then slowly return to the starting position.

DON'T

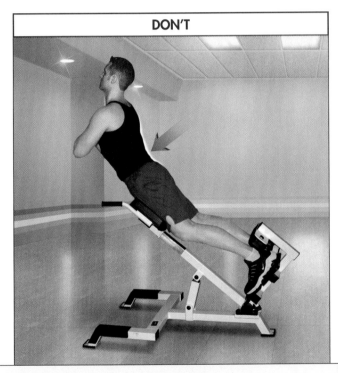

- Do not hunch or arch your back.
- Do not bend your neck. Keep your head, neck and back in a straight line.
- Do not lock your knees. Keep your knees slightly bent.

MUSCLES TARGETED

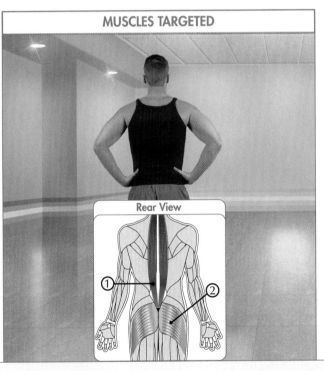

Rear View

Targeted muscles:
① lower back (*erector spinae*)

Additional muscles:
② buttocks (*gluteus maximus*)

seated cable row

The seated cable row is a great exercise for defining your upper back, as well as adding shape and mass to your upper and middle back. This exercise focuses mainly on your back, but also works your biceps and the rear of your shoulders. Performing the seated cable row can also help improve your posture.

Perform the exercise in a slow, controlled manner. If you find it difficult to perform the exercise in a controlled manner or if you are slamming the weight against the stack between repetitions, consider using less weight.

If you have neck, shoulder, elbow or back problems, be careful when performing the seated cable row. To prevent back injuries, do not round your back as you perform the exercise.

If a cable row machine is not available, you can perform a similar exercise sitting on the floor and using a cable machine. Position the cable of a cable machine slightly above the lowest setting and attach a straight bar. You also need to position a step directly next to the base of the cable machine and place your feet against the step.

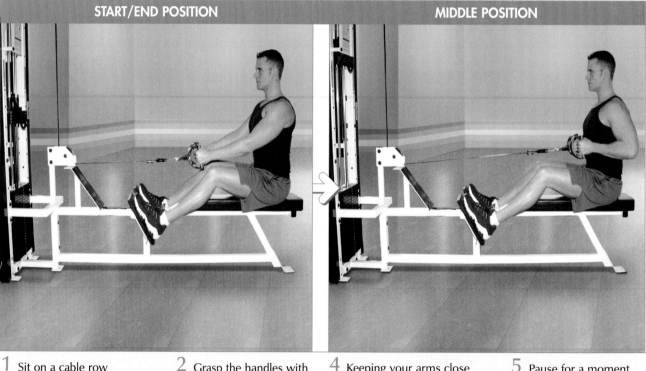

START/END POSITION   **MIDDLE POSITION**

1 Sit on a cable row machine with your feet on the foot platform.

2 Grasp the handles with your palms facing each other. Straighten your arms in front of you, but keep your elbows slightly bent.

3 Sit straight with your knees slightly bent.

4 Keeping your arms close to your sides, slowly bend your arms to pull the handles toward the top of your stomach.

• Make sure you keep your back straight, shoulders back and your abdominal muscles tight.

5 Pause for a moment and then slowly straighten your arms to return the handles to the starting position.

Can I use different attachments when performing the seated cable row?

Yes. You can attach a straight bar to put more emphasis on your upper and middle back and to work your forearms. Grasp the bar with your hands roughly shoulder width apart and your palms facing down. You can also grasp the bar with your palms facing up to add your biceps and the other side of your forearms to the muscles worked. You can attach a horseshoe handle to perform the exercise using one arm at a time, which helps correct muscle imbalances. Grasp the handle with your palm facing in.

I have lower back problems. Is there a safer way to perform seated rows?

You can perform the machine row, which is safer for people with lower back problems and is also great for beginners because of the added stability. Sit on a machine row facing the stack of weights and grasp the handles with your arms fully extended in front and your palms facing down. You may have to adjust the seat so that your arms are level with the handles. Slowly bend your arms to pull the handles toward you until your hands are alongside your chest.

DON'T

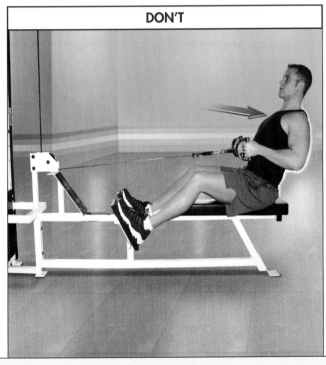

- Do not swing your upper body back and forth, lean back, arch your back or hunch your back to help you pull the weight.

- Do not bend your wrists.

- Do not lock your elbows or knees.

MUSCLES TARGETED

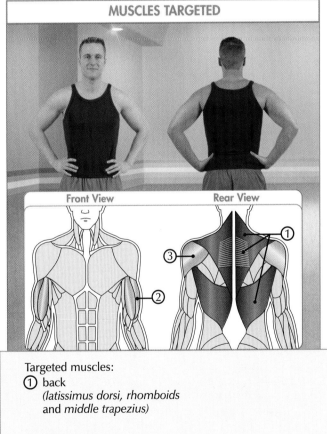

Front View   Rear View

Targeted muscles:
① back
   (*latissimus dorsi, rhomboids* and *middle trapezius*)

Additional muscles:
② biceps
③ rear shoulders
   (*posterior deltoids*)

bench dip

The bench dip primarily strengthens and shapes your triceps. Most tricep exercises only work your triceps, but the bench dip is a unique tricep exercise because it also works other muscles in your body, including your shoulders and upper back.

The bench dip is an arm exercise, so your arms should be raising and lowering your body weight as you bend and straighten your arms. Make sure you do not simply move your hips up and down as you perform the bench dip.

When performing a bench dip, only lower your body so that your upper arms are parallel to the floor. Lowering your body too far down can strain your shoulders. You can also strain your shoulders if you perform this exercise with your upper body too far away from the bench or chair.

You should use caution performing this exercise if you have neck or lower back problems. Do not perform this exercise if you have wrist, elbow or shoulder problems.

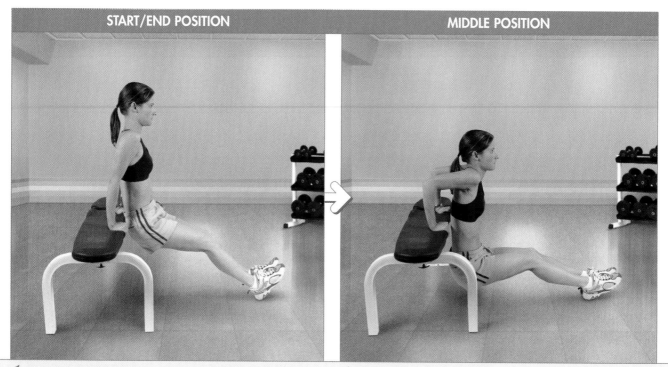

START/END POSITION → **MIDDLE POSITION**

1 Sit on the edge of a bench or chair with your legs straight and together and your toes pointing up.

2 Place your hands beside your hips on the edge of the bench or chair.

• Make sure you tighten your abdominal muscles to help protect your back.

3 Straighten your arms and lift your buttocks off the bench or chair and move your body forward slightly, supporting your weight on your arms.

4 Keeping your hips and back close to the bench or chair, slowly bend your arms and lower your body until your upper arms are parallel with the floor. Keep your elbows close to your sides.

5 Slowly straighten your arms and push yourself back up to the starting position.

What can I do if I find the bench dip too difficult?

You can perform a modified version of the bench dip to make the exercise easier. Perform the same movement as described below, except start with your knees bent at 90-degree angles and your feet flat on the floor. In this position, you will appear as if you are sitting on a chair as you perform the dips.

How can I make the bench dip more challenging?

To make the bench dip more challenging, perform the same movement as described below, except start with your feet up on another bench or chair of equal height. Position your hips close to the bench or chair that supports your arms and rest only your heels on the other bench or chair. You should tighten your abdominal muscles to help stabilize your body and make sure you do not lock your knees. To make the exercise even more difficult, you can place a weight plate on your thighs as you perform the dips.

DON'T

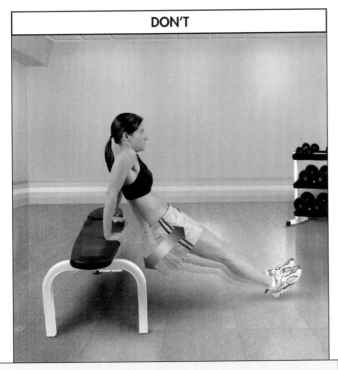

- Do not just move your hips up and down. Make sure you bend and straighten your arms.

- Do not lower your body too far down. Your upper arms should never be lower than parallel with the floor.

- Do not lock your elbows or move your body too far away from the bench or chair.

- Do not allow your elbows to flare out to the sides.

MUSCLES TARGETED

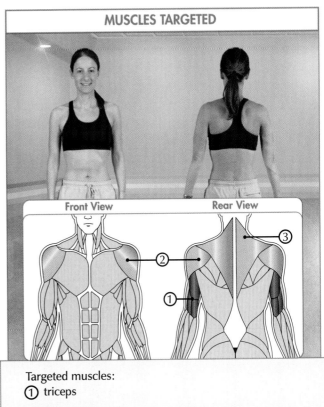

Front View   Rear View

Targeted muscles:
① triceps

Additional muscles:
② shoulders *(deltoids)*
③ upper back *(upper trapezius)*

tricep kickback

The tricep kickback helps tone and define your triceps, rather than build muscle mass in your triceps. This exercise is especially appropriate for beginners who can lift only a small amount of weight.

Correct arm movement is essential for ensuring the tricep kickback is effective. You must keep your upper arm stationary and parallel to the floor throughout the exercise. As you straighten your arm, make sure you do not lock your elbow. If you are doing the exercise correctly, you will feel a burning sensation in the back of your upper arm.

You should keep your head, neck and back in a straight line when performing the tricep kickback to avoid straining your neck or back. To help keep your neck straight, look down at the bench instead of looking up or to the side. You should also keep your abdominal muscles tightened throughout the exercise to help protect your back.

Make sure you use caution performing this exercise if you have shoulder, elbow or lower back problems.

START/END POSITION	MIDDLE POSITION

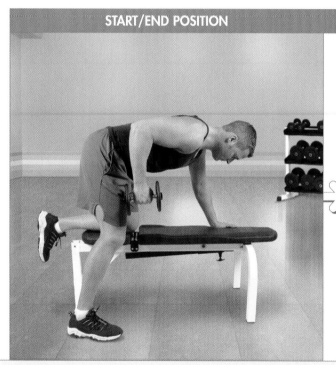

1 Position your right foot flat on the floor beside a bench with your knee slightly bent. Position your left knee on the bench.

2 Lean forward and position your left hand on the bench to support your upper body.

3 Reach down and pick up a dumbbell off the floor with your right hand, palm facing in. Position your upper arm parallel to the floor and bend your elbow at a 90-degree angle.

4 Keeping your upper arm stationary, slowly straighten your arm. Keep your arm close to your side.

- Make sure you tighten your abdominal muscles to help protect your back.

5 Slowly bend your arm to lower the dumbbell back to the starting position.

6 After completing a set with your right arm, position your right hand and right knee on the bench and repeat with your left arm.

Can I perform the tricep kickback using a cable machine?

Yes. Position a cable on a cable machine tower at the lowest setting and then attach a handle. Stand facing the tower, with your feet shoulder width apart and your knees slightly bent. Grasp the handle in your right hand, with your palm facing up, and then bend from your hips at a 45-degree angle, keeping your back straight. Rest your other hand on your thigh. Perform the same movement as described below, except face your palm forward to start the exercise. When you straighten your arm, your palm will face the floor. Perform a full set and then repeat the exercise with your left arm.

How can I make this exercise more challenging?

To make the tricep kickback more challenging, rotate your wrist as you straighten your arm so your palm ends up facing the ceiling. This modification allows more of your tricep muscle to work at the end of the movement.

DON'T

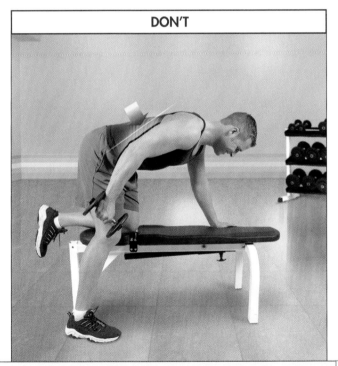

MUSCLES TARGETED

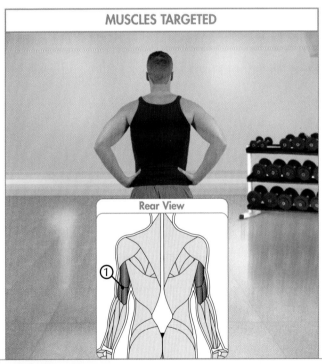

- Do not allow your upper arm to drop. Keep your upper arm parallel to the floor.

- Do not arch or hunch your back. Keep your back straight.

- Do not bend your neck. Keep your head, neck and back in a straight line.

- Do not lock the knee of the leg you are standing on or lock your elbow when you straighten your arm.

Targeted muscles:
① triceps

triceps pushdown

Performing the triceps pushdown using a cable machine is a good way to build mass in your triceps. The cable machine allows you to lift heavier weights when working your triceps.

When performing the triceps pushdown, lift and lower the weight with slow, controlled movements and take care not to lean forward or hunch your back. To help keep your back straight, keep your head up and look forward. Tightening your abdominal muscles can also help keep your back straight and protect your back.

As you push the bar down, remember to keep your elbows close to your sides.

If you find you have trouble maintaining your balance when performing this exercise, you can use a more stable stance. Stand with your feet shoulder width apart, but place one foot slightly in front of the other foot. You may find that this stance also helps you resist the temptation to use other muscles to lift the weight.

Use caution performing the triceps pushdown if you have back, neck, shoulder or elbow problems.

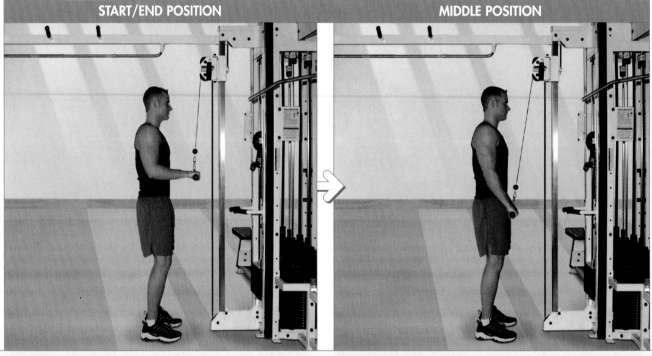

START/END POSITION   **MIDDLE POSITION**

1 Position a cable on a tower of a cable machine at the highest setting. Attach a straight or V-shaped bar to the cable.

2 Grasp the bar with your hands shoulder width apart and both palms facing down.

3 Stand a foot away from the machine with your feet flat on the floor, roughly shoulder width apart, knees slightly bent.

4 Position your elbows at your sides and bend your elbows so your forearms are parallel to the floor.

5 Slowly straighten your arms to lower the bar to the front of your thighs.

• Keep your back straight, head up and elbows close to your sides. Tighten your abdominal muscles to help protect your back.

6 Pause for a moment and then slowly bend your arms to raise the bar slightly above the starting position.

How can I vary the triceps pushdown to work my forearms as well as my triceps?

You can perform the reverse-grip pushdown. Attach a straight bar to the cable and grip the bar with your palms facing up. Then perform the exercise as described in the steps below.

Can I focus on one arm at a time?

Yes. Focusing on one arm at a time can help balance your triceps. Attach a horseshoe handle to the cable and grip the handle with your palm down. Facing your palm up will work the inner part of your tricep more. Then perform the exercise as described in the steps below.

How can I alter the triceps pushdown to work my entire tricep more?

To work your entire tricep more, you can perform this exercise using a rope attachment, instead of a straight or V-shaped bar. Grasp an end of the rope in each hand, with your palms facing each other. Then perform the same exercise as described in the steps below, except push the rope to the outside of your thighs.

DON'T

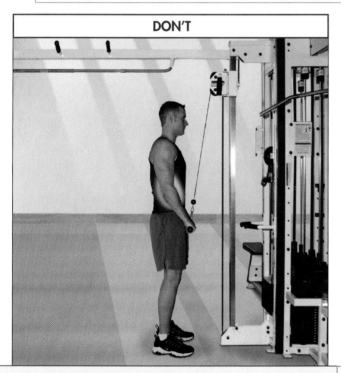

- Do not allow your elbows to move out to your sides as you push the bar down.
- Do not lock your elbows when you straighten your arms.
- Do not lean forward or hunch your back as you push the bar down. Keep your back straight and head up.
- Do not bend your wrists or lock your knees.

MUSCLES TARGETED

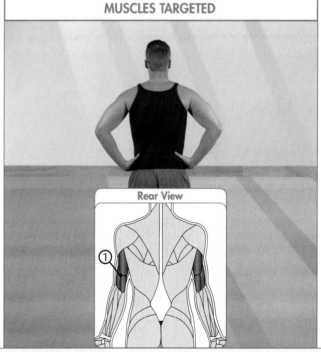

Rear View

Targeted muscles:
① triceps

barbell triceps press

The barbell triceps press provides an excellent way of building mass in your triceps. This exercise also works the front of your shoulders.

You may find the barbell triceps press is similar to the barbell bench press, which primarily works your chest. The major difference between the barbell triceps press and the barbell bench press is the position of your arms. When performing the barbell triceps press, your grip is narrower and your upper arms are closer to your body, which works your triceps instead of your chest. For information on the barbell bench press, see page 32.

If you find the barbell too heavy, you can perform this exercise using an EZ curl bar, which weighs less than a standard barbell. You should not hold the EZ curl bar on the curves though. Your hands should only be 6 inches apart on the bar. For more information on the EZ curl bar, see page 14.

Due to the arm movements in this exercise, you should use caution performing this exercise if you have shoulder problems. Avoid the exercise if you have elbow or wrist problems.

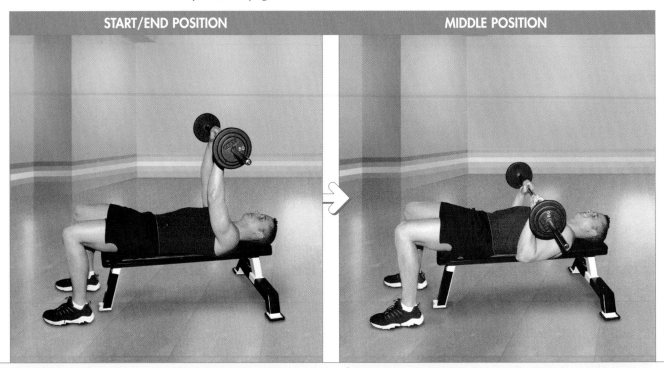

START/END POSITION   **MIDDLE POSITION**

1 Lie on your back on a bench and position your feet flat on the floor or on the bench. Tighten your abdominal muscles to help protect your back.

2 Hold the bar with your hands about 6 inches apart, both palms facing forward.

3 Straighten your arms to lift the bar over the middle of your chest. Keep your elbows slightly bent.

4 Slowly lower the bar until the bar is a few inches from the middle of your chest. Your elbows should end up slightly below your shoulders.

• Make sure you keep your elbows close to your body.

5 Pause for a moment and then slowly raise the bar back to the starting position. Push your shoulder blades into the bench while raising the bar.

Can I modify this exercise to work each arm separately?

Yes. You can perform a dumbbell triceps press to help you work out muscle imbalances between your triceps. Hold a dumbbell in each hand with your palms facing each other. Then perform the exercise as described in the steps below, lifting both dumbbells at the same time. To focus on one arm at a time, perform a full set with one arm and then a full set with your other arm. This exercise also works your biceps by controlling the weight on the way down.

Is there a way I can work my triceps without using weight?

Yes. Performing a push-up with your hands positioned closer together than normal will target your triceps. Lie on your stomach on the floor with your legs together and straight and the balls of your feet touching the floor. Bend your elbows and place your palms on the floor under your shoulders, fingers pointing forward. Slowly raise your body off the floor until your arms are straight. Then slowly lower your body until your chest is a few inches off the floor. If this is too difficult, you can rest on your knees rather than on your feet.

DON'T

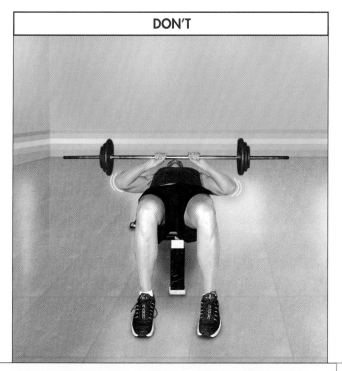

- Do not allow your elbows to flare out to the sides.
- Do not bend your wrists or lock your elbows when you straighten your arms.
- Do not lift your head off the bench.
- Do not arch your back or wiggle your body to help you lift the weight. Keep your back on the bench and your legs and feet stationary for better support.

MUSCLES TARGETED

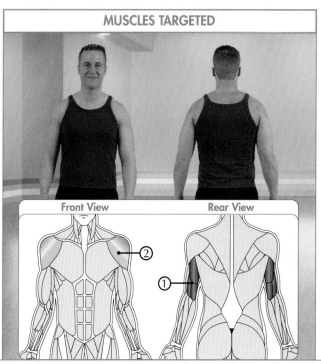

Targeted muscles:
① triceps

Additional muscles:
② front shoulders *(anterior deltoids)*

dumbbell overhead triceps extension

The dumbbell overhead triceps extension is one of the best exercises for strengthening your triceps.

You can perform the dumbbell overhead triceps extension while sitting or standing. If you prefer to stand, position your feet about shoulder width apart and bend your knees slightly. Whether sitting or standing, you should keep your head, neck and back in a straight line throughout the exercise. You should also keep your abdominal muscles tight to protect your back.

To keep the exercise focused on your triceps and to help avoid straining your shoulders, you should keep your elbows close to your head and pointed forward as you lift and lower the weight. You should also keep your upper arms as stationary as possible. If your elbows have a tendency to drift outwards, you can adjust your grip on the dumbbell to position your wrists closer together.

Do not perform this exercise if you have neck, shoulder or elbow problems and be careful if you have wrist problems.

START/END POSITION	MIDDLE POSITION

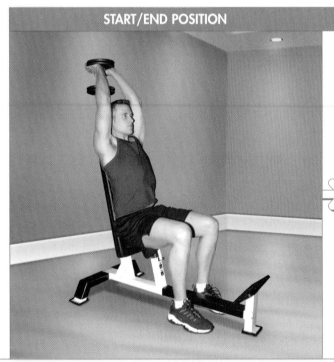
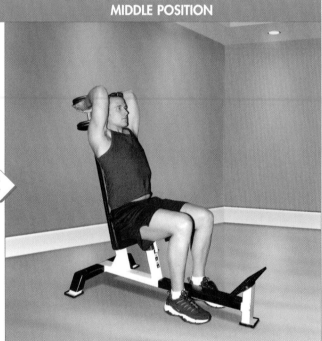

1 Hold a dumbbell in your hands.

2 Sit on a bench with back support and place your legs slightly apart, with your feet flat on the floor. Tighten your abdominal muscles to help protect your back.

3 Use both hands to grasp one end of the dumbbell, with your palms facing up and your fingers pointing back.

4 Raise the dumbbell above your head by extending your arms upwards, but keep your elbows slightly bent.

5 Keeping your elbows close to your head, slowly bend your arms to lower the dumbbell behind your head.

6 Pause for a moment and then slowly straighten your arms to raise the dumbbell above your head.

How can I work only one arm at a time?

Performing this exercise with one arm at a time can help correct any imbalances between the triceps of each arm. Grasp a dumbbell in one hand and raise the weight above your head so that your palm is facing in toward your head and your thumb is pointing down to the floor. Then lower the weight behind your head by bending your elbow. You can place your free arm below the elbow of the arm you are working for support. Complete a full set with one arm and then switch arms.

Can I perform overhead triceps extensions on a cable machine?

Yes. Position a cable on a tower of a cable machine at the highest setting and then connect the rope attachment to the cable. With your back to the tower, grasp an end of the rope in each hand with your palms facing each other and your upper arms beside your head. Move a step away from the tower and then place one foot in front of the other, about shoulder width apart. Lean forward from your hips slightly and then straighten your arms overhead.

DON'T	MUSCLES TARGETED
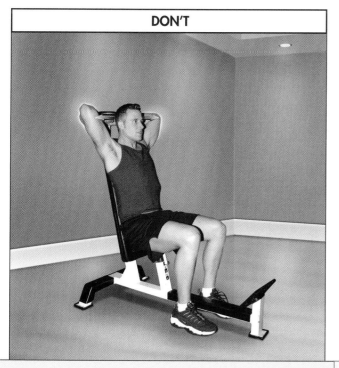	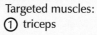Rear View

- Do not allow your elbows to move out to the sides. Keep your elbows close to your head and pointed forward to target your triceps, not your shoulders.

- Do not arch your back.

- Do not lock your elbows when you straighten your arms.

- Do not bend your neck. Keep your head, neck and back in a straight line.

Targeted muscles:
① triceps

lying barbell
triceps extension

The lying barbell triceps extension is an advanced exercise that works your triceps and forearms. This exercise, which is also known as the French press or the skull crusher, strengthens and builds mass in your triceps.

You should use a shorter barbell to perform this exercise. If you find the barbell too heavy, you can use an EZ curl bar instead. You will need to grasp the straight part of the EZ curl bar, just inside the curves.

As you perform the lying barbell triceps extension,

focus on keeping your upper arms stationary as you lower the bar. Stop lowering the bar a few inches above your forehead so that you do not accidentally hit your head. Do not lift your head or arch your back off the bench in order to lift and lower the bar.

Be careful performing the lying barbell triceps extension if you are a beginner or if you have problems with your shoulders or elbows. This exercise could make existing elbow problems worse if it is not performed properly.

START/END POSITION	MIDDLE POSITION

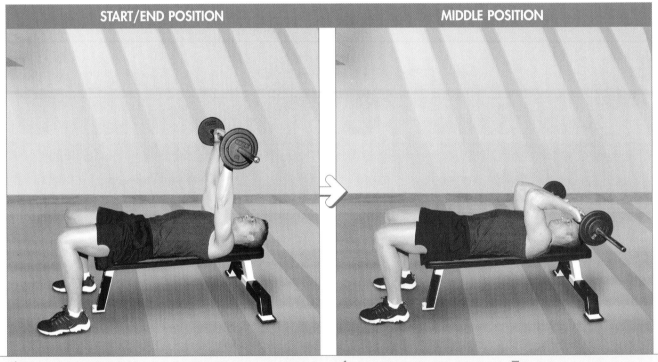

1 Pick up a barbell with your hands roughly shoulder width apart.

2 Lie on your back on a bench and position your feet flat on the floor or on the bench.

• Make sure you tighten your abdominal muscles to help protect your back.

3 Straighten your arms to lift the bar directly over your shoulders. Keep your elbows slightly bent.

4 Keeping your upper arms stationary, slowly bend your arms to lower the bar a few inches from your forehead. Keep your elbows pointing up and close to your body.

5 Pause for a moment and then slowly straighten your arms to raise the bar back to the starting position.

How can I make this exercise more intense?

For a more intense exercise, you can perform the seated barbell triceps extension. Pick up a barbell with your hands shoulder width apart and your palms facing down. Sit on a bench with a back support and place your feet together. Straighten your arms to lift the bar directly over your head, with your elbows pointing forward and slightly bent. Slowly lower the bar behind you by bending your elbows until they are at 90-degree angles.

How can I work one arm at a time?

To work one arm at a time, you can perform the lying dumbbell triceps extension. Pick up a dumbbell in one hand and lie on a bench. Straighten your arm to raise the weight directly over your shoulder, with your elbow slightly bent and your palm facing inward. Your other arm can rest at your side or support your raised upper arm. Slowly bend your arm to lower the weight beside your head. This variation helps correct any imbalances in your triceps and forearm muscles.

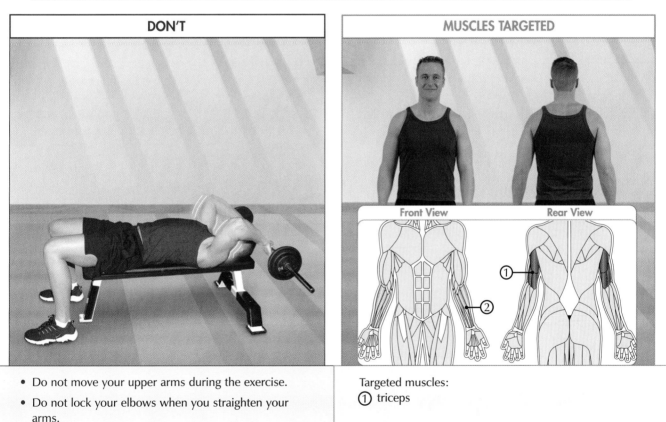

DON'T

- Do not move your upper arms during the exercise.
- Do not lock your elbows when you straighten your arms.
- Do not lift your head off the bench.
- Do not arch your back to help lift the weight.
- Do not bend your wrists.

MUSCLES TARGETED

Front View   Rear View

Targeted muscles:
① triceps

Additional muscles:
② forearm flexors

triceps extension machine

The triceps extension machine isolates and works your triceps. You should be careful using the triceps extension machine if you have elbow or wrist problems.

If you are new to weight training, using the triceps extension machine is a good way to start working your triceps. The machine isolates the triceps, provides stability and helps you maintain proper form so you can concentrate on working the muscle.

As you use the triceps extension machine, make sure

your elbows are pointed straight ahead, not out to the sides. Do not lock your elbows or bend your wrists as you straighten your arms to push the handles on the machine forward. You should also make sure you do not hunch your back or shrug your shoulders as you perform the exercise. Try to keep your back straight and your abdominal muscles tight to help protect your back.

To get the most out of this exercise, try to maintain a controlled and continuous flow of movement throughout the entire exercise.

START/END POSITION	MIDDLE POSITION
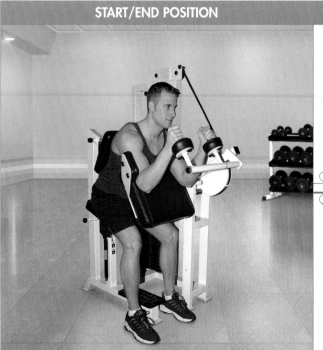	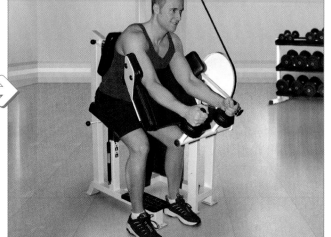

1 Sit on a triceps extension machine with your feet flat on the floor or on the foot rest, roughly shoulder width apart.

2 Rest your chest against the arm pad. The top of the pad should touch the middle of your chest.

• You can adjust the seat height to obtain the desired position.

3 Place your arms on the pad and grasp the handles with your palms facing each other.

4 Keeping your elbows pointing forward, slowly press the handles forward and down, straightening your arms in front of you.

• Make sure you keep your back straight and tighten your abdominal muscles to help protect your back.

5 Slowly bend your arms to return the handles to the starting position.

I find the triceps extension machine difficult to use. Is there another machine I can use to work my triceps?

Yes. You can use the triceps dip machine, which is easier to use than the triceps extension machine and allows you to push more weight. Sit on a triceps dip machine with your feet flat on the floor, about shoulder width apart. Grasp the handles on the machine with your palms facing in. Your elbows should not be higher than your shoulders. Straighten your arms to press the handles down, keeping your elbows slightly bent.

How can I work my triceps harder?

You can use the triceps machine to work your triceps harder. Although the triceps machine provides back support for people with back problems, the machine does not help you maintain proper form. To perform the exercise, press the arm pads on the machine down with your forearms. If you find you are pushing the arm pads down with your hands, adjust the height of the arm pads and seat until you are in the correct position.

DON'T

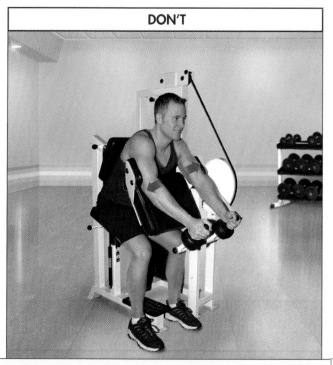

- Do not point your elbows out to the sides. Your elbows should always point straight ahead.
- Do not hunch your back or shrug your shoulders.
- Do not lock your elbows when you straighten your arms.
- Do not bend your wrists.

MUSCLES TARGETED

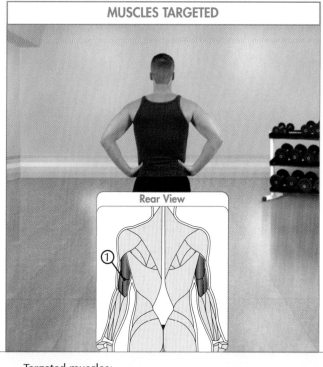

Rear View

Targeted muscles:
① triceps

seated dumbbell curl

The seated dumbbell curl isolates your biceps. This is a good exercise to start with when using free weights to work your biceps.

The seated position helps to stabilize your back, which is important for this exercise. To protect your back from strain, you should also tighten your abdominal muscles. If you find you are arching your back to lift the dumbbells, you need to reduce the amount of weight you are lifting.

As you perform the curl, keep your upper arms stable and your elbows close to your sides. As with all dumbbell exercises, you should make sure you lift and lower the dumbbells with slow, controlled movements. Due to the movement involved, you should use caution when performing the seated dumbbell curl if you have elbow or wrist problems.

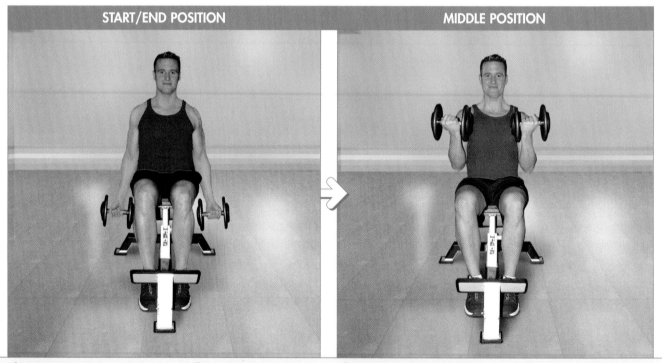

START/END POSITION | **MIDDLE POSITION**

1 Hold a dumbbell in each hand.

2 Sit on a bench with back support and place your legs slightly apart, feet flat on the floor. Tighten your abdominal muscles to help protect your back.

3 Start with your arms at your sides, elbows slightly bent, both palms facing forward.

4 Slowly bend your elbows to raise the dumbbells toward your shoulders.

• Make sure you keep your back straight, head up and your elbows close to your sides.

5 Slowly straighten your arms to lower the dumbbells back to the starting position.

Can I perform dumbbell curls while standing?

Yes. The standing dumbbell curl is a more advanced exercise because it requires you to keep your body stable as you work your biceps. Stand with your feet roughly shoulder width apart and then perform the same arm movements as you would when seated. Be careful not to strain your lower back as you perform this exercise.

How can I vary the seated dumbbell curl?

There are several variations you can try. You can focus on one arm at a time by alternating between your left and right arm to lift the dumbbells. For another variation, start with your palms facing in. Once your arms reach your thighs, start rotating your wrists so that your palms end up facing the ceiling when the lift is complete. This variation works the entire bicep muscle and your forearms.

DON'T

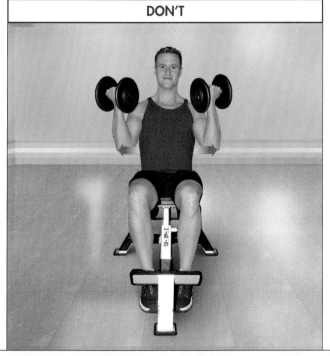

- Do not move your upper arms. Keep your upper arms stationary and close to your body.
- Do not dig your elbows into your sides or arch your back to help you lift the dumbbells.
- Do not shrug your shoulders or bend your wrists.
- Do not lock your elbows when you straighten your arms.

MUSCLES TARGETED

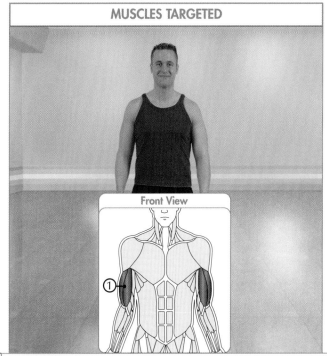

Front View

Targeted muscles:
① biceps

barbell curl

The barbell curl primarily works your biceps, with a secondary emphasis on your forearms. This classic biceps exercise is great for building mass in your biceps.

When performing barbell curls, it is important to keep your back straight to avoid straining your back. You can also protect your back by bending your knees slightly and tightening your abdominal muscles. If you have existing lower back problems, consider performing a seated biceps exercise instead, such as the seated dumbbell curl shown on page 92.

You should use caution performing barbell curls if you have elbow or wrist problems. If your grip is too wide or too narrow, you can strain your wrists and elbows. Your hands should be roughly shoulder width apart, with your elbows close to your sides. Your elbows should also remain stable as you lift the weight. You should not lift your elbows up or dig them into your sides.

If you find you are rocking back and forth to lift the bar, you are using too much weight. You should lighten the weight before continuing.

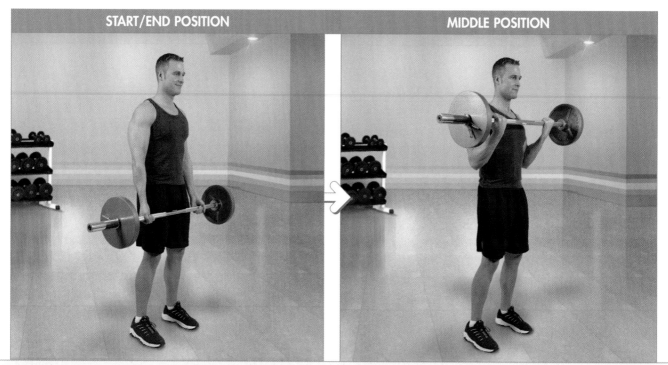

START/END POSITION **MIDDLE POSITION**

1 Stand straight with your feet roughly shoulder width apart. Bend your knees slightly and tighten your abdominal muscles to help protect your back.

2 Hold a barbell with both palms facing forward, roughly shoulder width apart. Allow your arms to hang straight down so the bar rests against the front of your thighs. Make sure your elbows are slightly bent.

3 Slowly bend your elbows to raise the bar almost to your shoulders.

- Make sure you keep your back straight, head up and elbows close to your sides.

4 Slowly straighten your arms to lower the bar back to the starting position.

QUESTION & ANSWER

How can I make the exercise more intense?

You can perform the following 21 repetitions to increase the intensity of the exercise. For the first seven repetitions, lift and lower the bar from your thigh to the mid point so that your elbows are bent at 90-degree angles. For the next seven repetitions, lift and lower the bar from the mid point almost to your shoulders. To finish the set, perform seven repetitions using the full range of motion. The half curls in this set help to isolate the upper and lower halves of your biceps.

How can I make the barbell curl more difficult?

You can perform a reverse-grip barbell curl, which isolates your forearms more, but still works your biceps. To perform the reverse-grip barbell curl, perform the same exercise as the barbell curl, except start by holding the bar with both palms facing your body. You may need to use a lighter weight for this exercise.

DON'T

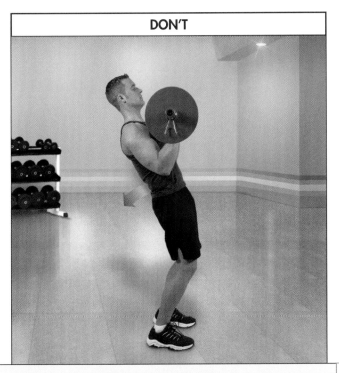

- Do not lean back, lean forward, arch your back or swing back and forth to help you lift the bar.

- Do not dig your elbows into your sides or shrug your shoulders when lifting the bar.

- Do not lock your elbows when you straighten your arms.

MUSCLES TARGETED

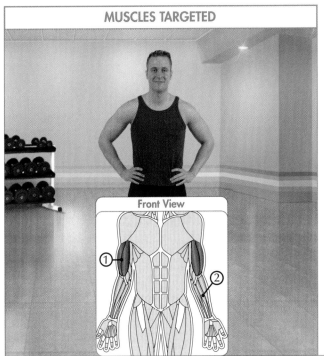

Front View

Targeted muscles:
① biceps

Additional muscles:
② forearm flexors

concentration curl

The concentration curl focuses on your biceps. Exercises that isolate your biceps are important for building strong arms, which can help make everyday activities, such as lifting and carrying, easier.

The concentration curl is slightly more difficult than the seated dumbbell curl shown on page 92. The movement required for the concentration curl forces you to use less weight than the seated dumbbell curl and to maintain perfect form throughout the exercise.

When you lean forward to perform the concentration curl, you should bend forward from your hips and keep your back straight, rather than bending at the waist and curving your lower back. Keeping your abdominal muscles tight when your back is straight will help protect your back during the exercise.

You should be very careful performing concentration curls if you have elbow, wrist or lower back problems. To avoid further injury, do not lean back, rock back and forth or move your leg to help lift the weight and do not use more weight than you can manage while maintaining good form.

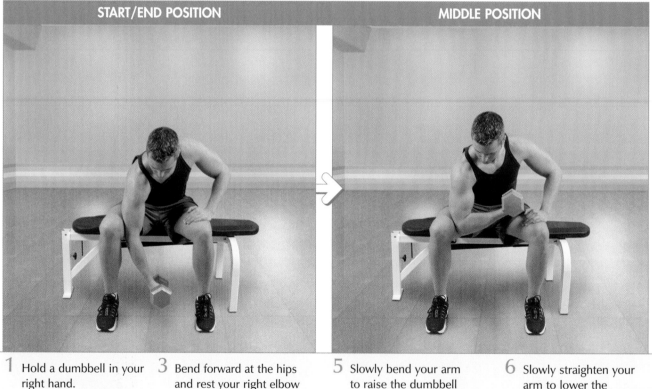

START/END POSITION　　　　　**MIDDLE POSITION**

1 Hold a dumbbell in your right hand.

2 Sit on the edge of a bench or chair with your feet slightly wider than shoulder width apart.

3 Bend forward at the hips and rest your right elbow on your right inner thigh just behind your knee.

4 Allow your arm to hang straight down, elbow slightly bent, palm facing your left leg. Position your left hand or elbow on your left thigh.

5 Slowly bend your arm to raise the dumbbell toward your shoulder.

- Keep your back straight and tighten your abdominal muscles to help protect your back.

6 Slowly straighten your arm to lower the dumbbell back to the starting position.

7 After completing a set with your right arm, repeat the exercise with your left arm.

How can I isolate my forearms and the outer edges of my biceps?

You can isolate your forearms and the outer edges of your biceps by rotating your wrist during the first part of the movement. Start by holding the dumbbell with your palm facing back. As you raise the dumbbell, rotate your wrist so that your palm is facing up when you are halfway through the movement. This variation also helps give a better overall shape to your biceps.

How can I make the exercise more intense?

You can increase the intensity of this exercise by using a cable machine instead of dumbbells. Position a cable on a tower of a cable machine at the lowest setting and attach a handle to the cable. With your right side facing the tower, kneel on your right knee with your left foot flat on the floor. Grip the handle with your left hand and use the inside of your left knee as a support. Then perform the exercise as described below. After completing a set, switch sides and repeat the exercise with your right arm. For more information on cable machines, see page 17.

DON'T	MUSCLES TARGETED
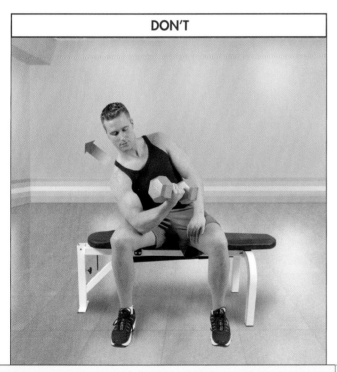	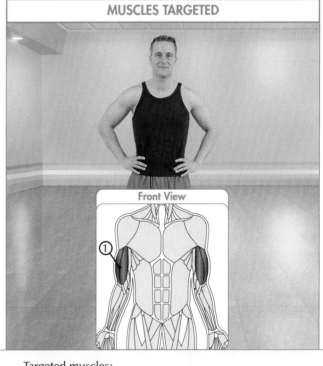 Front View

- Do not lean back, rock back and forth or move your leg to help lift the weight.

- Do not hunch your back. Keep your back straight.

- Do not lock your elbow.

- Do not bend your neck. Keep your head and neck in line with your body.

Targeted muscles:
① biceps

preacher curl

The preacher curl focuses on your biceps, but also strengthens your forearms. This exercise provides an excellent way to build strength and mass in your biceps, since you cannot easily cheat and use other muscles to lift the weight.

To perform the preacher curl, you should use an EZ curl bar, although a straight bar is also acceptable. As the name implies, the EZ curl bar is easier on your elbow and wrist joints than a straight bar. Although the EZ curl bar helps to reduce the stress on your elbow and wrist joints, you should still take care performing this exercise

if you have elbow or wrist problems.

While performing the preacher curl, you should maintain proper form and use slow, controlled movements. You may need to adjust the seat or pad height to make sure you are sitting in the proper position and your armpits are resting near the top of the pad. As you lift the bar, keep your body stable and do not lean back or wiggle your body. As you lower the bar, make sure you keep your body on the bench and avoid locking your elbows since this can place stress on your elbow joints.

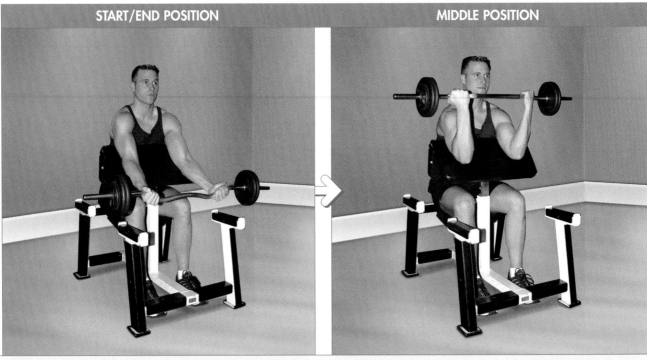

| START/END POSITION | MIDDLE POSITION |

1 Place an EZ curl bar on the rack of a preacher curl bench.

2 Sit on the bench with your feet flat on the floor, roughly shoulder width apart.

3 Place your arms on the pad. Your armpits should rest near the top of the pad.

4 Grasp the EZ curl bar on the outside curves of the bar, both palms facing up and elbows slightly bent.

5 Slowly bend your elbows to raise the bar toward your shoulders.

• Make sure you keep your back straight and tighten your abdominal muscles to help protect your back.

6 Slowly straighten your arms to lower the bar back to the starting position.

Can I exercise each arm separately?

Yes. You can use a dumbbell with a preacher curl bench to work one arm at a time. This will provide a more difficult workout and can help balance the strength between your arms. Sit on the preacher curl bench as you would to perform the exercise with an EZ curl bar, but instead hold a dumbbell with your palm facing up and allow your other arm to rest on the pad. Perform a full set with one arm and then perform a set with the other arm.

How can I vary the preacher curl exercise?

Using a cable machine with a preacher curl bench allows you to vary the resistance offered by this exercise. Position a cable on a tower of a cable machine at the lowest setting and then connect an EZ curl bar attachment to the cable. Position the preacher curl bench facing the tower and then perform the exercise as described in the steps below. You will need to have someone hand you the EZ curl bar attachment. For more information on cable machines, see page 17.

DON'T

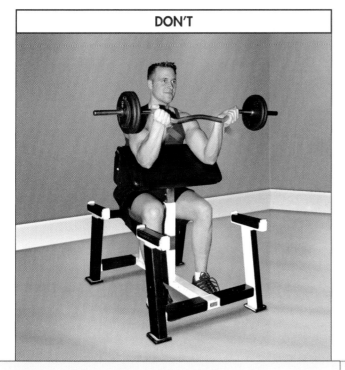

- Do not bend your wrists.
- Do not lean back or wiggle your body to help you lift the bar.
- Do not lock your elbows when you straighten your arms since this can place stress on your elbow joints.
- Do not allow your body to lift off the bench when you lower the bar.

MUSCLES TARGETED

Front View

Targeted muscles:
① biceps

Additional muscles:
② forearm flexors

hammer curl

The hammer curl is a great exercise for working your biceps and forearms. In addition to strengthening your biceps and giving shape to your upper forearms, this exercise can also help you build strength in your elbow joints.

The hammer curl is similar to the seated dumbbell curl, except you keep your palms facing each other when you perform the hammer curl, which focuses more on your forearms and works a different part of your biceps. For information on the seated dumbbell curl, see page 92. While performing the hammer curl, you can visualize yourself hammering in nails using two hammers at the same time.

As you perform the exercise, make sure you do not lean back or forward to help you lift the dumbbells. You should also resist the temptation to swing back and forth or arch your back in an effort to lift the dumbbells. You must be very careful performing the hammer curl if you have elbow or wrist problems.

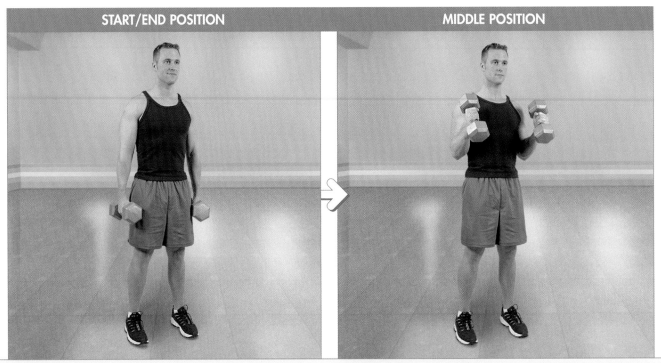

START/END POSITION	MIDDLE POSITION

1 Hold a dumbbell in each hand.

2 Stand straight with your feet roughly shoulder width apart. Bend your knees slightly and tighten your abdominal muscles to help protect your back.

3 Start with your arms straight at your sides, elbows slightly bent, both palms facing each other.

4 Slowly bend your elbows to raise the dumbbells toward your shoulders, keeping your palms facing each other.

• Make sure you keep your back straight, your head up and your elbows close to your sides.

5 Slowly straighten your arms to lower the dumbbells back to the starting position.

How can I protect my back when performing the hammer curl?

To protect your back, you can perform the hammer curl when seated on a bench with a back support. The seated hammer curl also helps isolate your biceps and forearms by making it more difficult to use other muscles to lift the weight.

Can I focus on one arm at a time?

Yes. You can focus on one arm at a time by alternating between your left and right arm to lift the dumbbells. Keep alternating arms until you finish a set.

How can I use the hammer curl to add definition to my biceps?

Stand with your feet shoulder width apart and hold a dumbbell in your right hand. Position your right arm straight at your side with your palm facing in. Then bend your elbow to sweep the dumbbell across the front of your body until your right palm faces your right shoulder. Sweep the dumbbell back down across your body to the starting position. When you complete a set with your right arm, repeat this exercise with your left arm.

DON'T

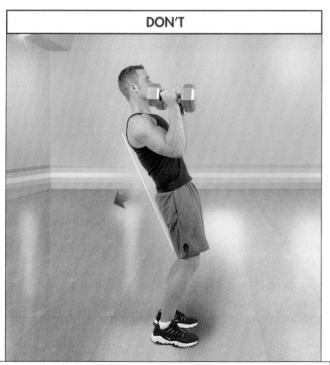

- Do not lean back, lean forward, arch your back or swing back and forth to help you lift the dumbbells.

- Do not move your upper arms. Keep your upper arms stationary and close to your body.

- Do not lock your elbows when you straighten your arms.

MUSCLES TARGETED

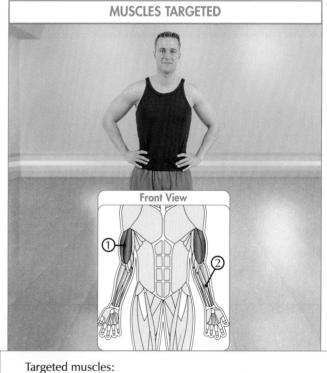

Front View

Targeted muscles:
① biceps

Additional muscles:
② forearm flexors

cable biceps curl

The cable biceps curl is an excellent exercise for building mass in your biceps. Although this exercise primarily works your biceps, it also strengthens your forearms. This exercise is very similar to the barbell curl, which is discussed on page 94. You may want to perform the cable biceps curl instead of the barbell curl to add variety to your workout routine.

To maintain proper form when performing the cable biceps curl, make sure you do not lean back or arch your back to help you lift the bar. You should also keep your head, neck and back in a straight line. Concentrate on keeping your shoulders down and your elbows close to your sides when you lift the bar, but do not dig your elbows into your sides. When you lower the bar back to the starting position, make sure you do not lock your elbows.

You should be careful performing this exercise if you have elbow, wrist or lower back problems.

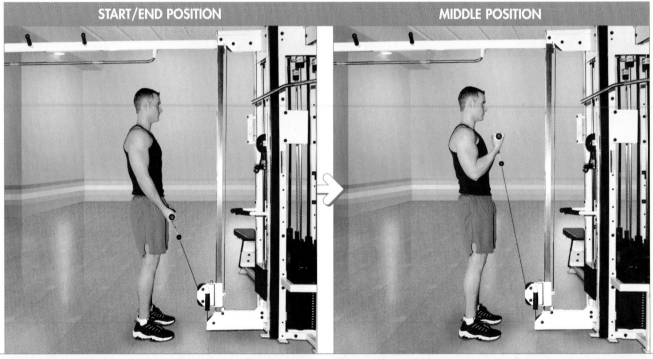

START/END POSITION **MIDDLE POSITION**

1 Position a cable on a tower of a cable machine at the lowest setting. Attach a straight bar to the cable.

2 Grasp the bar with your hands roughly shoulder width apart and both palms facing up.

3 Stand a foot away from the machine with your feet flat on the floor, roughly shoulder width apart, knees slightly bent.

4 Allow your arms to hang straight down so your hands rest against the front of your thighs.

5 Slowly bend your elbows to raise the bar almost to your shoulders.

• Make sure you keep your back straight, head up and elbows close to your sides. Tighten your abdominal muscles to help protect your back.

6 Pause for a moment and then slowly straighten your arms to lower the bar back to the starting position.

One of my arms is stronger than the other. How can I work them equally?

To make sure your stronger arm does not compensate for your weaker arm, you can perform the exercise using only one arm at a time. Attach a horseshoe handle, instead of a straight bar, to the cable and then perform a full set with one arm. Then switch arms and perform a set with your other arm.

How can I work my forearms and the outside of my biceps more?

To work your forearms and the outside of your biceps more, you can perform this exercise using a rope attachment instead of a straight bar. Attach the rope to the cable and then grasp an end of the rope in each hand. Your palms should be facing each other and your thumbs should be closest to the ends of the rope. As you pull the rope up, move your hands closer together so that they end up just inside your shoulders. This modification gives you more freedom of movement so you can work your muscles more efficiently.

DON'T

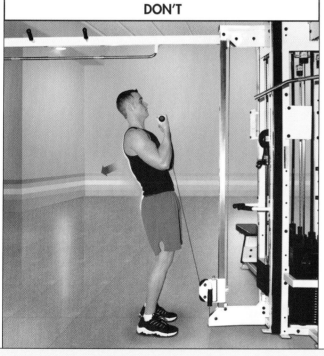

- Do not lean back, arch your back or swing back and forth to help you lift the bar.

- Do not dig your elbows into your sides or shrug your shoulders when lifting the bar.

- Do not lock your elbows when you straighten your arms.

- Do not bend your neck. Keep your head, neck and back in a straight line.

MUSCLES TARGETED

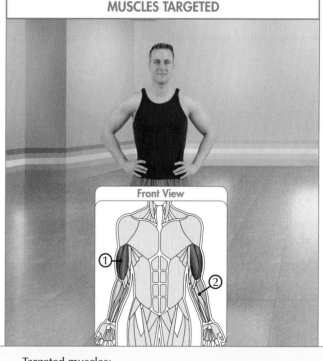

Front View

Targeted muscles:
① biceps

Additional muscles:
② forearm flexors

arm curl machine

The arm curl machine isolates your biceps. Unlike performing bicep exercises using free weights, using the arm curl machine ensures that you use only your biceps and not any other part of your body to lift the weight. The arm curl machine also helps keep your body stable, which is more difficult to do with free weights.

It is important to maintain good form when using the arm curl machine. You should be sitting up straight, rather than leaning back. As you lift and lower the weight, keep your wrists straight and make sure you do not lock your elbows when you straighten your arms. You should not shrug your shoulders to try to help lift the weight or lift your body off the seat when you lower the weight.

Due to the arm movements required when using the arm curl machine, you should use caution if you have elbow or wrist problems.

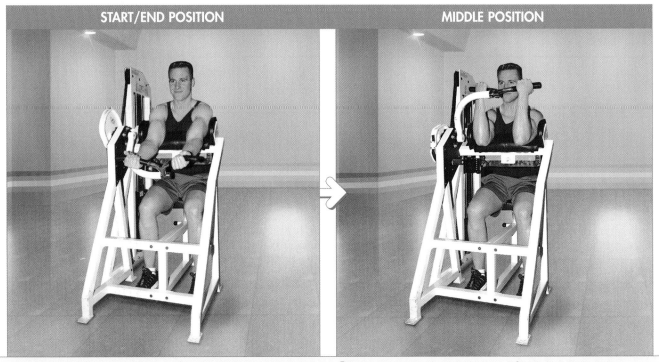

START/END POSITION　　　**MIDDLE POSITION**

1 Sit on an arm curl machine with your feet flat on the floor, roughly shoulder width apart. Make sure your back is straight and tighten your abdominal muscles to help protect your back.

2 Place your arms on the pad and grasp the handles with both palms facing up. The top of the pad should touch the middle of your chest.

 • You can adjust the seat height to obtain the desired position.

3 Slowly bend your arms to raise the handles toward your shoulders.

4 Slowly straighten your arms to lower the handles back to the starting position.

Where should I position the seat on the arm curl machine?

Make sure you adjust the seat on the arm curl machine so that the top of the arm pad is touching the middle of your chest. If the seat is too high, you may work muscles other than your biceps, such as your shoulders, and put unnecessary strain on your back and neck. If the seat is too low, you may hyperextend your elbows, causing injury.

Is there an arm curl machine that simulates the use of dumbbells?

Yes. You can find arm curl machines that have two independent handles for working each of your arms separately. This type of arm curl machine closely simulates the use of dumbbells. Since each of your arms must lift the weight separately, this machine ensures that you balance the strength between your arms.

DON'T	MUSCLES TARGETED

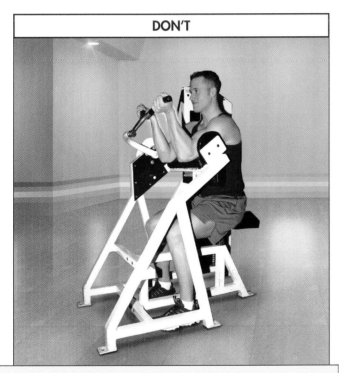

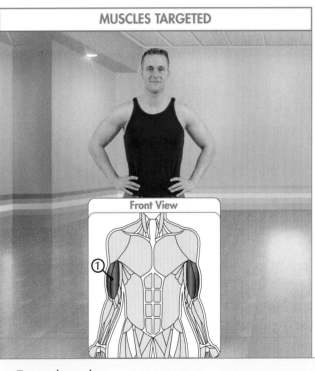

Front View

- Do not bend your wrists. Keep your wrists straight at all times.
- Do not lean back or shrug your shoulders when lifting the weight.
- Do not lift your body off the seat when you lower the weight.
- Do not lock your elbows when you straighten your arms.

Targeted muscles:
① biceps

wrist curl and reverse wrist curl

The wrist curl and reverse wrist curl are great exercises for strengthening your wrist muscles, which span the entire length of your forearm from your elbows to your wrists. You should be very careful performing wrist exercises if you have elbow problems and you should not perform either of these exercises if you have wrist problems.

Strong wrists can help improve your ability to grip objects and are important for preventing injury caused from lifting or carrying objects. You will also find these wrist exercises particularly beneficial if you participate in sports that involve extensive wrist movements, such as golf or tennis.

When you perform reverse wrist curls, you may need to use less weight than you use to perform wrist curls. As you curl your wrists up and down, make sure you do not lift your forearm off your thigh or twist your arm out to the sides. You should concentrate on performing the movements at a slow, even pace, keeping your abdominal muscles tight and your back straight.

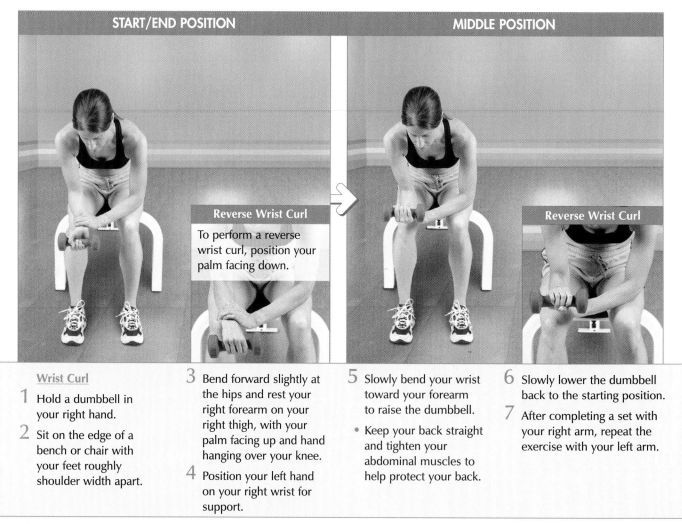

START/END POSITION

MIDDLE POSITION

Reverse Wrist Curl

To perform a reverse wrist curl, position your palm facing down.

Reverse Wrist Curl

Wrist Curl

1 Hold a dumbbell in your right hand.

2 Sit on the edge of a bench or chair with your feet roughly shoulder width apart.

3 Bend forward slightly at the hips and rest your right forearm on your right thigh, with your palm facing up and hand hanging over your knee.

4 Position your left hand on your right wrist for support.

5 Slowly bend your wrist toward your forearm to raise the dumbbell.

• Keep your back straight and tighten your abdominal muscles to help protect your back.

6 Slowly lower the dumbbell back to the starting position.

7 After completing a set with your right arm, repeat the exercise with your left arm.

How do I use a barbell to perform wrist curls?

To use a barbell to perform wrist curls, sit on a bench and hold the barbell in both hands with your palms turned up. Position your forearms on your thighs with your hands hanging over your knees and then perform the exercise as described in the steps below. For reverse wrist curls, turn your palms down instead of up. Using a barbell to perform wrist curls allows you to work both arms at once. You can also lift heavier weight when using a barbell than you would when using dumbbells.

Can I use a cable machine to perform wrist curls?

Yes. Set the cable on a cable machine tower at the lowest setting and attach a horseshoe handle to the cable. Sit on a bench facing the tower and hold the handle in your left hand with your palm facing up for wrist curls or down for reverse wrist curls. Bending forward, place your left forearm on your left thigh and let your hand hang over your knee. Using your right hand to support your left wrist, perform the exercise as described in the steps below. For more information on cable machines, see page 17.

DON'T	MUSCLES TARGETED

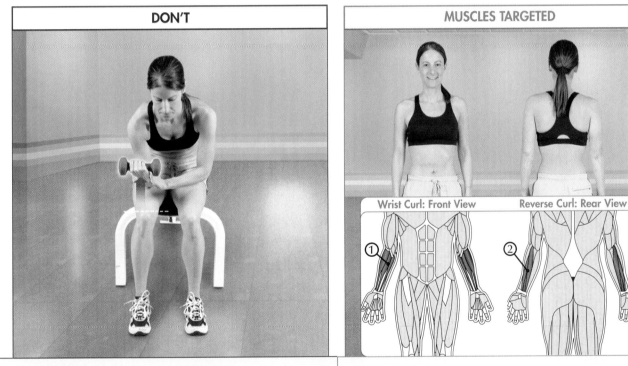

- Do not lift your forearm off your thigh.
- Do not twist your forearm to the left or right. Curl the dumbbell straight up.

Wrist Curl
Targeted muscles:
① forearm flexors

Reverse Wrist Curl
Targeted muscles:
② forearm extensors

abdominal crunch

The abdominal crunch is the most basic and one of the most effective exercises you can perform to strengthen and tone your abdominal muscles. Abdominal muscle strength is a key component of a flatter, firmer stomach.

When performing abdominal crunches, proper form is extremely important in the prevention of injury and in ensuring you get the most out of the exercise. To avoid straining your neck, do not bend your neck or pull on your head with your hands as you curl up. Keeping

your movements slow and controlled, use the upper part of your abdominal muscles to slowly lift your head and shoulders off the floor. You should also keep your lower back pressed to the floor and your elbows pointed out to the sides throughout the exercise.

If you perform the exercise properly, you should feel a burning sensation in your abdominal muscles by the time you complete about 12 repetitions.

People with neck problems should be careful when performing this exercise.

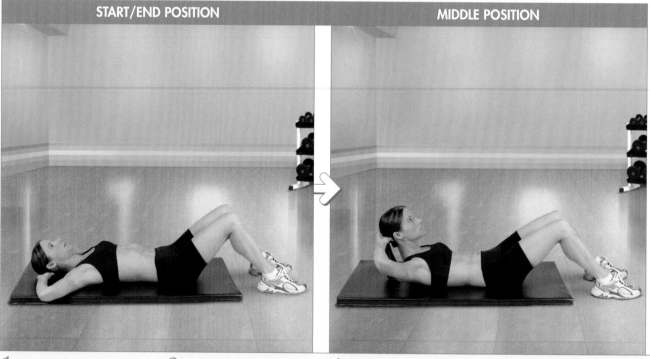

| START/END POSITION | MIDDLE POSITION |

1 Lie on your back on a mat, with your knees bent and your feet flat on the floor, roughly shoulder width apart.

2 Place your hands behind your head and move your elbows out to the sides. Do not interlock your fingers.

3 Push your lower back into the floor and tighten your abdominal muscles.

4 Slowly curl your head and shoulders a few inches off the floor, without pulling on your head with your hands. Keep your elbows out to the sides.

5 Pause for a moment and then slowly lower your head and shoulders back to the starting position.

Is there a way to make abdominal crunches easier?

To help make abdominal crunches easier, you can cross your arms on top of your chest or keep them at your sides with your palms facing the floor. If your neck feels strained while performing one of these modifications, you can place one hand behind your head for support while keeping the other arm on top of your chest or at your side.

How can I make abdominal crunches more challenging?

As your abdominal muscles grow stronger, regular crunches will become easier. For more challenging abdominal crunches, you can stretch your arms out over your head so they are parallel to the floor and then perform the exercise. You can also perform crunches with your legs lifted straight up so your body forms an "L" shape or with your legs lifted and your knees bent at 90-degree angles. Holding a light weight plate on your chest as you curl up and down can also increase the difficulty of the exercise.

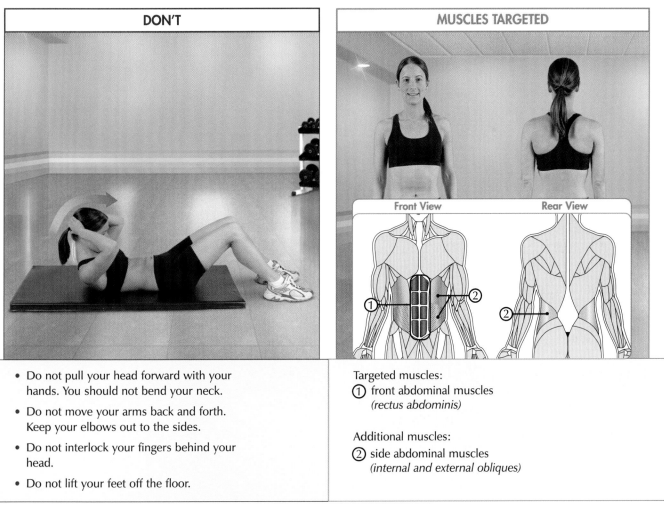

DON'T

- Do not pull your head forward with your hands. You should not bend your neck.

- Do not move your arms back and forth. Keep your elbows out to the sides.

- Do not interlock your fingers behind your head.

- Do not lift your feet off the floor.

MUSCLES TARGETED

Front View   Rear View

Targeted muscles:
① front abdominal muscles
   (rectus abdominis)

Additional muscles:
② side abdominal muscles
   (internal and external obliques)

twist crunch

The twist crunch is a good exercise for strengthening and toning the sides and front of your abdominal muscles. One important benefit of developing strong abdominal muscles is that these muscles help to support your back.

Proper form is essential to prevent injury and to get the most out of the exercise. To protect your lower back, do not lift your hips off the mat at any point during the exercise. Also avoid bending your neck or pulling your head with your hands.

When you lift your head and shoulders off the mat, do not immediately lower back to the starting position. Instead, contract your abdominal muscles and hold the position for at least one count before lowering. Focus on lifting using your abdominal muscles, keeping your elbows out to the sides instead of simply swinging your elbow toward your knee. Imagine that your goal is to lift your shoulder, not your elbow, toward your knee.

If you have existing back or neck problems, you should be careful performing twist crunches.

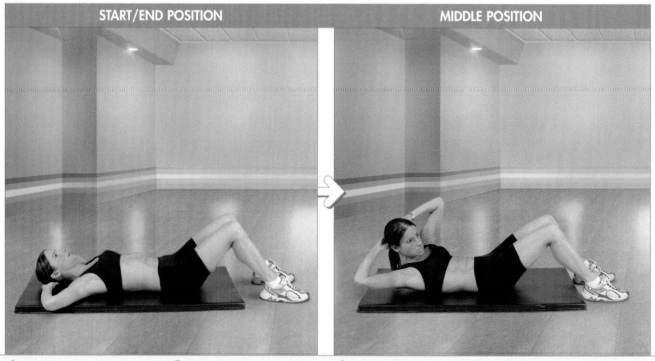

START/END POSITION **MIDDLE POSITION**

1 Lie on your back on a mat, with your knees bent. Position your feet flat on the floor, roughly shoulder width apart.

2 Place your hands behind your head and position your elbows out to the sides. Do not interlock your fingers.

3 Press your lower back into the floor and tighten your abdominal muscles.

4 Slowly curl your head and shoulders a few inches off the floor toward your right knee, without pulling on your neck with your hands. Keep your elbows out to the sides.

5 Pause for a moment and then slowly lower your head and shoulders back to the starting position.

6 After completing a set on one side, repeat the exercise on your other side.

Can I make the exercise easier?

Yes. Try crossing your arms on top of your chest as you perform the exercise. If your neck feels strained, place one hand behind your head for support. For another variation that also works the sides of your abdominal muscles more, lie on your back on the mat with your knees together and bent. Drop both knees to one side, keeping your shoulders flat on the floor. Then with your hands behind your head, lift your head and shoulders straight up. After completing a set, drop your knees to the other side and repeat the exercise.

How can I work the front of my abdominal muscles more?

You can perform the exercise as described in the steps below, except raise your legs and bend your hips and knees 90 degrees, keeping your knees together. To make this variation even more challenging, straighten your right leg as you lift your head and shoulders toward your left knee. Then straighten your left leg as you crunch toward your right knee and continue alternating legs until you complete the exercise. The last exercise looks like you are pedaling a bike.

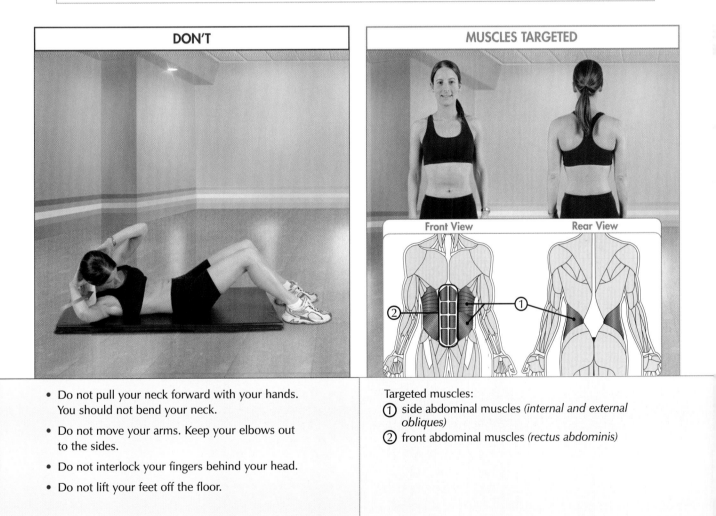

DON'T

MUSCLES TARGETED

Front View   Rear View

- Do not pull your neck forward with your hands. You should not bend your neck.

- Do not move your arms. Keep your elbows out to the sides.

- Do not interlock your fingers behind your head.

- Do not lift your feet off the floor.

Targeted muscles:
① side abdominal muscles *(internal and external obliques)*
② front abdominal muscles *(rectus abdominis)*

reverse crunch

The reverse crunch focuses on your front abdominal muscles, but also gives your side abdominal muscles a good workout. This is an excellent exercise for flattening and toning the lower portion of your front abdominal muscles. Be careful performing this exercise if you have lower back problems.

Your upper body should not move as you perform reverse crunches. To maintain proper form and help stabilize your upper body, you can grasp an edge of a secure object, such as the underside of a sturdy couch

or chair. You can also lie on a bench, instead of the floor, and hold the edges of the bench.

When performing the exercise, focus on using your lower abdominal muscles to lift your buttocks off the floor. To keep the focus on your abdominal muscles, do not jerk your legs or thrust your hips to lift your buttocks.

Once you are comfortable with the exercise, you can make it a bit harder by performing the exercise with your legs straight instead of bent.

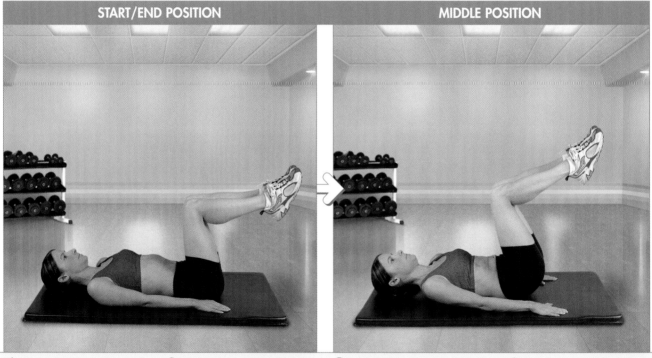

START/END POSITION	MIDDLE POSITION

1 Lie on your back on a mat and place your arms at your sides, with your palms facing the floor. Rest your head on the mat and tighten your abdominal muscles.

2 Position your legs together with your knees bent at 90-degree angles. Lift up your legs until your thighs are perpendicular to the floor.

3 Keeping your lower back on the floor, slowly lift your buttocks a few inches off the floor so your legs lift up and tilt slightly back towards your head.

4 Pause for a moment and then slowly lower your buttocks back to the starting position.

I find the reverse crunch too difficult. Is there an easier version of the exercise?

The pelvic tilt is an easier version of the reverse crunch. Lie on your back on a mat with your arms at your sides and your palms facing the floor. Bend your knees at 90-degree angles, keeping your feet flat on the floor, about shoulder width apart. Tighten your abdominal muscles as you tilt your hips toward your head and lift your lower buttocks off the floor slightly. Focus on lifting with your lower abdominal muscles, not your buttocks.

How can I make this exercise more difficult?

You can use a vertical bench. A vertical bench allows you to support your body on your forearms while your legs hang. Lift yourself into position with your forearms on the arm pads and your back pressed flat against the back pad. Bend your knees until your thighs are parallel with the floor. Then tighten your abdominal muscles and curl your buttocks up slightly, keeping your back against the back support. This exercise is more difficult because you are working against gravity.

DON'T

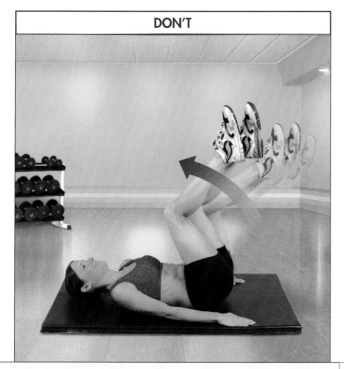

- Do not swing your legs. Focus on lifting just your buttocks.
- Do not allow your lower back to lift off the mat as you lift your buttocks.
- Do not lift your head off the mat.

MUSCLES TARGETED

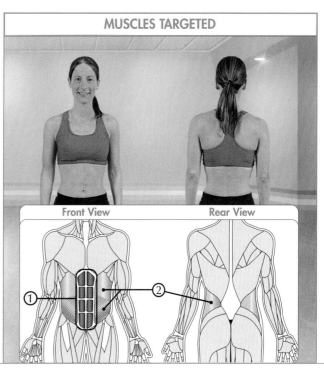

Front View   Rear View

Targeted muscles:
① front abdominal muscles *(rectus abdominis)*

Additional muscles:
② side abdominal muscles *(internal and external obliques)*

abdominal machine

The abdominal machine targets your front abdominal muscles, but also works your side abdominal muscles. If you have neck or back problems, using the abdominal machine is an ideal way for you to safely strengthen and tone your abdominal muscles. Since the machine allows you to use weight, this exercise can also help you build up your abdominal muscles.

There are a variety of abdominal machines available. Although abdominal machines may look different, they all allow you to crunch your abdominal muscles.

Depending on the type of machine you are using, you may have to position your arms on a chest pad or grasp handles or straps situated beside your head.

As you push the pad down in the exercise, concentrate on tightening your abdominal muscles and keeping your buttocks on the seat of the machine. Reduce the weight you are using if you find that your buttocks are lifting off the seat or if you are inadvertently slamming the weight onto the stack when you return to the starting position.

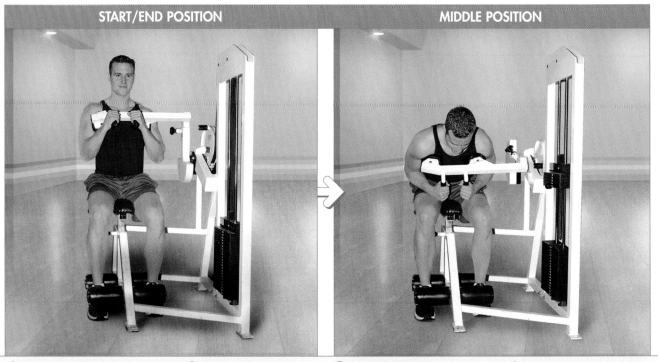

START/END POSITION   **MIDDLE POSITION**

1 Sit on an abdominal machine with your feet flat on the floor or on the footplate, roughly shoulder width apart.

• You may be able to adjust the footplate height to ensure your knees are bent at 90 degrees.

2 Rest your chest on the pad and grasp the handles in front of the pad.

• You can adjust the seat height to obtain the desired position.

3 Bend at your hips and slowly push the pad down toward your knees.

• Make sure you keep your back straight and tighten your abdominal muscles.

4 Slowly raise your upper body back to the starting position.

How can I change the intensity of the exercise?

You can adjust the angle of the pad to change the intensity of the exercise. To make the exercise easier, angle the pad away from you. To make the exercise more difficult, angle the pad toward you.

How can I put more focus on my side abdominal muscles?

You can use a rotary torso machine to put more focus on your side abdominal muscles. Sit on the seat of the rotary torso machine and then wrap your arms around the arm pads. If your arms do not feel comfortable, you can adjust the height of the seat. To perform the exercise, twist your torso to one side and then return to the starting position. After completing a set on one side, perform the same exercise on your other side. Be careful not to swing your body to the side to perform the exercise.

DON'T

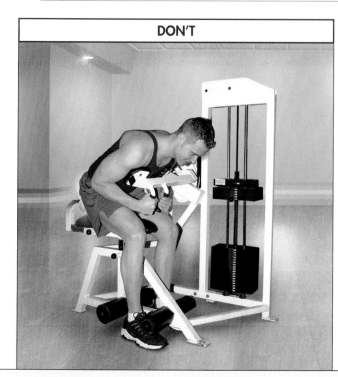

- Do not lift your buttocks off the seat when you push the pad down.
- Do not arch your back.
- Do not use your shoulders to push the pad down. Focus on using your abdominal muscles.
- Do not push the pad down too quickly. Keep the movement slow and controlled.

MUSCLES TARGETED

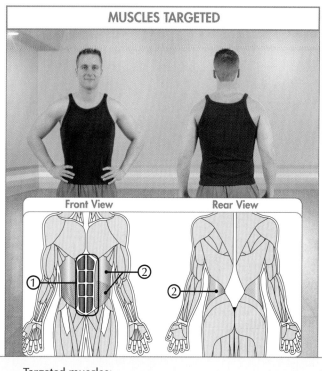

Targeted muscles:
① front abdominal muscles
   (rectus abdominis)

Additional muscles:
② side abdominal muscles
   (internal and external obliques)

leg raise

The leg raise works the front of your abdominal muscles, as well as the sides of your abdominal muscles and your hip flexors. This is a great exercise for strengthening your entire abdominal area, and is particularly useful for flattening the lower portion of your stomach.

You can perform this exercise while lying on a mat or on a flat bench. If you prefer to use a bench, lie flat on the bench and grasp the edges of the bench above your head for support.

To get into the starting position for this exercise, lie on your back and raise your legs a few inches off the floor. If you find this too difficult or your lower back feels strained, you can start with your legs a bit higher off the floor.

As you perform the exercise, focus on using your abdominal muscles to raise and lower your legs. You should also keep your lower back pressed to the floor and your head flat on the mat.

You should avoid leg raises if you have lower back problems.

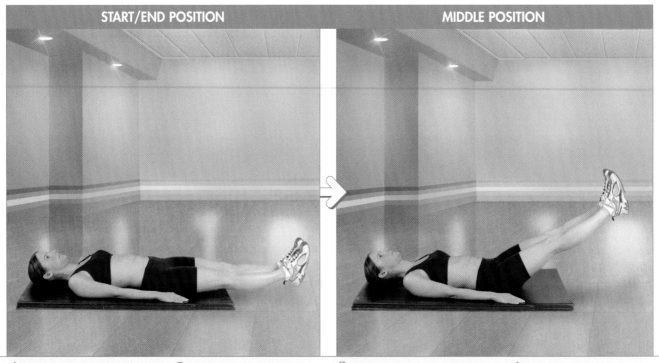

START/END POSITION

MIDDLE POSITION

1 Lie on your back on a mat and place your arms at your sides or under your buttocks, with your palms facing down. Rest your head on the mat and tighten your abdominal muscles.

2 Straighten your legs and position them together. Lift your legs a few inches off the floor.

3 Slowly raise your legs until they are at a 45-degree angle to the floor.

4 Pause for a moment and then slowly lower your legs back to the starting position.

How do I perform leg raises on a decline bench?

Lie on the decline bench with your head at the higher end of the bench and grasp the top of the bench for support. Start with your legs raised a few inches off the bench pad. Then lift your legs up until they form a 60-degree angle with the bench pad. Pause for a moment and then lower your legs to the starting position. In this variation of the exercise, you are working against gravity at a different angle, which makes it more difficult.

How can I work the upper part of my abdominal muscles more?

To work the upper part of your abdominal muscles more, sit on the long edge of a flat bench with your feet together on the floor. Grip the edge of the bench behind you with your palms facing your body. Leaning your upper body back by bending your elbows, extend your legs straight out in front of you so your body is almost parallel to the floor. Raise your legs and upper body until they form a "V" shape. Then return to the starting position.

DON'T

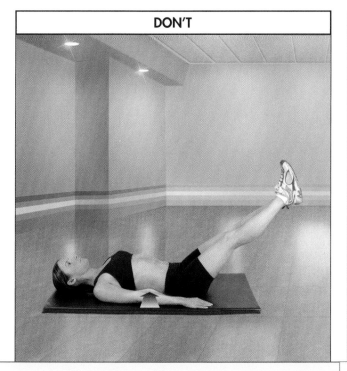

- Do not arch your back.
- Do not lift your head off the mat.
- Do not move your legs too quickly. Keep the movement slow and controlled.

MUSCLES TARGETED

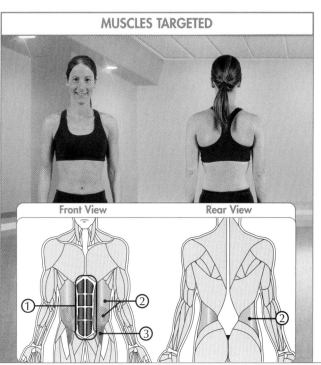

Targeted muscles:
① front abdominal muscles *(rectus abdominis)*

Additional muscles:
② side abdominal muscles *(internal and external obliques)*
③ hip flexors

plank

The plank works all of your abdominal muscles, your lower and middle back and your shoulders. The plank is a core stability exercise as it helps to strengthen your abdominal and lower back muscles, which are at the center, or core, of your body. Core stability exercises are important for improving your posture and making you less prone to injury when lifting heavy objects or bending.

When you lift your hips off the floor, try to hold the position for about 15 seconds. Then lower your hips and rest for about 10 seconds before repeating. When you begin practicing the plank, you may not be able to perform more than 2 repetitions of the exercise, but you can increase the duration and number of repetitions as you progress. When you are able to keep your body off the floor for more than 2 minutes, you should try a more challenging variation of the exercise. For more challenging variations, see the top of page 119.

You should be careful performing the plank if you have shoulder, elbow or lower back problems.

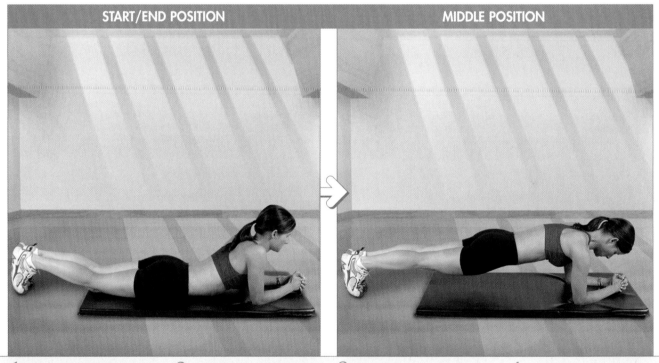

START/END POSITION　　　　**MIDDLE POSITION**

1 Lie on your stomach on a mat with your legs together and the balls of your feet on the floor. Tighten your abdominal muscles.

2 Lift your upper body off the mat and then use your forearms to support your upper body. Position your elbows directly under your shoulders, with your hands clasped.

3 Supporting your weight on your forearms and the balls of your feet, slowly lift your hips off the mat until your body is parallel to the floor.

4 Hold the position for about 15 seconds and then slowly lower your hips back to the mat.

Can I make the plank easier?

Yes. To make the plank easier, you can keep your knees on the floor as you perform the exercise. This is useful if you are a beginner or have a weak back.

How can I make the plank harder?

To make the plank harder, place the balls of your feet on a stable bench, instead of on the floor. You can vary the height of the bench to change the level of difficulty. Then perform the exercise as described in the steps below.

How can I work my buttocks more when performing the exercise?

To work your buttocks more, perform the steps below, except lift your left leg off the floor as you lift your hips and keep your leg raised for the entire 15 seconds. Then return to the starting position and repeat with your right leg raised. This is an advanced variation of the plank, since you are balancing on one foot instead of two. You can further increase the difficulty of this variation by extending the arm opposite to your raised leg.

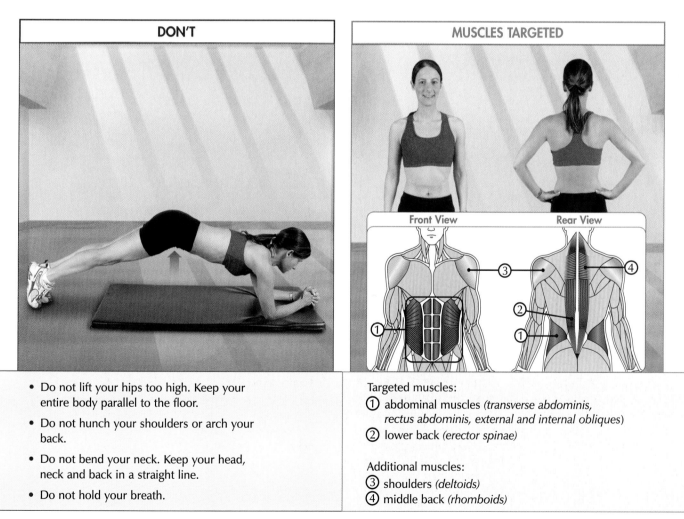

DON'T

MUSCLES TARGETED

Front View   Rear View

- Do not lift your hips too high. Keep your entire body parallel to the floor.
- Do not hunch your shoulders or arch your back.
- Do not bend your neck. Keep your head, neck and back in a straight line.
- Do not hold your breath.

Targeted muscles:
① abdominal muscles (*transverse abdominis, rectus abdominis, external and internal obliques*)
② lower back (*erector spinae*)

Additional muscles:
③ shoulders (*deltoids*)
④ middle back (*rhomboids*)

side plank

The side plank targets your abdominal muscles and lower back, as well as your shoulders and upper back. This exercise helps improve core stability, which makes you less prone to injury caused by lifting heavy objects or twisting your body. Core stability exercises, such as the side plank, can also shape and tone your waistline.

When you lift your hip off the floor, try to hold the position for about 10 seconds. Then lower your hip and rest for about 10 seconds before repeating. When you first try the side plank, you may not be able to

perform more than 2 repetitions of the exercise, but you can increase the number of repetitions and duration as you progress until you can perform 3 repetitions and hold the side plank for 2 minutes. Once you have mastered the side plank, you should try a more challenging variation of the exercise. For more challenging variations, see page 121.

You should be careful performing the side plank if you have back or shoulder problems.

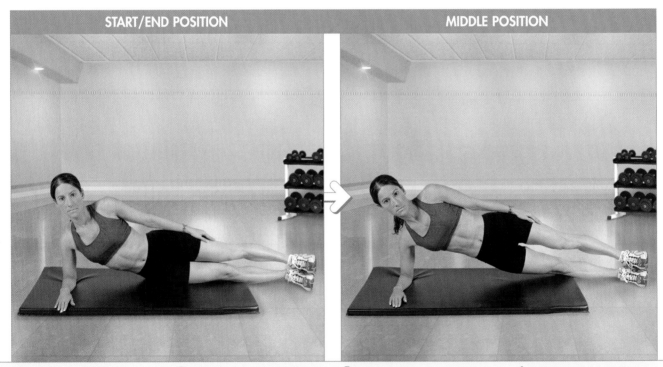

| START/END POSITION | MIDDLE POSITION |

1 Lie on your right side on a mat, with your legs together and straight. Tighten your abdominal muscles.

2 Lift your upper body off the mat and use your right forearm to support your upper body. Position your elbow directly under your shoulder. Rest your left arm straight at your side.

3 Supporting your weight on your forearm and the side of your right foot, slowly lift your hip off the mat until your entire body forms a straight line.

4 Hold the position for about 10 seconds and then slowly lower your hip back to the mat.

5 After completing a set on your right side, repeat the exercise on your left side.

How can I make the exercise easier?

If you find the side plank too difficult, you can modify the exercise. To perform a modified version of the side plank, lie on your side on a mat with your legs together and bent 90 degrees. Lift your upper body off the mat and then use your right forearm to support your upper body. Keeping your knees on the floor, raise your hip off the floor until your body forms a straight line from your knees to your shoulders.

I don't find side planks challenging enough. Are there harder variations of the exercise?

To make side planks harder, you can perform the exercise with your feet elevated on a step. For an even greater challenge, after you lift your hip off the mat, you can raise your top leg so that the leg is parallel to the floor or raise your top arm so the arm is perpendicular to the floor. You can also make the exercise harder by straightening your supporting arm so you are resting on your hand instead of your elbow and forearm.

DON'T

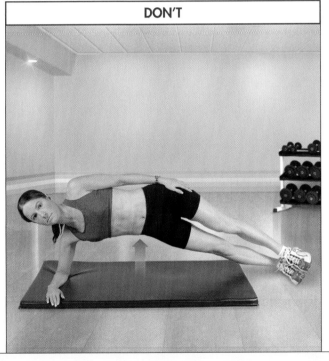

- Do not lift your hips too high or let your hips drop. Keep your entire body in a straight line.
- Do not lean your body back or forward.
- Do not hunch your shoulders.
- Do not bend your neck. Keep your head, neck and back in a straight line.

MUSCLES TARGETED

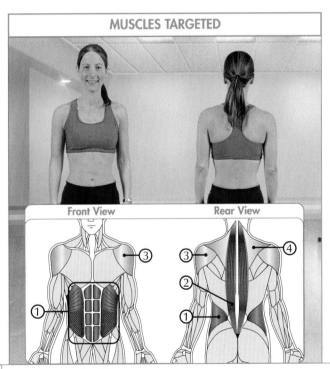

Targeted muscles:
① abdominal muscles *(transverse abdominis, rectus abdominis, external and internal obliques)*
② lower back *(erector spinae)*

Additional muscles:
③ shoulders *(deltoids)*
④ upper back *(trapezius)*

bridge

The bridge focuses on your buttocks and hamstrings, but also works your deep abdominal muscles and your lower back. This exercise strengthens your back and abdominal muscles, which can help make you less prone to injury when performing activities that involve heavy lifting or twisting your body. Your back and abdominal muscles are considered core muscles and strengthening these muscles is referred to as developing core stability.

When you lift your buttocks off the floor in this exercise, try to hold the position for about 10 seconds.

Then lower your buttocks back to the floor and rest for about 10 seconds before repeating the exercise. Once you develop strength in your core, you can increase the amount of time you hold your buttocks off the floor to as long as 2 minutes. If you are a beginner, you may not be able to perform more than 2 repetitions of the bridge, but you can increase the number of repetitions as you progress.

You should be careful performing the bridge if you have upper back problems.

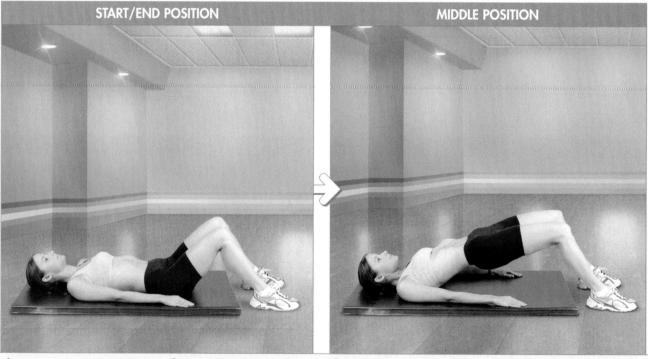

START/END POSITION

MIDDLE POSITION

1 Lie on your back on a mat with your knees bent. Position your feet flat on the floor, roughly shoulder width apart.

2 Place your arms at your sides with your palms facing down. Tighten your abdominal muscles.

3 Slowly lift your buttocks off the mat by pushing through your heels until your body and thighs form a straight line.

4 Hold the position for about 10 seconds and then slowly lower your buttocks back to the mat.

How can I make the exercise more difficult?

To make the exercise more difficult, you can place your feet flat on a step or bench so that you will have to lift your buttocks higher off the floor and at a greater angle to make your upper body and thighs form a straight line. Make sure the step or bench is secure and stable.

Can I work my hamstrings and buttocks more?

To work your hamstrings and buttocks more, straighten one leg while holding your buttocks off the floor. Straightening one leg makes the exercise more difficult since you have to balance all your weight on one leg.

How can I alternately work my left and right sides in this exercise?

To alternately work your left and right sides, perform the exercise as described below and then lift one foot slightly off the floor for 2 seconds, keeping your knee bent 90 degrees. Then lower the foot for 2 seconds and repeat using your other leg. You can make this variation more difficult by attaching ankle weights to your legs.

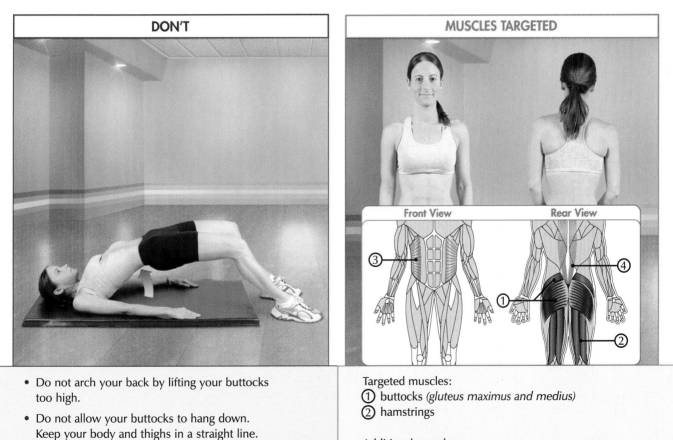

DON'T

- Do not arch your back by lifting your buttocks too high.

- Do not allow your buttocks to hang down. Keep your body and thighs in a straight line.

- Do not point your knees in or out. Keep your knees pointed straight ahead.

- Do not hold your breath.

MUSCLES TARGETED

Front View   Rear View

Targeted muscles:
① buttocks *(gluteus maximus and medius)*
② hamstrings

Additional muscles:
③ deep abdominal muscles *(transverse abdominis)*
④ lower back *(erector spinae)*

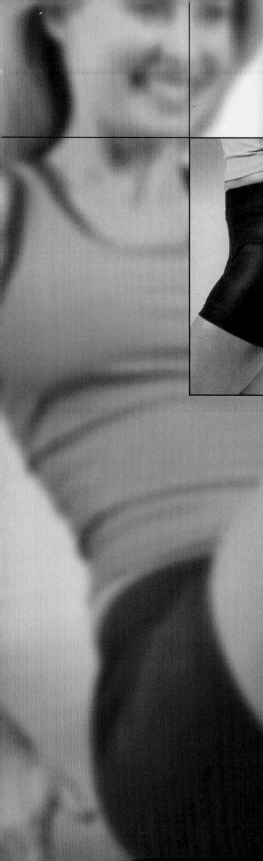

Section 3

Training your lower body involves working your legs, buttocks and calves. Building strength in your lower body can make everyday activities, such as walking, climbing stairs and lifting items off the floor, much easier.

A strong lower body also helps improve your balance and your ability to perform sports that primarily use lower body muscles, such as running, squash, skating and skiing. Section 3 takes you through the exercises you can perform to work your lower body.

Work Your Lower Body

In this Section...

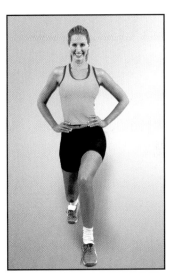

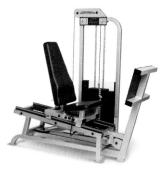

dumbbell squat

The dumbbell squat works most of the muscles in your lower body, including your quadriceps, hamstrings, buttocks, hip flexors and inner thighs. This is an excellent exercise for developing strong, well-toned legs, which can make many everyday activities, such as walking, climbing stairs or lifting things off the ground, easier to perform.

If you have trouble maintaining your balance while squatting, try to keep your head up, look straight ahead and focus on an object directly in front of you, instead of looking down at the floor. When you look straight down, you will be more likely to lose your balance and fall forward.

To improve your form, you can place a bench behind you and then lightly touch the bench with your buttocks each time you squat. As you come out of the squat, concentrate on pushing yourself up through your heels rather than the balls of your feet.

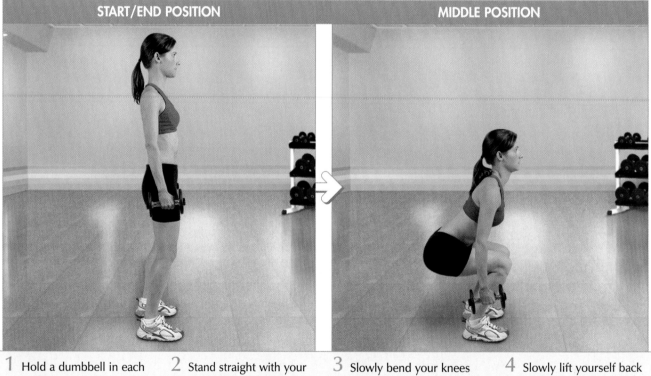

| START/END POSITION | MIDDLE POSITION |

1 Hold a dumbbell in each hand at your sides with both palms facing inward.

2 Stand straight with your feet shoulder width apart and your head up. Tighten your abdominal muscles to help protect your back.

3 Slowly bend your knees until your thighs are parallel to the floor. Your knees should not extend past your toes. Imagine you are sitting down in a chair.

• Make sure you keep your back straight and your feet flat on the floor.

4 Slowly lift yourself back to the starting position, pushing through your heels.

How can I focus the exercise more on my inner thighs and buttocks?

To focus the exercise more on your inner thighs and buttocks, place your feet roughly double shoulder width apart.

Can I perform squats without dumbbells?

Yes. If you find squatting with dumbbells difficult or if you do not have weights handy, you can simply place your hands on your hips or straight out in front of you to help maintain your balance while you squat.

How can I make the exercise harder?

Slowing down your movements can make the exercise harder and increase muscular and tendon strength. To slow down your movements, you can take 4 seconds to get down into the squat, pause at the bottom for 2 seconds and then take 4 seconds to get back up. This technique can be performed with or without weights.

DON'T

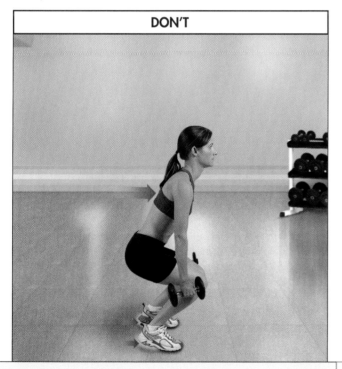

- Do not shift your body weight forward and allow your heels to lift off the floor.
- Do not hunch or excessively arch your back.
- Do not tilt your head up or down. Keep your head and neck in line with your back.
- Do not lock your knees.

MUSCLES TARGETED

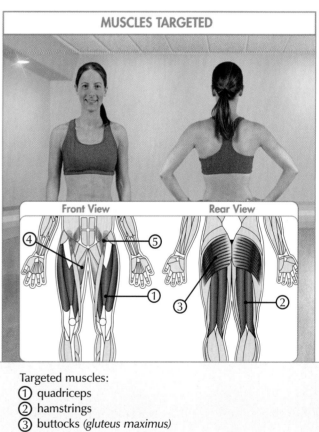

Front View   Rear View

Targeted muscles:
① quadriceps
② hamstrings
③ buttocks (*gluteus maximus*)

Additional muscles:
④ inner thighs (*adductors*)
⑤ hip flexors

barbell squat

The barbell squat is an important exercise for building stronger leg muscles, which can help make everyday activities, such as climbing stairs and lifting objects off the floor, easier. This exercise primarily works your quadriceps, hamstrings and buttocks, but it also strengthens your inner thighs, hip flexors and lower back.

Before performing this exercise, you should be sure to warm up properly, as you may get injured if your legs are too stiff. The barbell squat is more difficult to perform than the dumbbell squat and you typically use more weight when performing the barbell squat. If you have a weak or injured back, you should not perform this exercise.

Whenever possible, you should work with a spotter, who should be standing close by and ready to assist you if you get in trouble while lifting the weight. If a spotter is not available, perform this exercise using a power cage, which is designed to catch the barbell if you have trouble rising from the squatting position.

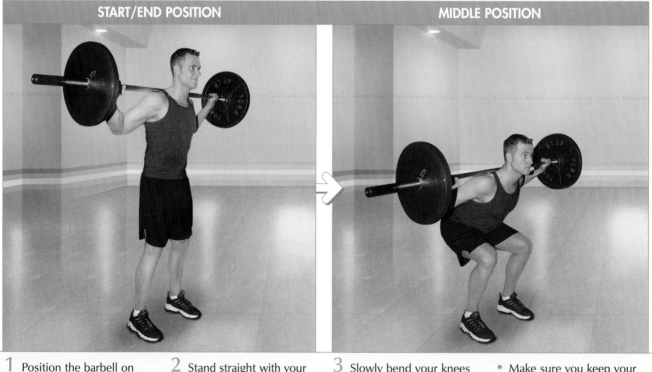

START/END POSITION | **MIDDLE POSITION**

1 Position the barbell on your upper back, not on your neck. Make sure the bar is centered on your back. Hold the bar with your hands almost double shoulder width apart and both palms facing forward.

2 Stand straight with your feet roughly shoulder width apart. Tighten your abdominal muscles to help protect your back.

3 Slowly bend your knees until your thighs are parallel to the floor. Your knees should not pass over your toes. Imagine you are sitting down in a chair.

• Make sure you keep your back straight and your feet flat on the floor. Your elbows should always be directly under your wrists.

4 Slowly lift yourself back to the starting position, pushing through your heels.

How can I work my quadriceps harder?

To work your quadriceps harder, you can perform a more advanced barbell squat by holding the barbell in a different manner. Position the bar across the front of your collar bone and shoulders. With your palms facing towards your chest, make an "X" with your forearms and hold the bar. When you hold the barbell in this manner, you should use less weight and take extra care to maintain your balance.

I am having difficulty keeping my balance when performing barbell squats. What can I do?

You can use the Smith machine to guide your movement so you feel more stable and balanced when performing squats. The Smith machine features a bar that travels straight up and down a vertical track. If you lose control of the weight, the machine has a safety stop that will catch the bar to prevent you from becoming injured. When using the Smith machine, start with your feet slightly in front of your body and your knees slightly bent. For more information on Smith machines, see page 16.

DON'T

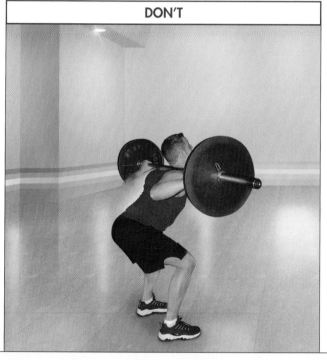

MUSCLES TARGETED

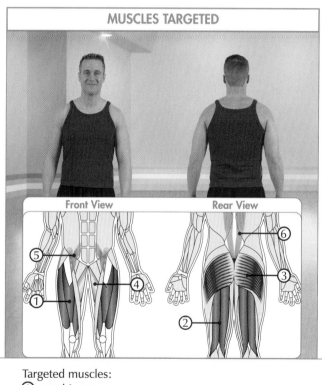

Front View   Rear View

- Do not hunch or excessively arch your back.

- Do not shift your body weight forward and allow your heels to lift off the floor.

- Do not tilt your head up or down. To help maintain your balance, look straight ahead and keep your head and neck in line with your back.

- Do not lock your knees.

Targeted muscles:
① quadriceps
② hamstrings
③ buttocks (gluteus maximus)

Additional muscles:
④ inner thighs (adductors)
⑤ hip flexors
⑥ lower back (erector spinae)

hack squat

The hack squat is an excellent exercise for helping you gain strength and mass in your quadriceps and buttocks. The hack squat also strengthens your hamstrings and hip flexors. Building strength in these muscles can help make many everyday activities, such as walking, running and lifting objects off the floor, easier.

When you perform the hack squat, you should keep the following things in mind. As you lower the weight, make sure you bend your knees to form a 90-degree angle. Your knees should not hang past your toes when they are bent. When you push the weight back up, focus on lifting the weight up through your heels rather than the balls of your feet. Also, make sure you do not lock your knees when you return to the starting position.

Due to the movement involved in the hack squat, you must be very careful performing this exercise if you have knee or lower back problems.

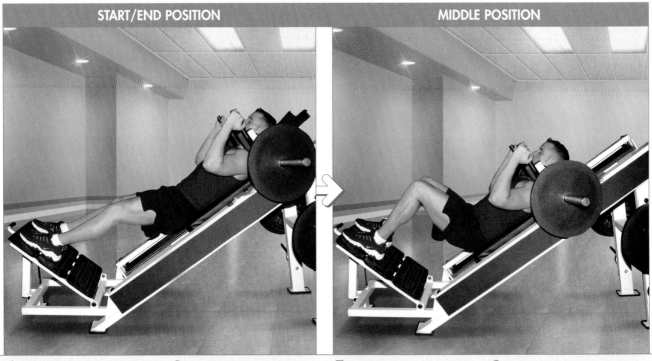

START/END POSITION   **MIDDLE POSITION**

1 Lie on your back on a hack squat machine. Your shoulders should fit firmly under the shoulder pads.

2 Position your feet slightly in front of your body on the platform, roughly shoulder width apart.

3 Grasp the handles on the machine. Tighten your abdominal muscles to help protect your back.

4 Release the lock to allow you to lower the weight.

5 Slowly lower the weight until your knees are bent at a 90-degree angle.

- Make sure you keep your back flat against the back pad.

6 Pause for a moment and then slowly push the weight back up through your heels to the starting position.

7 After completing a set, engage the lock to once again secure the weight in place.

How can I make sure my stronger leg does not compensate for my weaker leg in this exercise?

To prevent your stronger leg from compensating for your weaker leg, you can perform the exercise using one leg at a time. Perform the exercise the same way you would if you were using both legs, except lift the leg you are not working slightly in front of your body so it does not rest on the platform during the exercise. When working one leg at a time, you will need to reduce the weight you use. Working each leg separately is especially helpful if you participate in sports, such as high jump or basketball, where you need explosive power in both legs.

Can I change this exercise to work my buttocks and inner thighs more?

Yes. To work your buttocks and inner thighs more when performing this exercise, you can position your feet slightly wider than shoulder width apart on the platform.

DON'T

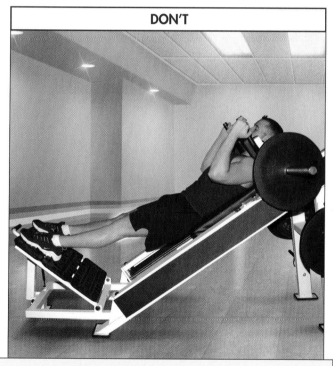

- Do not lock your knees.
- Do not lift your head off the pad.
- Do not allow your knees to go past your toes.
- Do not arch your back. Keep your back flat against the back pad.

MUSCLES TARGETED

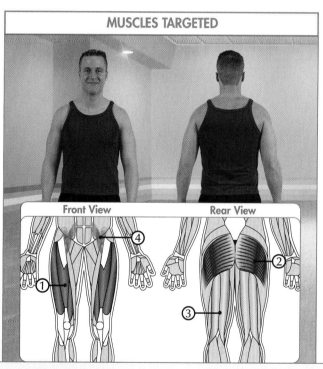

Targeted muscles:
① quadriceps
② buttocks (*gluteus maximus*)

Additional muscles:
③ hamstrings
④ hip flexors

leg press

The leg press helps build strength and endurance in your legs. The exercise focuses on your quadriceps and hamstrings, but also gives your hip flexors, buttocks and inner thighs a great workout.

If you have trouble performing squats or lunges because of lower back problems, the leg press is a good alternative. However, you may want to avoid the leg press if you have an existing knee problem or if your knees begin to hurt during the exercise.

There are different types of leg press machines available. Some machines require you to add weight plates to a bar, while others allow you to insert a pin into a stack of weights to select the amount of weight you want to lift. Depending on the machine, either the foot plate or the body pad will move as you perform the exercise. Your position on the machine and the angle at which you press your legs to raise the weight may also be different. However, the concept of the exercise is the same for each leg press machine.

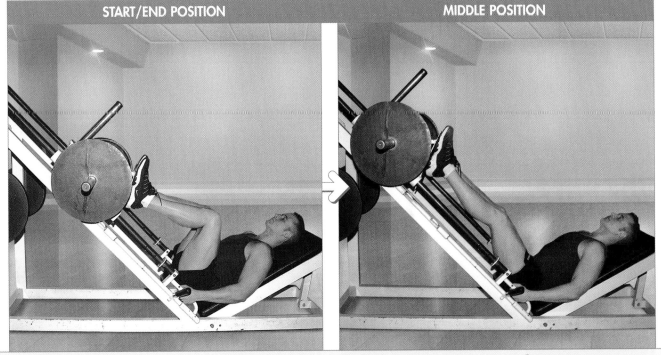

START/END POSITION | **MIDDLE POSITION**

1 Lie on your back on a leg press machine and position your feet flat on the foot plate about shoulder width apart with your toes pointing up.

2 If the machine has a brake, press the weight up through your heels just enough to be able to release the brake.

3 Grasp the handles on the machine. Tighten your abdominal muscles to help protect your back.

4 Lower the weight until your knees are bent at 90-degree angles.

5 Slowly push the weight through your heels, not your toes, until your legs are almost straight.

6 Pause for a moment and then slowly lower the weight to return to the starting position.

7 If the machine has a brake, use the brake to once again secure the weight in place when pushing the weight up for the last time.

Can I work one leg at a time?

Yes. Place your right leg on the floor as you perform the exercise with your left leg. After completing a full set with your left leg, repeat the exercise with your right leg. You will need to reduce the amount of weight used when working one leg. Working one leg at a time is useful if one of your legs is stronger than the other and you do not want the stronger leg compensating for the weaker leg.

Is there a way to change which muscles the exercise targets?

You can adjust the position of your feet on the foot plate to change the muscles targeted. To work your inner thighs and buttocks more, position your feet about 3 to 5 inches wider than shoulder width apart. To emphasize your hamstrings and buttocks more, place your feet about 2 to 3 inches higher than normal on the foot plate. You should be careful when performing these modifications if you have knee problems.

DON'T

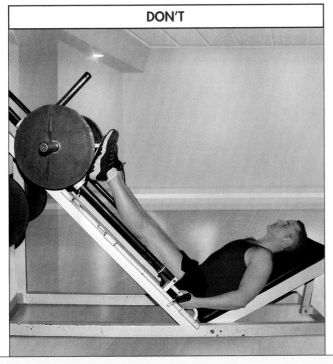

MUSCLES TARGETED

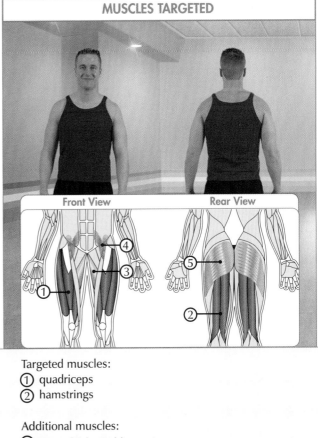

- Do not lock your knees when you straighten your legs.
- Do not raise your head off the head rest. Keep your head and neck in line with your back.
- Do not arch your back to help push the weight. Make sure your back remains flat against the back pad.

Targeted muscles:
1. quadriceps
2. hamstrings

Additional muscles:
3. inner thighs (adductors)
4. hip flexors
5. buttocks (gluteus maximus)

leg extension

The leg extension focuses on your quadriceps and is one of the best ways to develop strong thighs. In addition to giving you stronger and more toned thighs, the leg extension helps strengthen your knee joints. You require the use of a leg extension machine to perform this exercise.

To ensure that you get the most out of performing this exercise, you should try to complete the full range of motion by raising the weight all the way up and

lowering the weight all the way down. You should also make sure you concentrate on performing the movements slowly.

To prevent injuries, avoid jerking your legs up rapidly or locking your knees at the top of the movement. You should also avoid using more weight than you can control. If you are using too much weight, you may have a tendency to inadvertently slam the weight down onto the stack between repetitions.

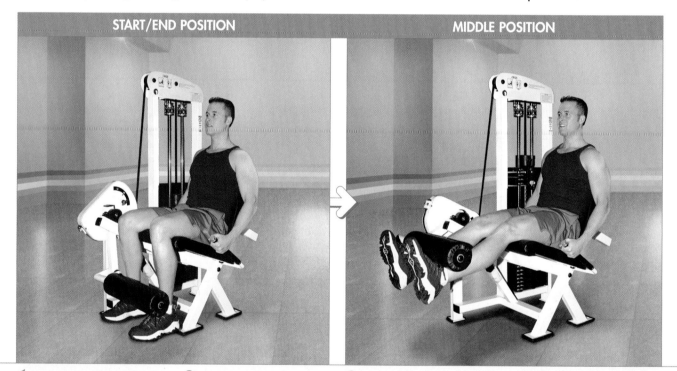

| START/END POSITION | MIDDLE POSITION |

1 Sit on a leg extension machine and position your feet below the foot pad. Make sure your back is flat against the back pad and the tops of your ankles rest against the foot pad.

• You can usually adjust the back pad and foot pad to obtain the desired position.

2 Grasp the handles on the machine or the edges of the seat lightly to keep your hips from lifting up. Tighten your abdominal muscles to help protect your back.

3 Slowly lift the weight with your legs until your knees are straight, but not locked.

4 Pause for a moment and then slowly lower your legs back to a 90-degree bend at the knees.

One of my legs is stronger than the other. How can I balance the strength in my legs?

To prevent the stronger leg from compensating for the weaker leg when you perform leg extensions using both legs, you can perform the exercise with less weight using one leg at a time. Developing equal strength in both legs is beneficial for athletes, such as runners and tennis players, who need good coordination between their legs.

How do I focus on strengthening the inner part of my quadriceps around the knees?

To focus on strengthening the inner part of your quadriceps around the knees, you can pause for about 3 to 5 seconds while your legs are fully extended and then take about 5 seconds to slowly lower the weight. Since the inner part of your quadriceps around the knees tends to be weaker than the outer part of your quadriceps, this variation works well.

DON'T

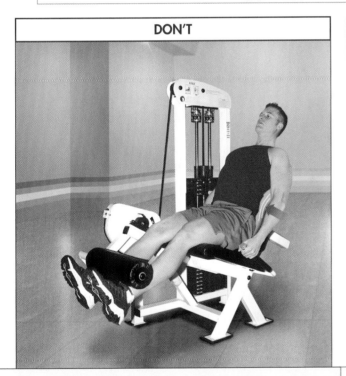

MUSCLES TARGETED

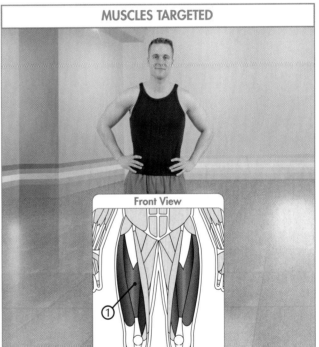

Front View

- Do not arch your back or raise your hips off the seat to help you lift the weight. Make sure your back and hips remain against the pads.

- Do not jerk your legs up or quickly release the weight. Make sure you maintain a constant motion during the entire exercise.

- Do not turn your toes in or out. Keep your feet straight as you perform the exercise.

Targeted muscles:
① quadriceps

leg curl

Using the leg curl machine is a popular way to work your hamstrings. While primarily strengthening your hamstrings, this machine also builds strength in your calves and buttocks.

Many people focus on building up their quadriceps and place less emphasis on their hamstrings. Working your hamstrings using the leg curl machine can improve the shape of your legs by giving your quadriceps and hamstrings a more balanced appearance.

Try to keep the movement in the exercise smooth and

continuous, making sure the weights do not slam down between repetitions. You should also keep your hips on the pad while performing this exercise. If your hips lift off the pad, your hamstrings will not work as hard and you may put stress on your lower back. It is also important that you do not lock your knees when you bring your legs back to the starting position.

Take extra caution using the leg curl machine if you have or previously had a knee injury or lower back problems.

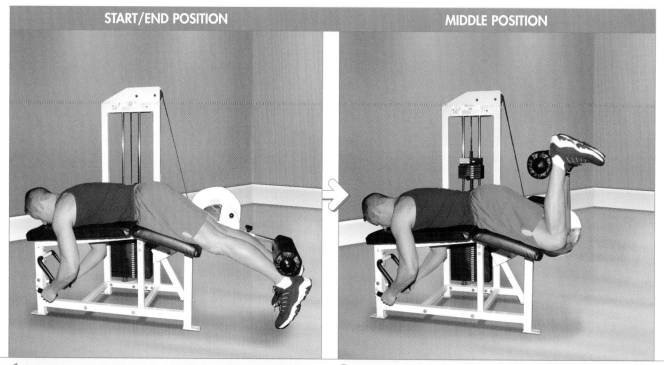

| START/END POSITION | MIDDLE POSITION |

1 Lie on your stomach on a leg curl machine and position your feet below the foot pad. Your knees should be just off the pad and the backs of your ankles should touch the foot pad.

• You should be able to adjust the foot pad to obtain the desired position.

2 Grasp the handles on the machine to help keep your hips from lifting up. Tighten your abdominal muscles to help protect your back.

3 Slowly bend your knees to lift your heels toward your buttocks, keeping your toes pulled toward your shins.

4 Pause for a moment and then slowly lower your legs back to the starting position.

How can I further protect my back when performing leg curls?

You can use a seated leg curl machine, which offers additional support and protection for your back. Sit on the seated leg curl machine with the back of your ankles resting on the foot pad. Secure the thigh pad across your thighs and grasp the handles on the pad to prevent your hips and lower back from lifting. Bring your heels toward your buttocks and then return to the starting position.

One of my legs is stronger than the other. How can I make sure each leg works equally?

To prevent your stronger leg from compensating for your weaker leg when you perform leg curls, you can perform the exercise using one leg at a time. Perform the exercise the same way you would if you were using both legs, except leave one of your legs straight as you work the other leg for an entire set. You will need to reduce the weight you use when working one leg at a time.

DON'T

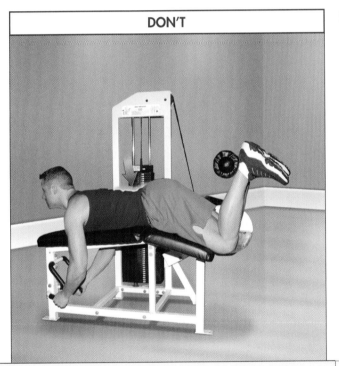

- Do not arch your back or lift your hips to help you lift the weight since this puts stress on your lower back.
- Do not lift your head off the pad.
- Do not lock your knees.
- Do not jerk your legs up or quickly release the weight. Make sure you maintain a constant motion during the entire exercise.

MUSCLES TARGETED

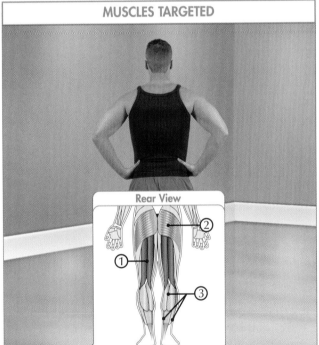

Rear View

Targeted muscles:
① hamstrings

Additional muscles:
② buttocks
   (gluteus maximus)
③ calves
   (gastrocnemius and soleus)

lunge

Lunges firm and tone your quadriceps, hamstrings and buttocks, as well as your hip flexors, inner thighs and calves.

This exercise strengthens your legs and helps improve your balance, which is particularly beneficial for activities that require vigorous legwork, such as tennis or squash. Since lunges involve deep knee bending, you should avoid this exercise if you have knee problems.

Depending on your fitness level, you may want to use weights while performing lunges. When using

dumbbells, hold a dumbbell in each hand with your arms at your sides and your palms facing your legs. To use a barbell, hold the bar across your upper back with your palms facing forward. When using a barbell, remember to keep the wrist and elbow of each arm in a straight line. Keep in mind that adding weights increases the intensity of the exercise and may make maintaining your balance more difficult.

When performing lunges, try to keep your back straight and look straight ahead to help maintain your balance.

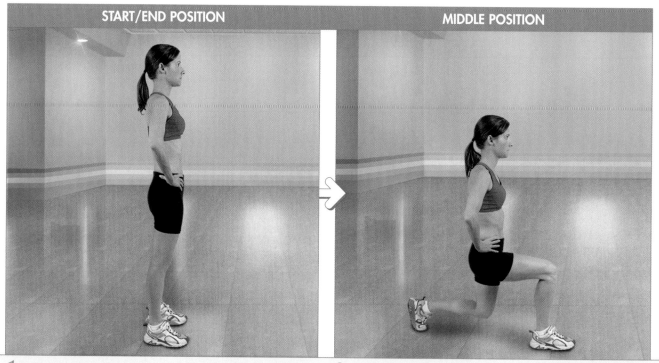

START/END POSITION   **MIDDLE POSITION**

1 Stand straight with your hands on your hips, your feet roughly shoulder width apart and your toes pointed forward.

- Make sure you keep your head up and your back straight. Tighten your abdominal muscles to help protect your back.

2 Take a large step forward with your right leg. Slowly bend your knees until your right thigh is parallel with the floor. Both knees should be bent at 90-degree angles and your right knee should not pass the front of your right foot.

3 Slowly lift your body and step back to the starting position, pushing through the heel of your right foot.

4 When you complete a set with your right leg, repeat the exercise with your left leg.

QUESTION & ANSWER

I have trouble keeping my balance when I perform lunges. What can I do?

You can perform a stationary lunge, which you may find more stable. Start with your right foot flat on the floor about one stride length in front of your left foot. Your feet should be shoulder width apart. Bend your knees and lower your body for two seconds, pause for one second and then raise your body for two seconds. Make sure you do not move your feet. After you complete a set, switch legs and repeat the exercise.

How can I add some variation to the exercise?

After you have mastered the basic lunging technique, you can perform variations, such as reverse lunges and walking lunges. You perform reverse lunges the same way you perform regular lunges except you step backward instead of forward. To perform a walking lunge, instead of returning your front leg to the starting position after your first lunge, lean your weight forward on your front leg, lift your back leg in and lunge forward with your back leg. Then continue alternating legs as you travel forward.

DON'T	MUSCLES TARGETED

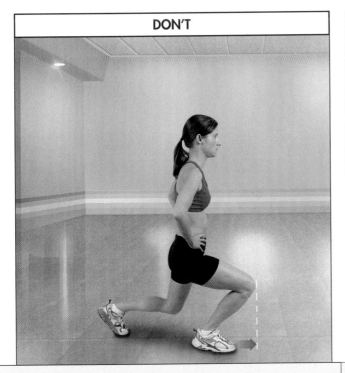

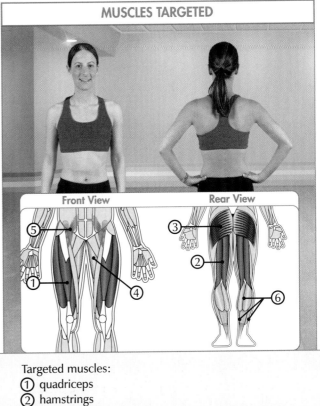

Front View   Rear View

- Do not allow your front knee to pass your toes.
- Do not twist your body or lean forward. Your shoulders should be square and face forward.
- Do not point your toes in or out. Your toes should point straight ahead.
- Do not land on the toes of your front foot when stepping forward. Make sure your front foot is flat on the floor.

Targeted muscles:
① quadriceps
② hamstrings
③ buttocks (*gluteus maximus*)

Additional muscles:
④ inner thighs (*adductors*)
⑤ hip flexors
⑥ calves (*gastrocnemius* and *soleus*)

step-up

Step-ups focus on your quadriceps and hip flexors, but also strengthen your hamstrings and buttocks. Step-ups are a good way to improve the shape and definition of your legs. Performing this exercise can help make activities that involve a lot of climbing less difficult.

When performing step-ups, make sure the step or bench is large enough to accommodate your entire foot, so you can pull yourself up onto the step or bench with your entire foot instead of just the ball of your foot.

Use caution when performing this exercise if you have

knee problems. You can lessen the pressure on your knees and make this exercise easier by using a lower step or bench.

You can also reduce the strain on your elbows and shoulder joints and get better balance by holding the dumbbells on your shoulders. When holding the dumbbells on your shoulders, your elbows should be bent and off to the sides. Your palms should be facing the ground. Since this position will make the exercise more difficult, be sure to use lighter weights.

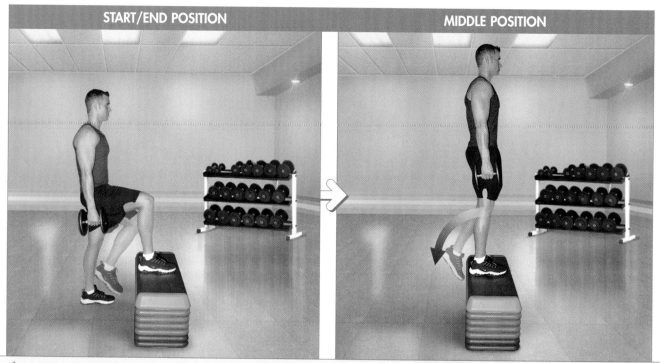

START/END POSITION   **MIDDLE POSITION**

1 Hold a dumbbell in each hand at your sides, palms facing in.

2 Stand in front of a step or bench with your feet roughly shoulder width apart. Tighten your abdominal muscles to help protect your back.

• The step or bench should be high enough so that your upper leg is parallel to the ground when you step up.

3 Step up by placing your right leg on top of the step or bench. Lean forward slightly and pull yourself up through the heel of your right foot.

4 When both feet are flat on the step or bench, step down with your left leg and then your right leg.

5 After completing a set stepping up with your right leg, repeat the exercise and step up with your left leg.

How can I work my hamstrings and buttocks more?

You can perform step-ups that work your hamstrings and buttocks more by positioning yourself farther away from the step or bench. Since you will have to stretch your leg and lean forward more in order to bring yourself up onto the step or bench, you should take extra care not to lose your balance. Make sure the step or bench is secured next to a wall or a sturdy object so it does not slide away from you.

Can I perform step-ups that further target my buttocks?

Yes. You can perform step-ups that further target your buttocks by stepping up onto the step or bench with your right foot and then kicking back your left leg to extend it behind you. Your left leg should then come down onto the floor. After completing a set kicking back with your left leg, repeat the exercise kicking back with your right leg. This variation also helps build balance and strength in your legs.

DON'T

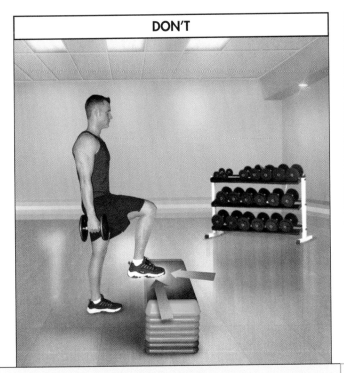

- Do not step up onto the ball of your foot. Make sure your entire foot steps up onto the step or bench and you pull yourself up through your heel.

- Do not hunch or arch your back. Make sure your head, neck and back form a straight line during the entire exercise.

MUSCLES TARGETED

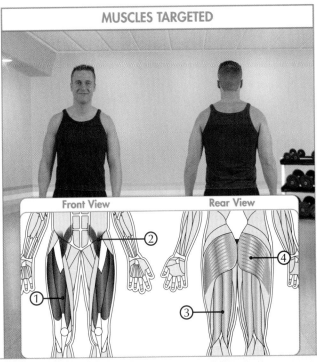

Front View   Rear View

Targeted muscles:
① quadriceps
② hip flexors

Additional muscles:
③ hamstrings
④ buttocks (*gluteus maximus*)

barbell deadlift

The barbell deadlift focuses on your hamstrings and buttocks, but also works your lower back and abdominal muscles.

The barbell deadlift is considered one of the best overall body exercises, but it is an advanced exercise that must be performed with perfect form in order to avoid injury. Throughout the exercise, you must keep your back straight and your abdominal muscles tight. Do not lean back to help lift the weight or bend your neck as you move. You should keep your head,

neck and back in a straight line at all times.

As you perform the barbell deadlift, lower the barbell to about knee height or you can go lower if you are more flexible. When lifting the weight, visualize pushing through your feet to the floor to work your legs thoroughly.

Due to the increased difficulty and risk of injury, beginners and people with lower back, hip or knee problems should consider excluding this exercise from their training program.

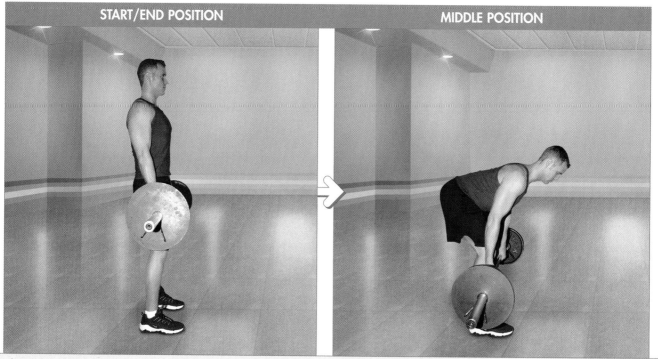

START/END POSITION

MIDDLE POSITION

1 Grasp a barbell with your hands roughly shoulder width apart and your palms facing your body.

- When lifting a heavy weight, grasp the bar with one palm facing your body and the other palm facing forward to prevent forearm fatigue.

2 Stand straight with your feet roughly shoulder width apart, knees slightly bent. Rest the bar against the top of your thighs.

3 Keeping your elbows slightly bent, slowly bend forward at your hips to lower the bar to about knee level.

- Make sure you tighten your abdominal muscles to help protect your back.

4 Pause for a moment and then slowly lift the bar back to the starting position by raising your upper body.

How can this exercise be made easier for beginners?

If you are a beginner, you can position your feet slightly wider than shoulder width apart and bend your knees a little more to make this exercise easier. This stance will also place more emphasis on your inner thighs. You can also use less weight by using dumbbells instead of a barbell to perform this exercise. Grasp the dumbbells with your palms facing your body and then perform the exercise as described below.

How can I make the barbell deadlift more intense?

To make the barbell deadlift more intense, you can stand on a platform or step and try lowering the bar below your feet, while still maintaining proper form. Standing on a platform or step gives you a greater range of motion. You need to be quite flexible to perform this variation.

DON'T

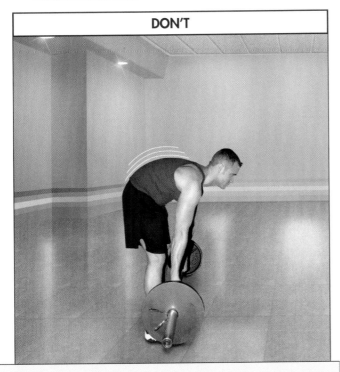

- Do not arch or hunch your back.
- Do not lean back when you lift the bar.
- Do not lock your elbows or knees.
- Do not bend your neck. Keep your head, neck and back in a straight line.

MUSCLES TARGETED

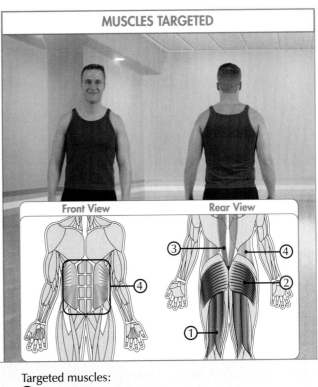

Front View   Rear View

Targeted muscles:
① hamstrings
② buttocks (*gluteus maximus*)

Additional muscles:
③ lower back (*erector spinae*)
④ abdominal muscles (*rectus abdominis, internal and external obliques and transverse abdominis*)

side-lying inner thigh lift

The side-lying inner thigh lift focuses on toning and firming your inner thighs. You should be careful performing this exercise if you have lower back or hip problems.

Your flexibility and strength will determine how high you can lift your leg when performing the side-lying inner thigh lift. However, you should not lift your leg higher than your bent knee. When you start to feel tension in the muscles of your inner thigh, stop lifting your leg,

hold the position and then lower your leg slowly.

Remember to maintain proper form as you perform the side-lying inner thigh lift. You must keep your abdominal muscles tight to help protect your back and avoid bending your neck throughout the entire exercise. You should keep your head, neck and back in a straight line.

As with other exercises, perform the side-lying inner thigh lift in a slow, controlled manner to avoid injury and to receive the full benefit of the exercise.

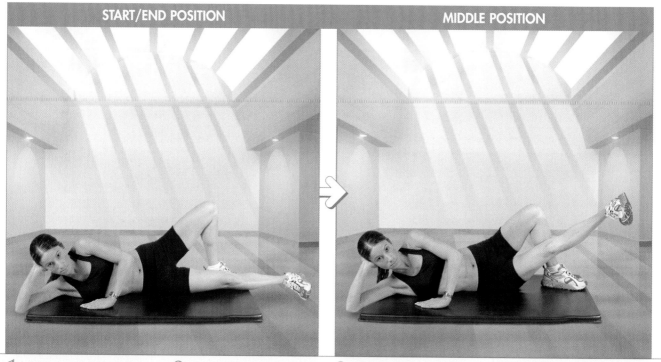

| START/END POSITION | MIDDLE POSITION |

1 Lie on your right side on a mat with your right leg straight. Bend your left knee and place your left foot flat on the floor behind your right knee, toes pointing toward your right foot.

2 Rest your head in your right hand or on your outstretched right arm. Rest your left hand in front of you on the mat for support.

3 Keeping your right leg straight and your toes pulled toward your shin, slowly raise your right leg no higher than your left knee. Tighten your abdominal muscles to help protect your back.

4 Pause for a moment and then slowly lower your right leg back toward the floor.

5 After completing a set with your right leg, switch sides and repeat the exercise with your left leg.

How can I work my inner thighs harder?

To work your inner thighs harder, you can lie on your right side on a mat and bend your left leg 90 degrees at the hip and knee. Place your left knee in front of you on the mat. For more comfort, you can place your left knee on a rolled-up towel or on a step aerobics platform. Keeping your right leg straight, lift your right leg off the floor, pause for a moment and then lower your leg back to the starting position. After completing a set with your right leg, repeat the exercise with your left leg.

How can I change the intensity of the side-lying inner thigh lift?

To make the side-lying inner thigh lift a little easier, you can keep your leg slightly bent as you raise it. To make the exercise harder, you can attach an ankle weight to your leg for extra resistance. If you have knee problems, place the ankle weight on top of your inner thigh.

DON'T

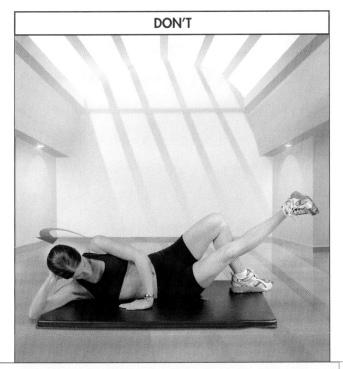

- Do not bend your neck. Keep your head, neck and back in a straight line.

- Do not lift your leg higher than your bent knee.

- Do not rapidly raise and lower your leg. Keep the movement slow and controlled.

- Do not rotate your leg so your toes point to the ceiling. Keep your toes pointed to the side.

MUSCLES TARGETED

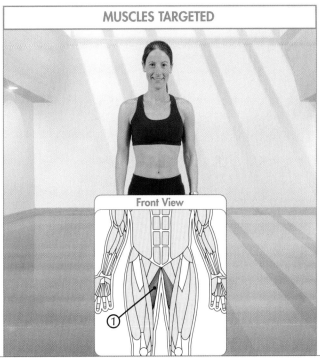

Front View

Targeted muscles:
① inner thighs *(adductors)*

hip adduction machine

The hip adduction machine strengthens and tones your inner thighs while helping to shape your legs. Using the hip adduction machine can also prevent injury caused by activities that overstretch and overuse your inner thigh muscles or that require extensive side-to-side movements.

Contrary to what many people believe, performing hundreds of repetitions of this exercise will not help burn fat and slim your thighs. In actuality, using the hip adduction machine adds mass and size to your inner thigh muscles if you are lifting a moderate to heavy weight.

When using the hip adduction machine, it is important that you maintain proper form to avoid injury and to obtain the full benefit of the exercise. Keep your back straight and your abdominal muscles tight to help protect your back. Avoid leaning forward or arching your back to help push the weight. You should keep your head and back on the back pad throughout the entire exercise.

To work your inner thigh muscles thoroughly and to prevent the weight from slamming onto the stack between repetitions, keep your movements slow and controlled as you use the hip adduction machine.

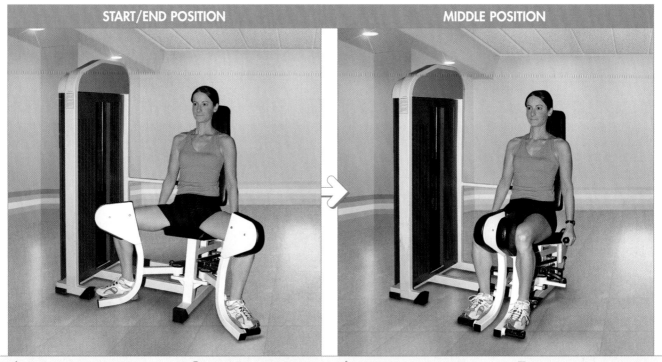

START/END POSITION   **MIDDLE POSITION**

1 Sit on a hip adduction machine. Position your back flat against the back pad with your feet flat on the footrests and your legs against the leg pads.

2 Adjust the machine so your legs are spread out as far apart as they can comfortably go.

3 Grasp the handles at your sides for support.

4 Slowly push your legs against the leg pads to bring your legs together.

- Make sure your back is straight and you tighten your abdominal muscles to help protect your back.

5 Pause for a moment and then slowly move your legs as far apart as you can to return to the starting position.

What other machines can I use to perform the same exercise?

Cable Machine

Position the cable on a cable machine tower at the lowest setting and attach an ankle strap to the cable. Stand with your right side facing the machine and wrap the ankle strap around your right ankle. Place your right leg slightly in front of your left leg and bend your left knee slightly. While keeping your right leg straight with a slight bend, lift your right ankle across the front of your left leg. Pause before returning to the starting position. After completing a set, repeat the exercise using your left leg.

Multi-Hip Machine

Adjust the roller pad of a multi-hip machine to the left side position and then stand on the platform, facing the machine and grasping the bars on the sides. Place the inside of your left thigh against the roller pad and with your left leg slightly bent, slowly push your left leg against the roller pad until your left leg crosses your right leg. Pause before returning to the starting position. After completing a set, repeat the exercise using your right leg.

DON'T	MUSCLES TARGETED

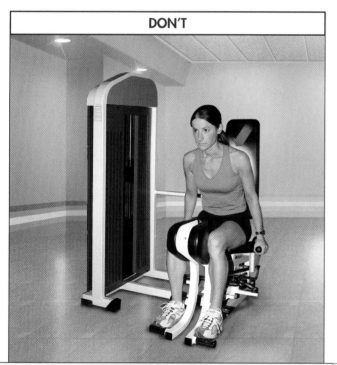

Front View

- Do not lean forward or arch your back to help you push the weight. Keep your head and back on the back pad at all times.

- Do not rapidly move your legs. Keep the movement slow and controlled.

Targeted muscles:
① inner thighs *(adductors)*

cable knee lift

The cable knee lift focuses on your hip flexors, but also works part of your quadriceps. Strengthening the front of your hip muscles can help make everyday activities, such as running, riding a bike and walking up stairs, easier.

You need to use a cable machine to perform this exercise. However, if a cable machine is not available, you can perform the same exercise using ankle weights. When performing the exercise with ankle weights, you need to stand beside a wall and hold on to the wall for support and balance. Using ankle weights instead of a

cable machine makes the exercise easier.

As with other exercises, remember to maintain proper form when performing the cable knee lift. Keep your back straight and your abdominal muscles tight to help protect your back. You should also keep your supporting knee slightly bent throughout the entire exercise and avoid rocking your body back and forth as you raise your knee.

You should be careful performing the cable knee lift if you have lower back or hip problems.

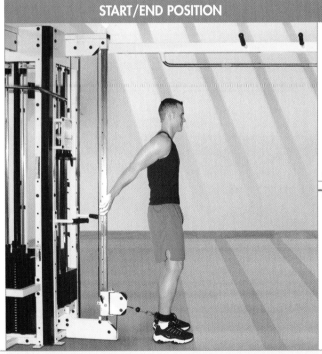

START/END POSITION **MIDDLE POSITION**

1 Set a cable on a cable machine tower to the lowest position. Attach an ankle strap to the cable and place the strap around your right ankle.

2 Stand with your back to the machine with your right leg directly in front of the cable, your left foot flat on the floor and knee slightly bent.

3 Grasp the machine for support.

4 Slowly raise your right knee until your thigh is parallel to the floor.

- Make sure you keep your back straight and you tighten your abdominal muscles to help protect your back.

5 Pause for a moment and then slowly return your leg to the starting position.

6 After completing a set with your right leg, repeat the exercise with your left leg.

Is there another way to work my hip flexors and quadriceps?

Yes. You can perform the walking lunge as described on the top of page 139, except modify the exercise by taking big steps and bringing your knee up to your chest with each step. You can place your hands on your hips as you perform the walking lunge. This exercise is great for working your entire lower body and can be performed with or without the use of ankle weights.

Can I use a multi-hip machine to perform knee lifts?

Yes. Adjust the roller pad of a multi-hip machine to a low position and then stand on the platform with your left side facing the machine, grasping the bar in front of you for support. Place the front of your left thigh, just above the knee, against the roller pad. With your left knee bent, slowly push your left leg against the roller pad until your thigh is parallel to the floor and pause before returning to the starting position. After completing a set, repeat the exercise using your right leg.

DON'T

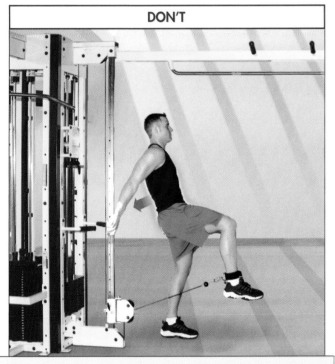

- Do not rock your body back and forth as you raise your knee.

- Do not lock your supporting knee. Keep your knee slightly bent at all times.

- Do not allow your hips to tilt forward and back. Keep your hips tucked under by keeping your abdominal muscles tight.

MUSCLES TARGETED

Front View

Targeted muscles:
① hip flexors

Additional muscles:
② quadriceps

kneeling kickback

The kneeling kickback is a great exercise for tightening and toning your buttocks as well as your hamstrings. You should be careful performing kneeling kickbacks if you have knee, shoulder or lower back problems.

As you perform the kneeling kickback, keep your back straight and your abdominal muscles tight to protect your lower back. You should also keep your neck aligned with your back and your shoulders relaxed. Instead of jerking your leg up and letting it drop back to the starting position, focus on performing the movement in a slow, controlled manner.

When you lift and lower your leg, try not to lean your body to the left or right. Also, avoid raising your knee higher than your hips as you perform the exercise.

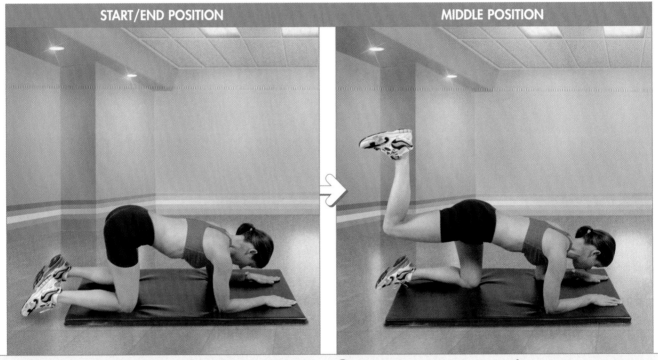

START/END POSITION **MIDDLE POSITION**

1 Kneel on a mat, resting your body weight on your knees and forearms. Position your knees roughly shoulder width apart and clasp your hands together or place your palms flat on the floor.

2 Position your elbows directly under your shoulders and your knees directly under your buttocks. Make sure you tighten your abdominal muscles to help protect your back.

3 Keeping your right knee bent at a 90-degree angle, slowly lift your right leg until your thigh is parallel to the floor.

4 Pause for a moment and then slowly lower your leg back to the floor.

5 After completing a set with your right leg, repeat the exercise with your left leg.

QUESTION & ANSWER

Can I use a machine to perform kneeling kickbacks?

You can use a glute machine to perform kneeling kickbacks. Kneel with your left knee on the knee pad of the machine. Place your forearms on the arm pads and grip the handles with your palms facing each other. Position your right foot against the foot plate and then press your leg up, focusing on pushing with your heel. After completing a set with your right leg, repeat the exercise with your left leg. Using a glute machine increases the intensity of kneeling kickbacks by adding resistance.

How can I make the exercise harder?

There are several ways to make the exercise harder. You can perform the exercise described below, except keep the leg you are lifting straight instead of bent and lift your leg until it is parallel to the floor. To add resistance, you can also add an ankle weight or squeeze a small dumbbell behind your bent knee while you lift your leg. Straightening your arms and resting your upper body weight on your hands instead of your forearms will also make the exercise harder.

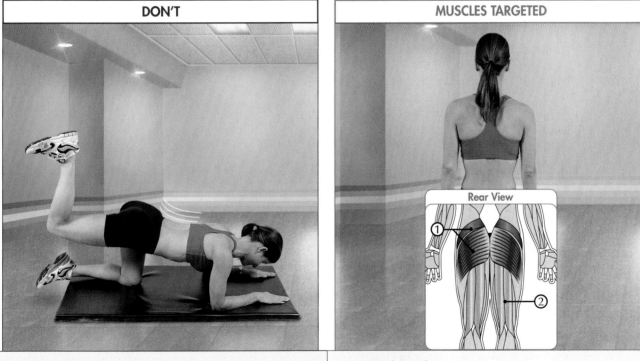

DON'T

- Do not arch your back as you lift your leg.
- Do not shrug your shoulders.
- Do not bend your neck. Keep your head, neck and back in a straight line.
- Do not raise your thigh above parallel to the floor.
- Do not lean your body to the left or right.

MUSCLES TARGETED

Rear View

Targeted muscles:
① buttocks (*gluteus maximus and medius*)

Additional muscles:
② hamstrings

side-lying leg lift

The side-lying leg lift strengthens and tones your outer hips and buttocks. You should be careful when performing this exercise if you have hip problems.

When performing side-lying leg lifts, your abdominal muscles should be tight to help stabilize your body and maintain the focus on your outer hip. You should concentrate on using your buttocks and outer hip muscles to slowly lift your leg and then slowly lower your leg back to the starting position without releasing the tension in the muscles. Try to avoid tightening your neck and shoulders as you lift and lower your leg. Do not twist your body or lean backward or forward. Instead, keep your hips vertically aligned with each other throughout the entire exercise.

If you find the side-lying leg lift too difficult, you can make the exercise a bit easier by performing the movements with your top leg bent 90 degrees at the hip and knee instead of straightening your leg.

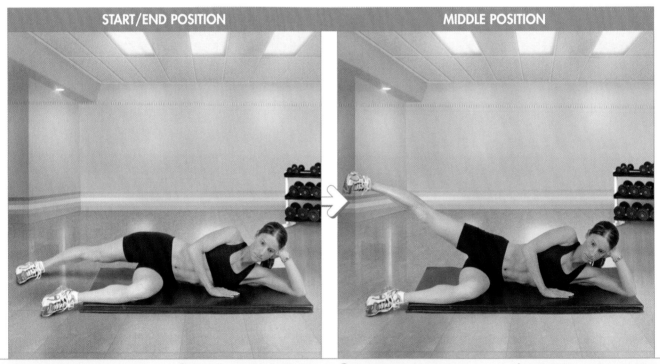

START/END POSITION	MIDDLE POSITION

1 Lie on your left side on a mat with your left leg bent at your hip and knee at 90-degree angles. Keep your right leg straight. Tighten your abdominal muscles to help protect your back.

2 Rest your head in the palm of your left hand or on your outstretched left arm. Rest your right hand on the mat in front of you for support.

3 Keeping your right leg straight and your toes pulled toward your shin, slowly raise your right leg until your right knee is slightly above shoulder height.

4 Pause for a moment and then slowly lower your right leg back toward the floor.

5 After completing a set with your right leg, switch sides and repeat the exercise with your left leg.

How can I make side-lying leg lifts more challenging?

To make the exercise more challenging, you can perform the leg lifts with your bottom leg straight rather than bent. Straightening your bottom leg requires more balance so you will need to keep your back straight and your abdominal muscles tight to maintain stability. You can also add an ankle weight to supply extra resistance. If you have knee problems, hold the weight on the top of your outer thigh instead of strapping it to your ankle.

Can I focus the exercise more on my buttocks than my outer hips?

Yes. To focus the side-lying leg lifts more on your buttocks, lie on your side with both knees bent at 90-degree angles. Lift your top leg to about a 45-degree angle and then turn your thigh outward so your knee points up toward the ceiling. Then turn your thigh inward and lower your leg back to the starting position. You will find this variation more difficult.

DON'T

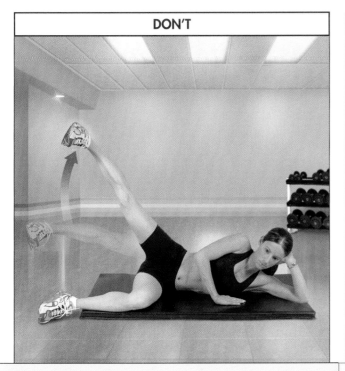

- Do not raise your knee higher than slightly above shoulder height.
- Do not lean your body back or forward.
- Do not bend your neck. Keep your head, neck and back in a straight line.

MUSCLES TARGETED

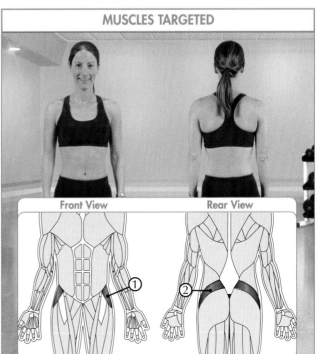

Front View   Rear View

Targeted muscles:
1. outer hips
2. buttocks (*gluteus medius*)

hip abduction machine

The hip abduction machine focuses on your buttocks and outer hips. In addition to helping shape your buttocks and tone your outer hips, using the hip abduction machine can help prevent injury caused by activities that require extensive side-to-side movements, such as skating, skiing and basketball. People with hip problems should be careful when using the hip abduction machine.

As with other exercises, it is important that you maintain proper form when using the hip abduction machine to avoid injury and to get the full benefit of the exercise. You must keep your back straight and your abdominal muscles tight to help protect your back. Do not lean forward or arch your back to help push the weight. You should keep your head and back on the back pad throughout the entire exercise.

When using the hip abduction machine, perform the exercise in a slow, controlled manner to work your muscles thoroughly and to prevent the weight from slamming onto the stack between repetitions.

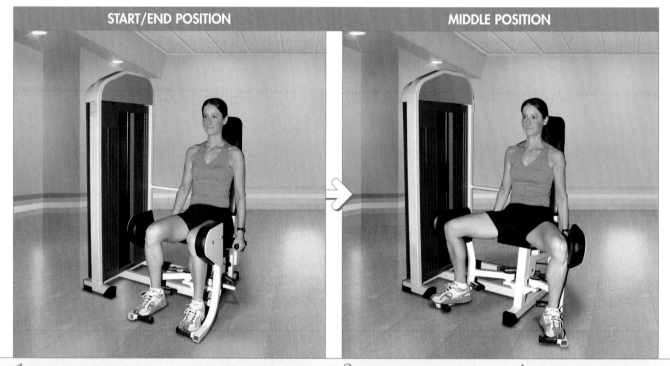

START/END POSITION **MIDDLE POSITION**

1 Sit on a hip abduction machine. Position your back flat against the back pad with your feet flat on the footrests and your outer legs against the leg pads.

• Make sure your back is straight and tighten your abdominal muscles to help protect your back.

2 Grasp the handles at your sides for support.

3 Slowly push your legs against the leg pads to move your legs as far apart as possible.

4 Pause for a moment and then slowly bring your legs back together to return to the starting position.

What other machines can I use to perform the same exercise?

Cable Machine

Position the cable on a cable machine tower at the lowest setting and attach an ankle strap to the cable. Stand with your left side facing the machine and wrap the ankle strap around your right ankle. Place your right leg slightly in front of your left leg and bend your left knee slightly. While keeping your right leg straight with a slight bend, lift your right ankle away from the machine, pause and then return to the starting position. After completing a set, repeat the exercise using your left leg.

Multi-Hip Machine

Adjust the roller pad of a multi-hip machine to a low position and then stand on the platform, facing the machine and grasping the bars on the sides. Place the outside of your left thigh against the roller pad and with your left leg slightly bent, slowly raise your left leg to the side by pushing your leg against the roller pad. Pause before returning your leg to the starting position. Make sure to also keep your supporting leg slightly bent. After completing a set, repeat the exercise using your right leg.

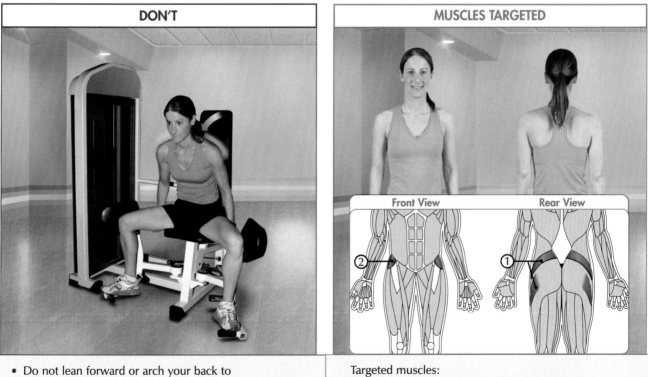

DON'T	MUSCLES TARGETED

Front View   **Rear View**

- Do not lean forward or arch your back to help you push the weight. Keep your head and back on the back pad at all times.

- Do not rapidly move your legs. Keep the movement slow and controlled.

Targeted muscles:
① buttocks *(gluteus medius and minimus)*
② outer hips

cable kickback

The cable kickback strengthens and tones your buttocks, but also works your hamstrings. You should not perform this exercise if you have lower back or hip problems.

Cable kickbacks not only help to shape and tone your buttocks and legs, but also strengthen and stabilize your abdominal muscles and back. To keep the focus on your buttocks, remember to maintain the muscle tension in your buttocks as you perform the movement. You should also try to avoid locking your knees or rocking your upper body forward as you push your leg back.

For a different variation of the exercise, you can change your starting position. Perform the exercise as described below, except start by bending your right knee at a 90-degree angle slightly in front of your body. Push your leg back until your leg is straight. Complete a set with your right leg and then repeat the exercise with your left leg.

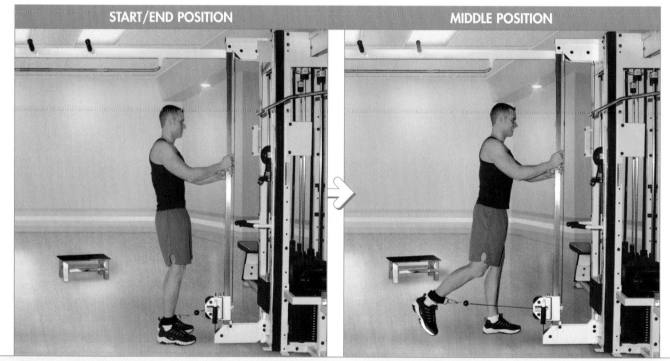

START/END POSITION **MIDDLE POSITION**

1 Set a cable on a tower of a cable machine to the lowest position. Attach an ankle strap to the cable and place the strap around your right ankle.

2 Stand facing the machine with your right foot directly in front of the cable and your left foot flat on the floor, knee slightly bent.

3 Grasp the machine for support.

4 Slowly push your leg straight behind you as far as you can without moving the rest of your body.

• Keep your back straight and tighten your abdominal muscles to help protect your back.

5 Pause for a moment and then slowly return your leg to the starting position.

6 After completing a set with your right leg, repeat the exercise with your left leg.

Can I use a multi-hip machine to perform this exercise?

Yes. Standing with your left side facing the machine, bend your left knee about 90 degrees so that the back of your left thigh touches the roller pad. You can adjust the roller pad to get the desired position. Push your left leg back against the pad as you straighten your leg behind you. Keep your right knee slightly bent as you perform the movement. Complete a set with your left leg and then repeat the exercise with your right leg. Performing kickbacks on the multi-hip machine works your hamstrings more.

How do I perform kickbacks without a machine?

If you do not have access to a machine, you can perform kickbacks using ankle weights instead. Attach the ankle weight to your ankle and then hold a wall or the back of a sturdy chair for support as you perform the exercise as described in the steps below.

DON'T	MUSCLES TARGETED
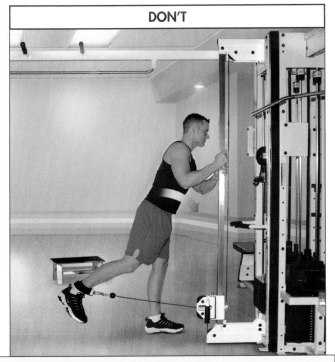	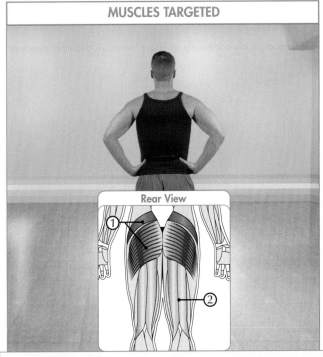

- Do not swing your upper body forward as you push your leg back.

- Do not lock your knees. Keep your knees slightly bent at all times.

Targeted muscles:
① buttocks
   (gluteus maximus and medius)

Additional muscles:
② hamstrings

standing calf raise machine

The standing calf raise machine is great for strengthening and shaping your calves. Strong calf muscles allow you to perform activities such as climbing stairs, running or jumping with more ease. You should not perform standing calf raises if you have back, knee, shoulder or ankle problems.

When you stand at the calf raise machine, position your shoulders in the middle of the shoulder pads

and bend your knees slightly. You can adjust the height of the shoulder pads if necessary.

As you perform the exercise, keep your abdominal muscles tight and your back and hips in a straight line. Make sure you perform the movements slowly, concentrating on using your calf muscles to lift your heels up.

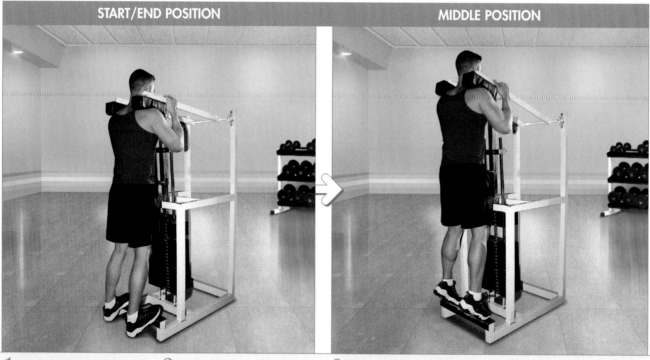

START/END POSITION   **MIDDLE POSITION**

1 Stand with your feet roughly shoulder width apart on a standing calf raise machine. Position the balls of your feet on the platform with your heels hanging over the edge.

2 Position your shoulders beneath the shoulder pads and grasp the handles or the top of the machine for support.

• You can adjust the height of the shoulder pads to obtain the desired position.

3 While keeping your body straight, slowly raise your heels as high as you can until you are standing on your toes.

• Make sure you tighten your abdominal muscles to help protect your back.

4 Pause for a moment and then slowly lower your heels slightly below the platform.

QUESTION & ANSWER

Can I use a barbell to perform this exercise?

Set a barbell on a barbell rack at about shoulder height and then position your body so the bar sits across your upper back. Position your feet shoulder width apart and bend your knees slightly. Grasp the bar with your hands slightly wider than shoulder width apart with your palms facing forward. Then lift the bar off the rack and slowly raise your heels. To make the exercise more challenging, stand with the balls of your feet on a block or step as you perform the exercise. This variation provides a greater range of movement and requires more balance.

How do I perform standing calf raises without weights?

If you find standing calf raises difficult or you do not have access to a machine or barbell, you can perform this exercise without weights. Stand at the edge of a block or step with the balls of your feet on the block or step and your heels hanging off the edge. Grasp a sturdy object or wall for support and then slowly raise and lower your heels to perform the exercise.

DON'T	MUSCLES TARGETED
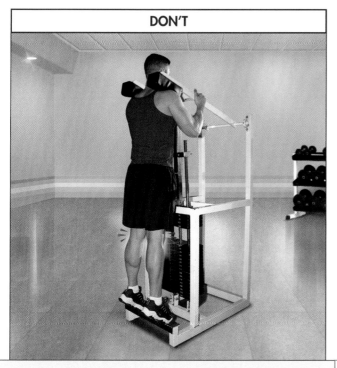	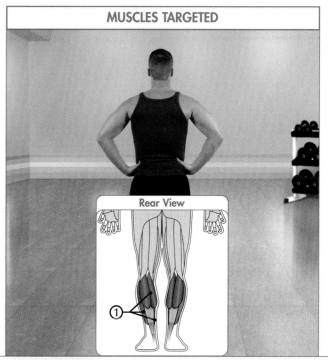

- Do not lift the weight by bending and straightening your knees. Keep your legs straight, without locking your knees.

- Do not hunch your back. Keep your back straight.

- Do not bend at your hips.

Targeted muscles:
① calf muscles (*gastrocnemius* and *soleus*)

seated calf raise machine

The seated calf raise machine focuses on strengthening your calf muscles. This is a great exercise for people who are involved in sports that require lots of power and jumping, such as running, basketball, volleyball and squash. Compared to the standing calf raise machine, the seated calf raise machine works more of the deeper part of your calf muscles and helps enlarge your calf muscles. The seated calf raise machine is beneficial for people who do not want to lift weight on their shoulders due to shoulder problems.

When performing the exercise on the seated calf raise machine, make sure to keep your back straight and your abdominal muscles tight to help protect your back. To set yourself up properly on the machine, you should position the thigh pads closer to your knees. Do not place the thigh pads high up on your thighs. Perform the seated calf raise machine in a slow, controlled manner to help feel the burn in your calf muscles.

You should be careful performing this exercise if you have knee or ankle problems.

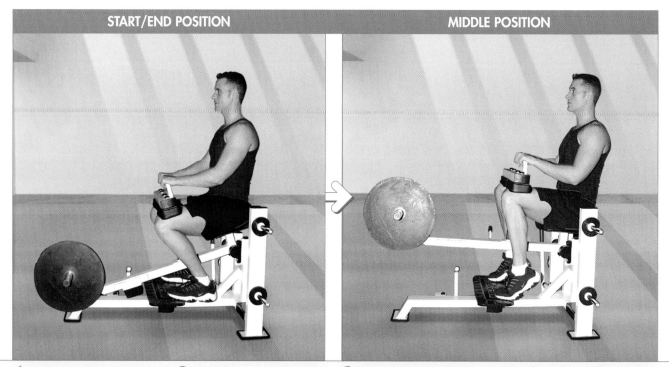

START/END POSITION	MIDDLE POSITION

1 Sit on a seated calf raise machine with your feet roughly shoulder width apart. Position the balls of your feet on the footrest and your heels hanging over the edge.

2 Position your thighs firmly under the thigh pads and grasp the handle or place your hands on top of the thigh pads for support.

- You can adjust the height of the thigh pads to obtain the desired position.

3 Slowly rise up on your toes as high as you can. The first time you rise up, you may have to release the brake that secures the weight in place.

- Make sure you tighten your abdominal muscles to help protect your back.

4 Pause for a moment and then slowly lower your heels slightly below the footrest.

5 When rising up on your toes for the last time, use the brake to once again secure the weight in place.

Can I perform this exercise using a barbell instead of a machine?

Yes. Sit on a bench with the balls of your feet on a step or platform and your thighs parallel to the floor. Grasping the barbell with your hands shoulder width apart and your palms facing down, place the barbell across your thighs, just above your knees. For comfort, you can pad the middle of the bar by rolling a towel around the bar. Then perform the same movement as described in the steps below. This exercise is harder than the seated calf raise machine because you have to balance the bar on your thighs.

How can I put more focus on specific parts of my calf muscles?

You can perform the exercise as described in the steps below, except change the position of your feet to put more focus on specific parts of your calf muscles. Turn your heels slightly out to put more focus on the inside of your calf muscles. You can also turn your heels slightly in to put more focus on the outside of your calf muscles.

DON'T

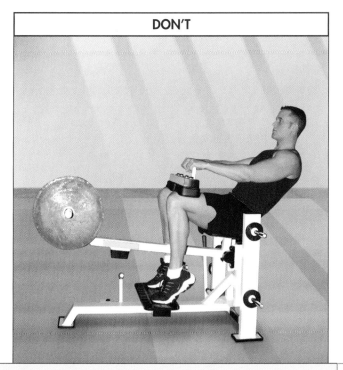

MUSCLES TARGETED

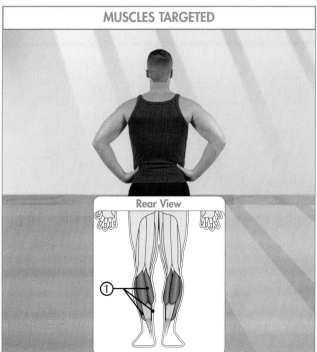

Rear View

- Do not rock your body back and forth to help lift the weight.
- Do not lower your heels too far below the footrest.
- Do not rapidly raise and lower your feet. Keep the movement slow and controlled.

Targeted muscles:
① calf muscles *(gastrocnemius and soleus)*

single-leg calf raise

The single-leg calf raise is a good way to work your calf muscles using free weights instead of a machine. This exercise targets your calves to help give you strong, well-toned legs, which can make daily activities, such as walking, running or climbing stairs, easier to perform. Be careful performing single-leg calf raises if you have ankle, lower back or knee problems.

Performing calf raises one leg at a time is useful when your calf muscles in one leg are stronger than the calf muscles in the other leg and you want to correct the imbalance. Since each leg works independently, the stronger calf muscles cannot compensate for the weaker muscles.

When performing the exercise, aim to raise your heel as high as it can go, but be careful not to lower your heel too far, as this can cause injury. Avoid lowering your heel beyond the point where the stretch feels comfortable. Throughout the exercise, keep the supporting knee slightly bent and your abdominal muscles tight to support your back.

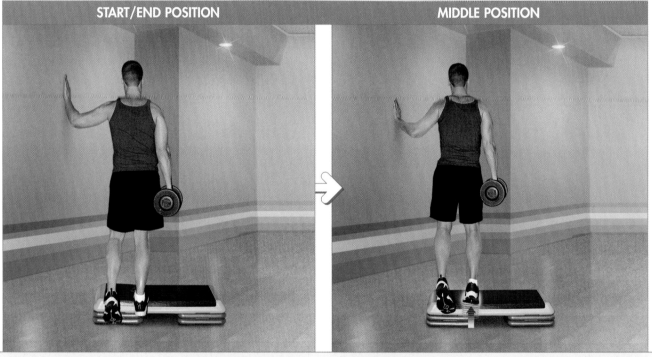

START/END POSITION   **MIDDLE POSITION**

1 Hold a dumbbell in your right hand at your side with your palm facing in.

2 Stand on a step or platform with the ball of your right foot on the step or platform and your heel hanging over the edge.

3 Slightly bend your left leg to keep the leg off the floor. Rest your left hand on a chair or wall for support.

4 While keeping your body straight, slowly raise your heel as high as you can until you are standing on your toes. Make sure you tighten your abdominal muscles to help protect your back.

5 Pause for a moment and then slowly lower your heel slightly below the step or platform.

6 When you complete a set with your right leg, hold the dumbbell in your left hand and repeat the exercise with your left leg.

Why am I able to complete only a few repetitions of the exercise?

When performing the single-leg calf raise, you may not be able to complete as many repetitions as other exercises, since the calf muscles tend to become fatigued more quickly than other muscles. If you are using moderate weight, your calf muscles may start aching by the time you complete about 10 repetitions. Keep in mind that even a few repetitions can effectively work your calf, but you can try stretching after each set to help relax the muscles and make it easier to perform the next set.

How can I make the exercise easier?

To make calf raises easier, you can perform the exercise with your foot flat on the floor instead of on a step or platform. Standing on a flat surface allows a shorter range of movement, so your calf muscles do not work as hard. You can also make the exercise easier by working both feet at once. If you can maintain your balance, you can challenge yourself by holding a dumbbell in each hand as you lift and lower your heels.

DON'T

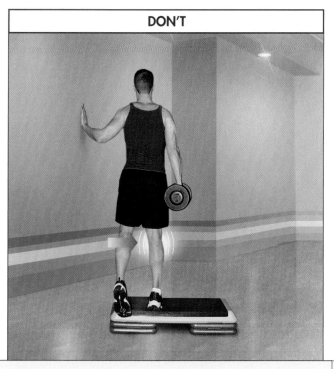

MUSCLES TARGETED

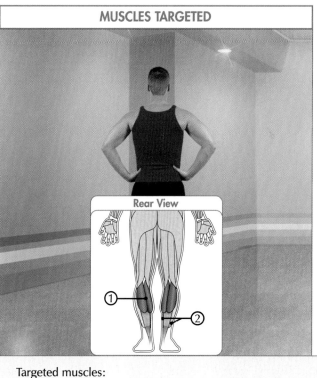

- Do not lock the knee of the leg you are standing on.
- Do not roll your foot toward your little toe when raising your heel.
- Do not bend your neck. Keep your head, neck and back in a straight line.
- Do not lower your heel too far below the step or platform.

Targeted muscles:
① calf muscles (*gastrocnemius*)

Additional muscles:
② calf muscles (*soleus*)

calf press

The calf press builds the size and strength of your calves, which can make daily activities, such as walking, climbing stairs and running, easier to perform. You can use a leg press machine to perform this exercise.

There are different types of leg press machines. Some machines require you to add weight plates to a bar, while others allow you to insert a pin into a stack of weights to select the amount of weight you want to lift. Your position on the machine and the angle at which you press your legs to raise the weight may also be different. A plate loaded machine is more difficult to use because your legs are positioned higher, which means you are pushing against gravity.

You should be careful when performing the calf press if you have knee or ankle problems. You should be especially careful of your knees when using a plate loaded machine since your legs tend to bear most of the weight during the exercise.

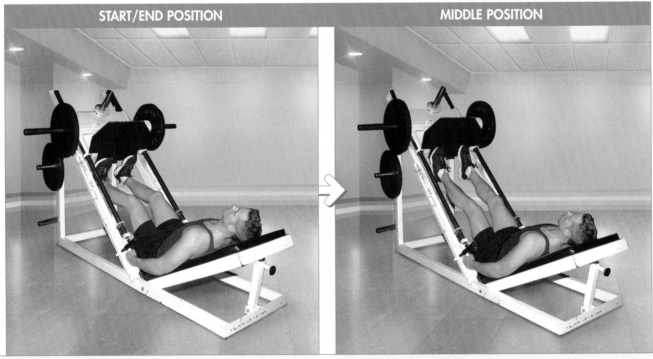

START/END POSITION   MIDDLE POSITION

1 Lie on your back on a leg press machine. Position the balls of your feet roughly shoulder width apart on the platform with your heels hanging over the edge.

2 Grasp the handles on the machine.

3 Slowly push the weight with the balls of your feet until your legs are almost straight.

4 Keeping your knees slightly bent, slowly push the weight with the balls of your feet as far as you can. Make sure you tighten your abdominal muscles to help protect your back.

5 Pause for a moment and then slowly lower the weight until your heels are slightly below the platform.

How can I work one calf at a time?

You can rest your right leg on the floor as you perform the exercise with your left leg. After completing a set, repeat the exercise with your right leg. You will need to reduce the amount of weight used when working one leg. Working one leg at a time is useful if one of your legs is stronger than the other and you want to strengthen your legs equally.

Can I work my calves differently?

You can adjust the position of your feet on the foot plate to work your calves differently. To target the inside of your calves, turn your heels out slightly. To target the outside of your calves, turn your heels in slightly. You will need to use less weight when performing this variation.

DON'T

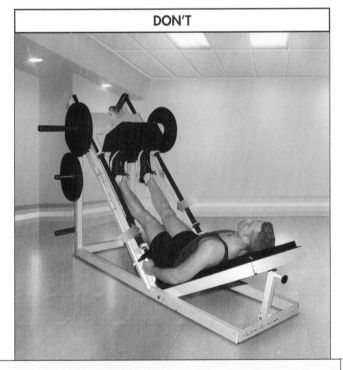

- Do not lock your knees.
- Do not raise your head off the head rest. Keep your head and neck in line with your back.
- Do not arch your back to help push the weight. Make sure your back remains flat against the back pad.

MUSCLES TARGETED

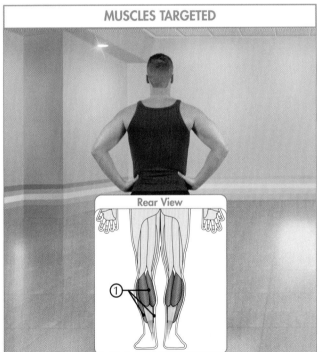

Rear View

Targeted muscles:
① calves (*gastrocnemius* and *soleus*)

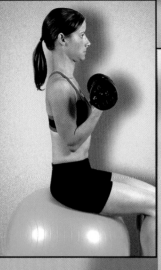

Section 4

An exercise ball and exercise tubing are accessories you can use to vary your normal weight training routine. An exercise ball is particularly useful for working your core muscles, which include your back and abdominal muscles. Exercise tubing is lightweight, portable and can be used in almost any location, which makes it especially handy when traveling. Section 4 provides a variety of strength training exercises you can perform using an exercise ball and exercise tubing.

Using an Exercise Ball and Tubing

In this Section...

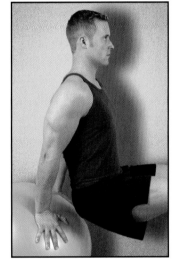

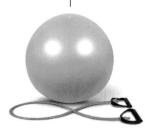

introduction to exercise balls

Exercise balls are a popular fitness tool that can be used in a variety of exercises, including stretching and strength training. Also known as fitness balls, Swiss balls or stability balls, exercise balls are generally large, inflatable vinyl balls that can make your workouts more interesting.

The main appeal of exercise balls is their instability, which requires your back and abdominal muscles to work at keeping your body balanced when using the ball, even if the exercise you are doing does not specifically target those muscles.

Exercise balls are relatively inexpensive and are readily available at most gyms or you can purchase your own at health, fitness or department stores. Be careful not to confuse exercise balls with medicine balls, which are smaller, weighted balls that are also used for fitness purposes, but in a different way than exercise balls.

If you have never exercised before and you are just starting an exercise program, you should not use an exercise ball without supervision.

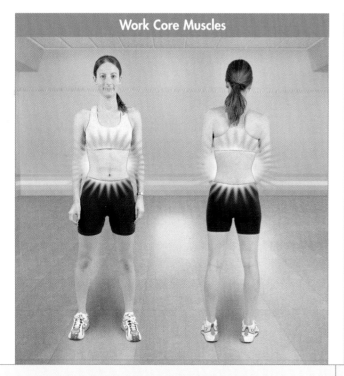

Work Core Muscles

- An exercise ball works your core muscles, which include your abdominal and back muscles. A ball provides an unstable platform on which you can perform exercises. Performing exercises on an unstable platform forces your core muscles to work to keep you balanced during the exercises.

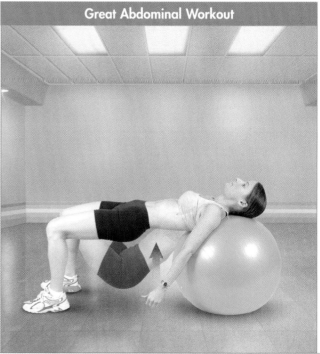

Great Abdominal Workout

- An exercise ball provides many ways to effectively work your abdominal muscles and offers an excellent range of motion when targeting these muscles.

What size exercise ball should I use?

The size of the exercise ball you should use depends largely on your height. As a general rule, when you sit on the ball, your hips should be level with or slightly higher than your knees. When you first inflate your new exercise ball, it is a good idea to measure the ball to make sure it is inflated to the correct size. You can use the following chart as a guideline for choosing a ball.

Height	Ball Size
Under 4'10"	17" or 45 cm
Under 6'	21" or 55 cm
6' and taller	25" or 65 cm

How can I get used to balancing on my exercise ball?

You can try some simple exercises to help you get used to balancing on your exercise ball. Sit on the ball with your feet flat on the floor and hold on to a sturdy object, if necessary. Then slowly move your hips forward, backward, left and then right. While sitting on the ball with your feet flat on the floor, also try raising one leg in front of you, keeping your knee bent and then lower the leg. Make sure your back stays straight. Do not lean back. Repeat with your other leg.

Use as Bench Replacement

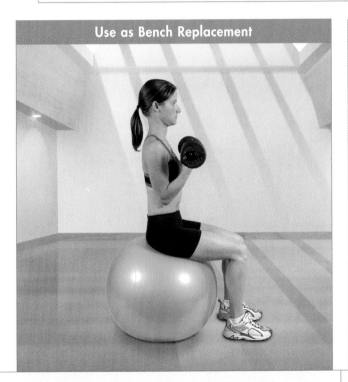

Improve Balance and Posture

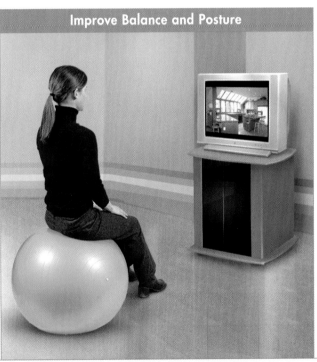

- You can use an exercise ball instead of a bench for many exercises. Performing exercises on a ball adds variety to your workouts and is more difficult since you also have to keep your body balanced on the ball.

- You can use an exercise ball as a chair at home or at work to improve your balance and posture. Try sitting on an exercise ball in front of your computer or when watching television.

- Maintaining proper posture can prevent and relieve lower back pain.

wall squat

The wall squat tones your entire lower body, strengthening your quadriceps, buttocks, hamstrings, hip flexors and inner thighs. This is an excellent exercise for developing strong, well-toned legs, which help increase your endurance when performing activities such as walking or riding a bike. If you have lower back or knee problems, be careful performing this exercise.

Using a ball makes wall squats easier and is a good way for beginners to start performing squats. For information on exercise balls, see page 168.

When you lower into the squat, make sure you do not move your buttocks forward as you squat and your knees do not extend past your toes. As you raise back to the starting position, concentrate on pushing up through your heels rather than through the balls of your feet. If you want to add an extra challenge, you can hold a dumbbell in each hand with both arms at your sides and your palms facing in as you perform the exercise.

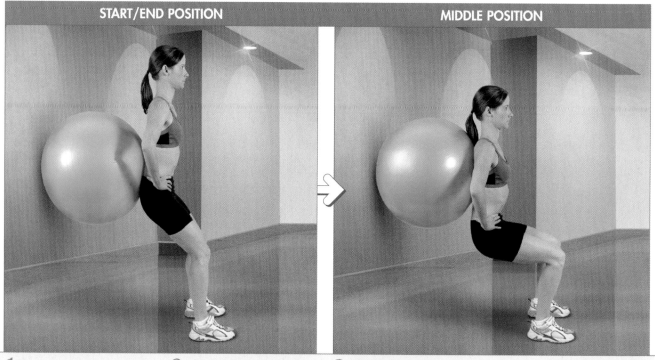

START/END POSITION

MIDDLE POSITION

1 Stand with your back facing a wall. Place a ball between you and the wall, positioning the ball against your lower back. Place your hands on your hips.

2 Stand straight with your feet roughly shoulder width apart and slightly in front of your body.

- Tighten your abdominal muscles to help protect your back.

3 Slowly bend your knees until your thighs are parallel to the floor. Your knees should not pass your toes. Imagine you are sitting down in a chair.

- As you bend your knees, the ball will move to the middle of your back.

4 Slowly lift yourself back to the starting position, pushing through your heels.

Can I make wall squats harder?

Yes. Perform the exercise described below, except extend your left leg straight out in front of you with your knee slightly bent before lowering into the squat position. To avoid putting too much pressure on your supporting leg, lower only about one-third of the distance you would normally lower for a full squat. After completing a set, repeat the exercise with your right leg extended. Performing wall squats on one leg focuses more on strengthening the muscles around your knee and is useful when you want to strengthen your legs equally.

Can I perform squats with the ball without using the wall for support?

Yes. Standing with your left side facing the ball, extend your left leg straight out to the side and place the inside of your left foot and ankle on top of the ball. Then lower about one-third the distance of a full squat, keeping your foot on the ball. After completing a set, switch legs and repeat the exercise.

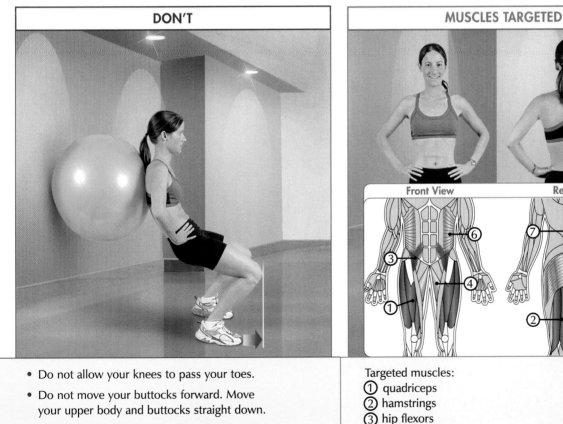

DON'T

MUSCLES TARGETED

Front View   Rear View

- Do not allow your knees to pass your toes.
- Do not move your buttocks forward. Move your upper body and buttocks straight down.
- Do not tilt your head up or down. Keep your head, neck and back in a straight line.
- Do not lock your knees.

Targeted muscles:
① quadriceps
② hamstrings
③ hip flexors

Additional muscles:
④ inner thighs
  (*adductors*)
⑤ buttocks
  (*gluteus maximus*)
⑥ deep abdominal muscles
  (*transverse abdominis*)
⑦ lower back
  (*erector spinae*)

lunge

The lunge focuses on your quadriceps, hamstrings and buttocks, but also works your deep abdominal muscles, lower back, inner thighs, hip flexors and calves. Performing this exercise helps you with balance and is great for people who participate in sports that require a lot of powerful movements, such as squash and tennis.

The lunge shown in the steps below requires the use of an exercise ball. For more information on exercise balls, see page 168. The use of an exercise ball helps you perform lunges with proper technique and form. Performing lunges using an exercise ball also works

your calves more than without the use of a ball.

As you perform lunges, avoid twisting or leaning your body ahead. You should always keep your shoulders square and facing forward and make sure your shoulders and hips are in a straight line. Do not let your front knee pass your toes or let your toes point in or out. Throughout the entire exercise, remember to keep your toes pointing straight ahead.

You should be careful performing this exercise if you have knee problems.

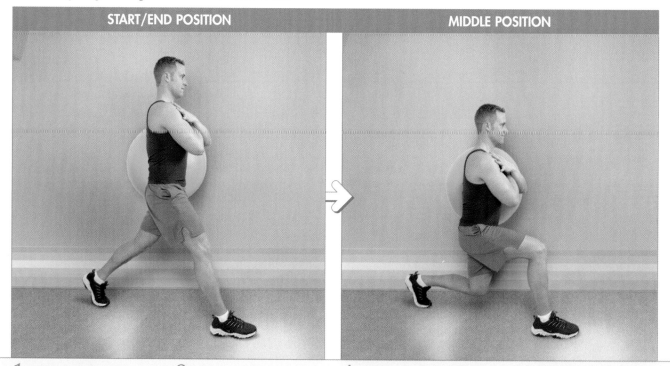

| START/END POSITION | MIDDLE POSITION |

1 Stand straight with your left side facing a wall. Position your feet roughly shoulder width apart and your toes pointed forward. Tighten your abdominal muscles to help protect your back.

2 Place a ball between you and the wall, with the ball against your hip and side. Cross your arms.

3 Take a step forward with your right leg and a small step back onto the ball of your left foot. Bend your knees slightly, keeping the ball at hip level.

4 Slowly bend your knees until your right thigh is parallel with the floor. Both knees should be bent at 90-degree angles and your right knee should not pass the front of your right foot.

5 Slowly lift your body by straightening your legs to return to the starting position.

6 When you complete a set with your right leg forward, repeat the exercise with your left leg forward.

How can I make this exercise harder?

You can try a couple of ways to make this exercise harder. You can position a step behind you and as you take a small step back with your left leg, place the ball of your left foot on the step. You can also make the exercise harder by using both arms to hold a weight plate across your chest for added resistance.

When performing the lunge, is there another way to position the exercise ball?

Yes. You can place your back leg on top of the exercise ball with the top of your toes on the ball. Then perform the exercise as described below. This is considered an advanced variation of the lunge and is more difficult since one of your legs is unstable. For this reason, take extra care to maintain your balance.

DON'T

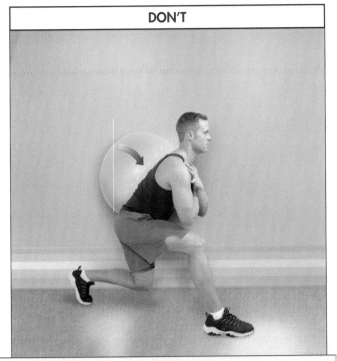

- Do not lean your body forward. Keep your shoulders and hips in a straight line.
- Do not allow your front knee to pass your toes.
- Do not twist your body. Your shoulders should be square and facing forward.
- Do not point your toes in or out. Your toes should point straight ahead.

MUSCLES TARGETED

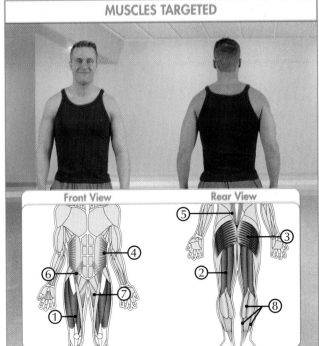

Targeted muscles:
1 quadriceps
2 hamstrings
3 buttocks *(gluteus maximus)*

Additional muscles:
4 deep abdominal muscles *(transverse abdominis)*
5 lower back *(erector spinae)*
6 hip flexors
7 inner thighs *(adductors)*
8 calves *(gastrocnemius and soleus)*

bridge

The bridge tightens and tones your buttocks and hamstrings, but also strengthens your deep abdominal muscles and lower back. You need to use an exercise ball to perform this exercise. For more information on exercise balls, see page 168.

When lifting your buttocks, try to hold the position for about 10 seconds. Then lower your buttocks back toward the floor and rest for 10 seconds before repeating the exercise. As your muscles become stronger, you can increase the amount of time you hold your buttocks up to as long as 2 minutes. Beginners may not be able to perform more than 2 repetitions, but as one progresses, the number of repetitions can be increased up to 10. When you can hold your buttocks up for 2 minutes and perform 5 repetitions, you can try a more advanced version of the bridge. For more information, see page 175.

If you have upper back problems, you should be careful performing this exercise.

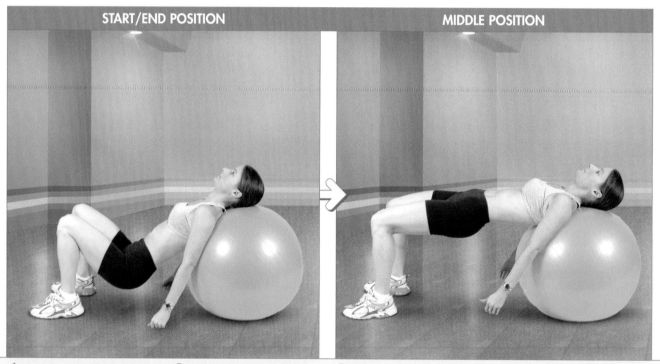

| START/END POSITION | MIDDLE POSITION |

1 Position your upper back and head on a ball. Place your arms at your sides and tighten your abdominal muscles to help protect your back.

2 Position your feet roughly shoulder width apart, with your knees bent, feet flat on the floor and toes pointing forward. Your buttocks should be slightly off the floor.

3 Slowly lift your buttocks by pushing through your heels until your thighs and upper body are in a straight line.

4 Hold the position for about 10 seconds and then slowly lower your buttocks back toward the floor.

How can I make the exercise more difficult?

To make the exercise more difficult, raise your arms with your fingers pointing to the ceiling, as you perform the exercise. You can also make the exercise more difficult by placing your back on the floor with your arms at your sides and positioning your calves on top of the ball with your legs together and your knees bent 90 degrees. Then lift your buttocks off the floor until your thighs and upper body form a straight line. You will need to work harder to maintain your balance. To increase the difficulty of this exercise even more, you can try placing just your heels on the ball.

How can I work my buttocks and hamstrings harder?

To work your buttocks and hamstrings harder, hold one leg straight out in front while moving your buttocks up and down. Straightening one leg also makes the exercise more difficult since you have to balance all your weight on one leg.

DON'T

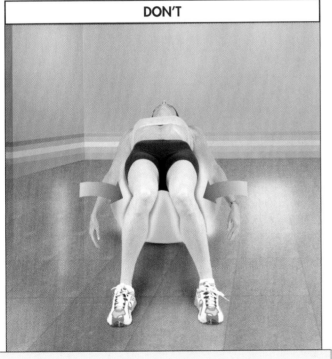

- Do not point your knees in or out. Keep your knees pointed straight ahead.
- Do not allow your hips to drop down while holding your buttocks up.
- Do not allow the ball to move during the exercise.
- Do not hold your breath.

MUSCLES TARGETED

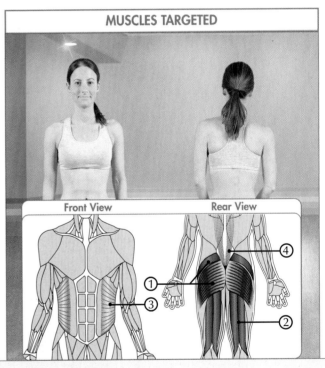

Front View Rear View

Targeted muscles:
① buttocks (*gluteus maximus and medius*)
② hamstrings

Additional muscles:
③ deep abdominal muscles (*transverse abdominis*)
④ lower back (*erector spinae*)

calf raise

The calf raise tones and strengthens your calves, focusing on the deeper part of your calf muscles. As with other ball exercises, when you perform calf raises while sitting on a ball, your deep abdominal and back muscles work to help keep your body balanced on the ball throughout the exercise. Using a ball also makes the exercise easier and is a good way for beginners to start performing calf raises. For more information on exercise balls, see page 168.

To get the maximum benefit from the exercise, you should perform the movements in a slow, controlled manner. Avoid jerking your heels up or allowing them to simply drop back to the floor. As you perform calf raises, keep your abdominal muscles tight to help protect your back and make sure your back remains erect throughout the exercise.

If you want to make the exercise more challenging, you can hold a weight on your lap as you lift and lower your heels.

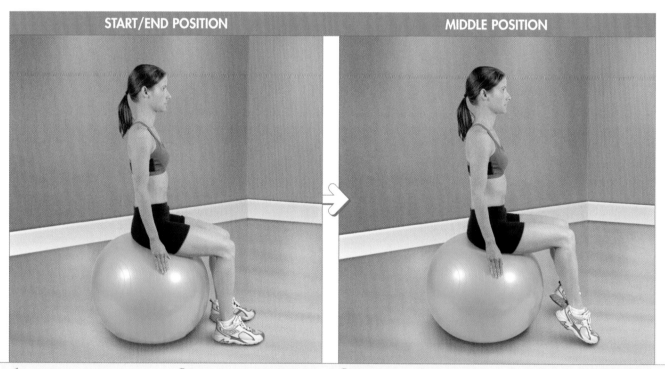

START/END POSITION **MIDDLE POSITION**

1 Sit on a ball with your legs roughly shoulder width apart, your knees bent at 90-degree angles and your feet flat on the floor. Make sure your toes are pointed forward.

2 Place your hands straight at your sides. Tighten your abdominal muscles to help protect your back.

3 Slowly raise your heels as high as you can until you are on your toes.

4 Pause for a moment and then slowly lower your heels back to the floor.

How can I work my calf muscles harder?

Perform the exercise as described below, except place the balls of your feet on a step or platform as you perform the exercise. Lower your heels slightly below the step or platform. Placing your feet on a step or platform provides a greater range of motion to raise and lower your heels, which works your calf muscles harder. When performing this variation, you should use a larger ball to ensure your hips are higher than your knees.

Can I use a ball to perform calf raises while standing?

Yes. Stand facing a wall and place the ball between your stomach and the wall. Position your feet shoulder width apart with your knees slightly bent. Hold your arms behind your back, lean forward slightly and then slowly raise and lower your heels. Performing calf raises while standing works your calf muscles more than when sitting. For another variation, with the ball positioned between your stomach and the wall, raise your right leg off the floor slightly by bending your knee and place your hands on the ball. Then perform calf raises with your left leg. After completing a set, switch legs and repeat the exercise.

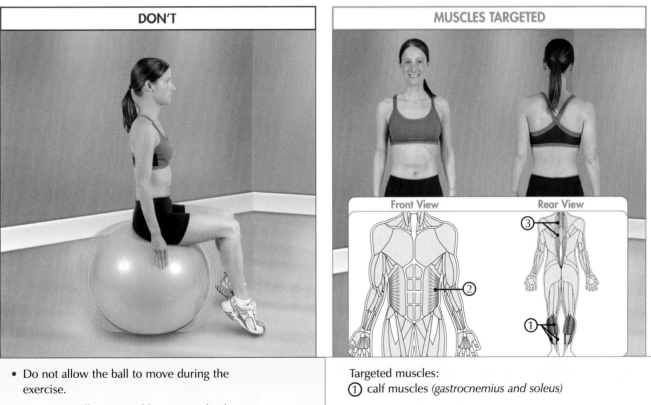

DON'T

- Do not allow the ball to move during the exercise.
- Do not rapidly raise and lower your heels. Keep the movement slow and controlled.

MUSCLES TARGETED

Front View   Rear View

Targeted muscles:
① calf muscles *(gastrocnemius and soleus)*

Additional muscles:
② abdominal muscles *(transverse abdominis)*
③ upper back *(erector spinae, rhomboids)*

chest press

The chest press works your chest, as well as your triceps and the front of your shoulders. Performing this exercise on a ball also forces your abdominal and back muscles to work to help keep your body balanced on the ball. This is a good exercise for helping you build upper body strength. If you have shoulder, wrist or elbow problems, you should be careful when performing this exercise.

Performing the chest press with dumbbells is useful when one of your arms is stronger than the other and you want to balance the strength in your arms. Since each arm must lift its own weight, the stronger arm cannot compensate for the weaker arm. People who tend to use one arm more than the other, such as tennis players, will benefit from this exercise.

Lying on an unstable ball, instead of a bench, makes the chest press more challenging because you also need to stabilize yourself on the ball while lifting the dumbbells. You should try to have the ball move as little as possible during the exercise. For more information on exercise balls, see page 168.

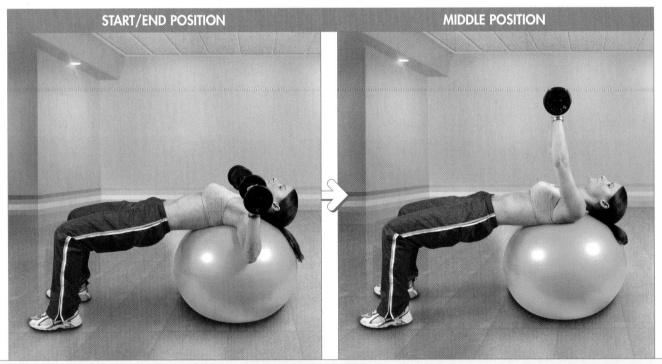

START/END POSITION — MIDDLE POSITION

1 Hold a dumbbell in each hand. Position your upper back and head on a ball.

2 Bend your elbows about 90 degrees, elbows pointing to the sides and both palms facing your feet.

3 Position your feet roughly shoulder width apart with your knees bent about 90 degrees and your feet flat on the floor. Your thighs and upper body should form a straight line.

4 Slowly push the dumbbells up above the middle of your chest. The dumbbells should almost touch.

• Make sure you tighten your abdominal muscles to help protect your back.

5 Slowly lower the dumbbells back to the starting position.

What other variation of the chest press can I perform?

Perform the exercise as described below, except hold a dumbbell only in your right hand and stretch your left arm toward the ceiling. As you press the dumbbell up, slightly lift your right shoulder so your body rotates on the ball and bend your left elbow so your elbow ends up slightly below shoulder level. Continue to alternate arms until you complete a full set, then hold the dumbbell in your left hand and repeat the exercise. This variation works your abdominal muscles and allows you to focus on one arm at a time.

How can I work the upper and outer edge of my chest more?

You can perform the Pec Fly. Holding a dumbbell in each hand, lie on the ball as shown in the steps below. With your palms facing each other, raise the dumbbells directly above your chest until your arms are almost straight and the dumbbells almost touch. Then slowly lower the dumbbells out to the sides in a semicircular motion, until your elbows are level with your shoulders. Pause for a moment and then slowly raise the dumbbells back to the starting position.

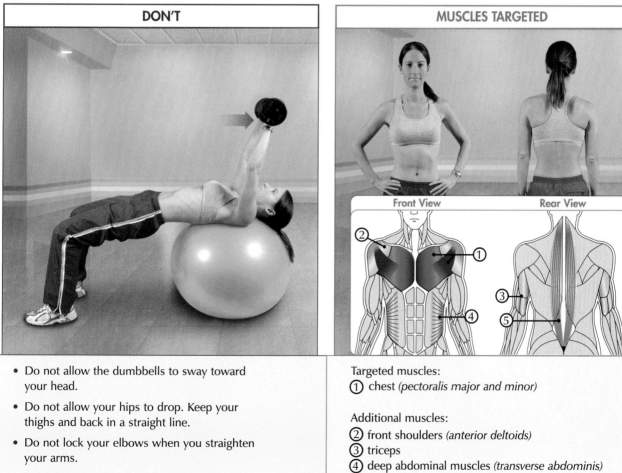

DON'T	MUSCLES TARGETED

DON'T

- Do not allow the dumbbells to sway toward your head.
- Do not allow your hips to drop. Keep your thighs and back in a straight line.
- Do not lock your elbows when you straighten your arms.
- Do not lift your head off the ball.

MUSCLES TARGETED

Front View   Rear View

Targeted muscles:
① chest (*pectoralis major and minor*)

Additional muscles:
② front shoulders (*anterior deltoids*)
③ triceps
④ deep abdominal muscles (*transverse abdominis*)
⑤ lower back (*erector spinae*)

front bridge

The front bridge is a great exercise that requires a number of your muscles to work together. This exercise focuses on your shoulders, chest, upper back and triceps, but also works your lower back, buttocks and deep abdominal muscles. You need to use an exercise ball to perform the front bridge shown in the steps below. For more information on exercise balls, see page 168.

As with other exercises, remember to maintain proper form when performing the front bridge. Do not arch your back, bend forward at your hips or hunch your shoulders as you perform the exercise. You should also avoid bending your neck forward or back. To keep the exercise ball moving in a straight line, do not allow your legs to move from side to side.

You should be careful performing the front bridge if you have shoulder, neck, back or elbow problems.

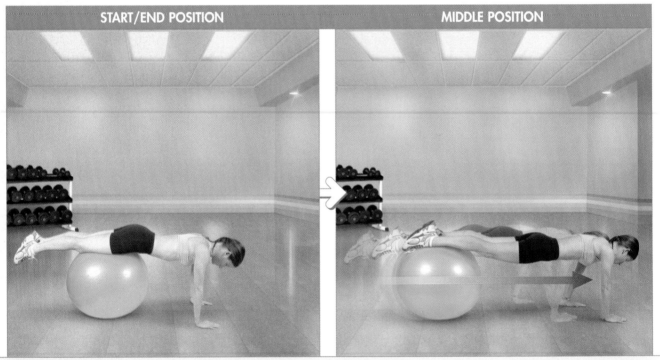

START/END POSITION **MIDDLE POSITION**

1 Position your thighs on a ball with your legs together and straight. Tighten your abdominal muscles to help protect your back.

2 Position your hands on the floor, roughly shoulder width apart.

3 Slowly walk your hands forward until the ball reaches your feet.

4 Slowly walk your hands backward to return to the starting position.

How can I make the exercise harder?

You can make the exercise harder by supporting your body in the starting position with only one arm. Keep your arm in line with the center of your body. Hold for 10 seconds before switching arms.

Can I put more emphasis on my abdominal muscles?

Yes. Position yourself on a ball as described below and then, without moving your hands, roll the ball in from your thighs to your shins by bringing your thighs toward your stomach. To return to the starting position, roll the ball from your shins back to your thighs.

How can I work the muscles of my upper body more?

To work the muscles of your upper body more, you can perform push-ups using an exercise ball. After positioning yourself on the ball as described below, bend your elbows until they are bent at about 90-degrees and then push your body back up to the starting position. To make this exercise more difficult, place your shins on the ball instead.

DON'T

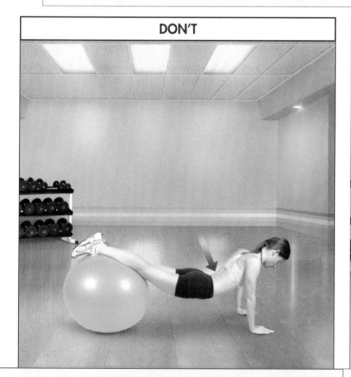

- Do not arch your back.
- Do not bend your neck forward or back or hunch your shoulders.
- Do not allow your legs to move from side to side. Keep the ball moving in a straight line.
- Do not bend forward at your hips.

MUSCLES TARGETED

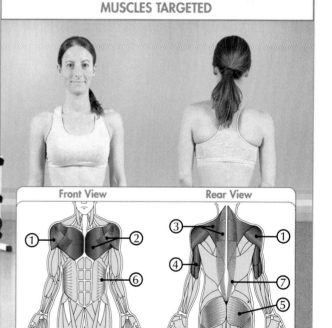

Front View   Rear View

Targeted muscles:
① shoulders *(deltoids)*
② chest *(pectoralis major and minor)*
③ upper back *(trapezius and rhomboids)*
④ triceps

Additional muscles:
⑤ buttocks *(gluteus maximus)*
⑥ deep abdominal muscles *(transverse abdominis)*
⑦ lower back *(erector spinae)*

bent over lateral raise

The bent over lateral raise focuses on your rear shoulders and your middle and upper back, but it also works your deep abdominal muscles and your lower back. This exercise can help improve your posture and make activities that involve lifting easier.

You need to use an exercise ball to perform this exercise. For more information on exercise balls, see page 168. Since you have to keep your body balanced on the ball, this exercise works your core muscles,

which includes your back and abdominal muscles.

When performing the bent over lateral raise, you should keep your head, neck and back in a straight line at all times. Also, as you raise and lower the weights, do not hunch your back or raise your elbows past your shoulders.

You should be careful performing the bent over lateral raise if you have shoulder or neck problems.

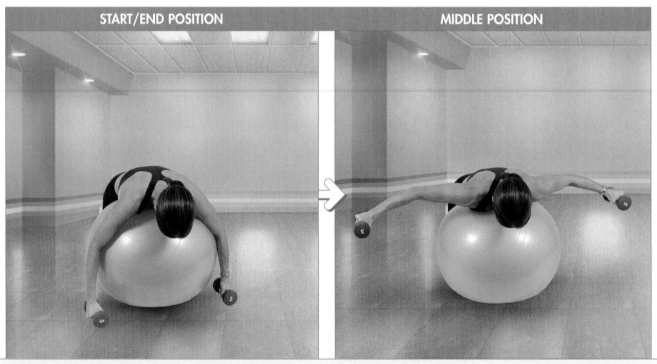

START/END POSITION   **MIDDLE POSITION**

1 Lie on your stomach on a ball with your feet roughly shoulder width apart, your knees bent at about a 90-degree angle and the balls of your feet on the floor.

2 Hold a dumbbell in each hand. Allow your arms to hang down with your elbows slightly bent and your palms facing each other.

3 Slowly raise the dumbbells out to your sides until your elbows are at shoulder height. Squeeze your shoulder blades together as you lift the dumbbells.

• Make sure you keep your elbows slightly bent and your palms facing down.

4 Pause for a moment and then slowly lower the dumbbells back to your sides.

Can I make the bent over lateral raise easier?

Yes. You can make the bent over lateral raise easier by holding the dumbbells with your palms facing your feet at the start of the exercise. Then, as you slowly raise the dumbbells, bend your arms to about 90-degree angles until your elbows pass slightly beyond your shoulders.

How can I work one arm at a time?

To work one arm at a time, rest one of your arms on the exercise ball and then with your other arm holding a dumbbell, perform the same arm movement as described below. It is more difficult to work one arm at a time because of the weight imbalance, which requires you to work harder to keep yourself on the exercise ball.

DON'T

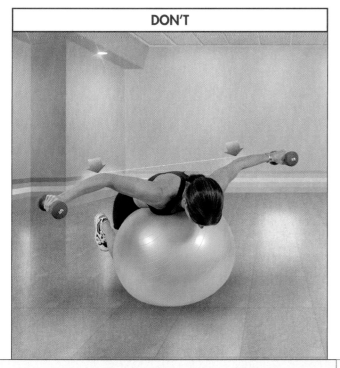

- Do not raise your elbows past your shoulders.
- Do not bend your neck up, down, left or right. Keep your head, neck and back in a straight line.
- Do not hunch or arch your back as you raise and lower the dumbbells.

MUSCLES TARGETED

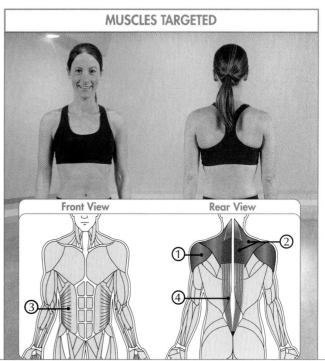

Front View   Rear View

Targeted muscles:
① rear shoulders (*posterior deltoids*)
② middle and upper back (*rhomboids* and *upper trapezius*)

Additional muscles:
③ deep abdominal muscles (*transverse abdominis*)
④ lower back (*erector spinae*)

external rotation

The external rotation works your rotator cuff muscles, located deep within your shoulders. Performing this exercise on a ball forces your abdominal and back muscles to work to help keep your body balanced on the ball. Strengthening the rotator cuff is particularly beneficial for people who participate in racquet sports, such as tennis or squash.

Using an exercise ball increases the level of difficulty of the exercise, since you are not only working against gravity, but you need to exert extra effort to stabilize

your body on the ball while you lift the dumbbells. For more information on exercise balls, see page 168.

As you perform the exercise, keep your head and back in a straight line and your abdominal muscles tight to protect your back. Try to avoid swinging your hands up or down. Instead, slowly raise and then lower the weights, maintaining the complete range of motion throughout the exercise.

You should be careful performing external rotations if you have a recent rotator cuff injury or if you have lower back problems.

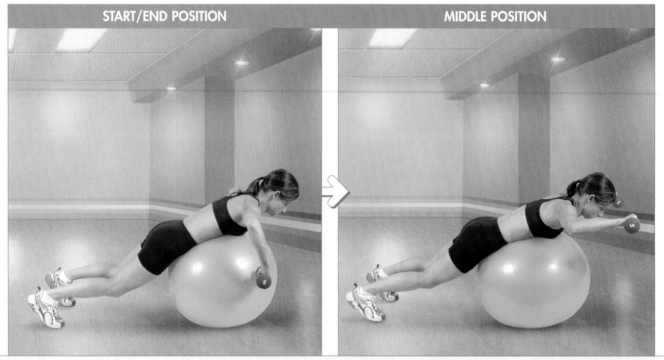

START/END POSITION	MIDDLE POSITION

1 Lie on your chest on a ball with your legs roughly shoulder width apart, your knees slightly bent and the balls of your feet on the floor.

2 Grasp a dumbbell in each hand. Bend your elbows at 90-degree angles, elbows pointing toward the ceiling, both palms facing your feet.

3 Slowly raise the dumbbells so both palms face the floor and your elbows point toward your feet.

• Make sure you tighten your abdominal muscles to help protect your back.

4 Slowly lower the dumbbells back to the starting position.

What other variation can I perform?

You can perform internal rotations. Holding a dumbbell in each hand, lie on your back on the ball with your feet straight in front of you and your knees bent. Hold the dumbbells with your elbows bent 90 degrees, your palms facing the ceiling and your elbows pointing to your toes. Raise the dumbbells so that your palms face your feet and your elbows point to the floor. Then lower the dumbbells and repeat the exercise. This variation works a different part of your rotator cuff.

Can I also work my back muscles when performing external rotations?

Yes. In addition to working your rotator cuff, you can work the muscles in the middle of your back by performing arm raises with your arms straight instead of bent. Lie on your chest on the ball as shown in the steps below. Hold a dumbbell in each hand with your arms by your sides, your elbows slightly bent and your palms facing forward. Slowly raise the dumbbells to shoulder level so your arms and back are in a straight line. Then lower the dumbbells and repeat the exercise.

DON'T

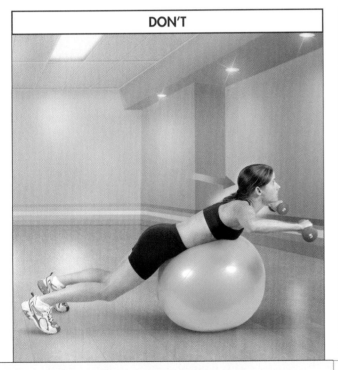

- Do not bend your neck forward or backward. Keep your head, neck and back in a straight line.

- Do not bend your wrists when raising or lowering the dumbbells.

- Do not lift the dumbbells higher than shoulder height.

MUSCLES TARGETED

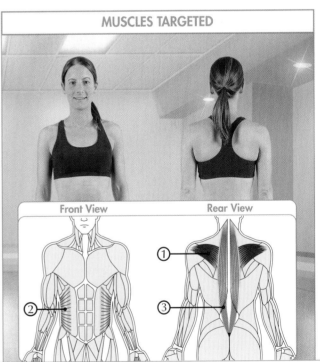

Front View   Rear View

Targeted muscles:
① deep shoulder muscles (*rotator cuff*)

Additional muscles:
② deep abdominal muscles (*transverse abdominis*)
③ lower back (*erector spinae*)

ball dip

The ball dip focuses on strengthening and giving shape to your triceps, but also works your shoulders, your upper and lower back and your deep abdominal muscles. The ball dip is ideal for fit individuals looking for a more challenging exercise.

You need to use an exercise ball to perform this exercise. For more information on exercise balls, see page 168. Due to the instability resulting from the use of an exercise ball, this exercise is more difficult than

the bench dip shown on page 78. You will need to work harder to keep your balance. However, working to keep your balance on the ball contributes to working your core muscles, which includes your back and abdominal muscles.

You should be careful performing the ball dip if you have neck or lower back problems. Do not perform this exercise if you have shoulder, elbow or wrist problems.

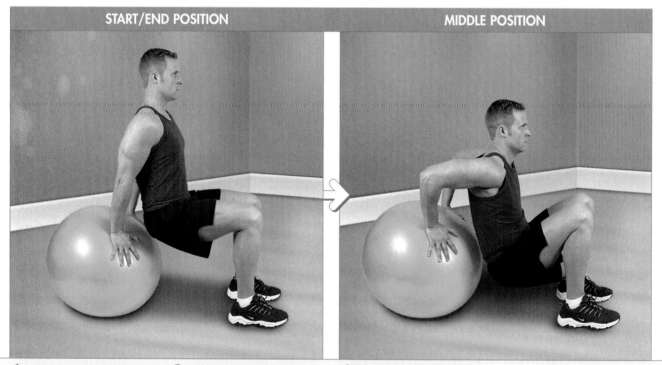

START/END POSITION

MIDDLE POSITION

1 Sit on the edge of a ball with your legs together, knees bent at 90-degree angles and your feet flat on the floor. Tighten your abdominal muscles to help protect your back.

2 Place your hands beside your hips with your fingers pointing to the sides.

3 Push the palms of your hands into the ball, straighten your arms and lift your buttocks off the ball, supporting your weight on your arms.

4 Slowly bend your arms and lower your body until your upper arms are parallel with the floor. Keep your elbows from flaring out to the sides.

5 Slowly straighten your arms and push yourself back up to the starting position.

How can I make the exercise easier?

You can place the exercise ball against a wall for better stability or change the position of your hands on the ball so that your thumbs are pointing forward with your other fingers pointing out. You can also sit on the ball with your knees shoulder width apart, bent at 90-degree angles. Place your palms slightly behind you, with your fingers pointing forward and your elbows slightly bent. Bend your elbows as you lean back to a 45-degree angle and then straighten your arms to return to the starting position. Make sure to keep your back straight in this last exercise.

Is there a way to make this exercise harder?

Yes. You can make the ball dip harder by sitting on the exercise ball with your legs straight and together. Then with your toes pointing up and your weight on your heels, perform the exercise as described in the steps below.

DON'T

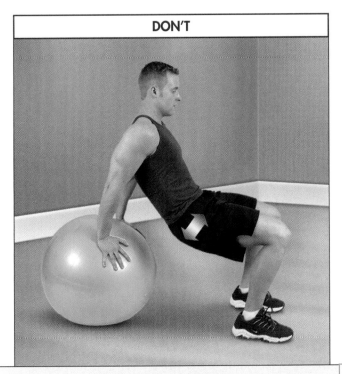

- Do not just move your hips up and down. Make sure you bend and straighten your arms.

- Do not lower your body too far down. Your upper arms should never be lower than parallel with the floor.

- Do not lock your elbows or allow your elbows to flare out to the sides.

- Do not shrug your shoulders.

MUSCLES TARGETED

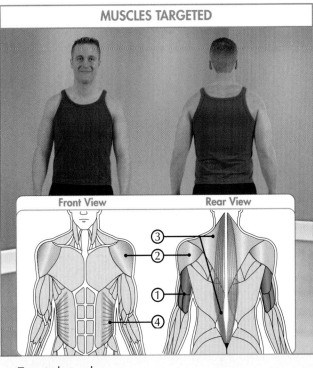

Front View   Rear View

Targeted muscles:
① triceps

Additional muscles:
② shoulders (*deltoids*)
③ upper and lower back (*trapezius, erector spinae*)
④ deep abdominal muscles (*transverse abdominis*)

seated dumbbell curl

The seated dumbbell curl works your biceps. You should be careful performing this exercise if you have elbow or wrist problems.

Performing dumbbell curls while sitting on an exercise ball also works your abdominal and back muscles, which helps to improve core strength. Using an exercise ball is a good way to vary your weight training routine to avoid boredom. The ball also adds an extra element of difficulty to the exercise, since you need to work at stabilizing yourself on the ball while you lift the dumbbells.

Pay close attention to your form as you perform the exercise. You should keep your elbows close to your body, but try not to dig your elbows into your body or arch your back to help you lift the dumbbells. If you need to arch your back, you should probably use lighter weights. To get the maximum benefit from the exercise, do not use momentum to swing the dumbbells up or allow them to simply drop. Instead, keep your movements slow and controlled throughout the entire exercise.

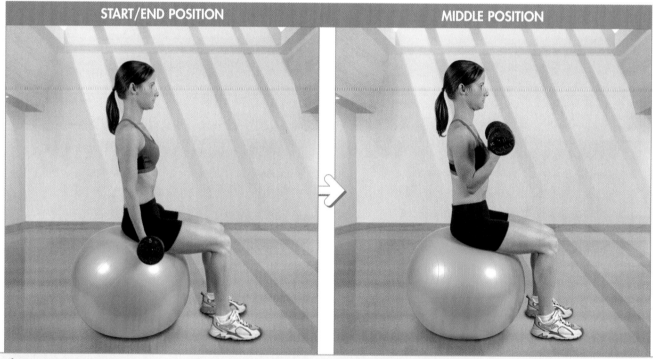

START/END POSITION | **MIDDLE POSITION**

1 Hold a dumbbell in each hand.

2 Sit on a ball with your knees bent, your legs a few inches apart and your feet flat on the floor. Tighten your abdominal muscles to help protect your back.

3 Start with your arms at your sides, elbows slightly bent, both palms facing forward.

4 Slowly bend your elbows to raise the dumbbells toward your shoulders.

- Make sure you keep your back straight, your head up and your elbows close to your sides.

5 Slowly straighten your arms to lower the dumbbells back to the starting position.

What other variations of the dumbbell curl can I perform?

There are several variations you can try. You can focus on one arm at a time by alternating between your left and right arm to lift the dumbbells. For another variation, start with your palms facing in. Once your arms reach your thighs, start rotating your wrists so that your palms end up facing the ceiling when the lift is complete. This variation works the entire bicep muscle and your forearms.

How can I make the exercise harder?

To make the dumbbell curl harder, perform the exercise as described in the steps below, except curl only your left arm and extend your right leg in front of you so you are supported by only one leg. After completing a set, repeat the exercise by curling your right arm with your left leg extended. When performing this variation, you will find it more difficult to maintain your balance on the ball. Take care not to hunch your back as you perform the exercise.

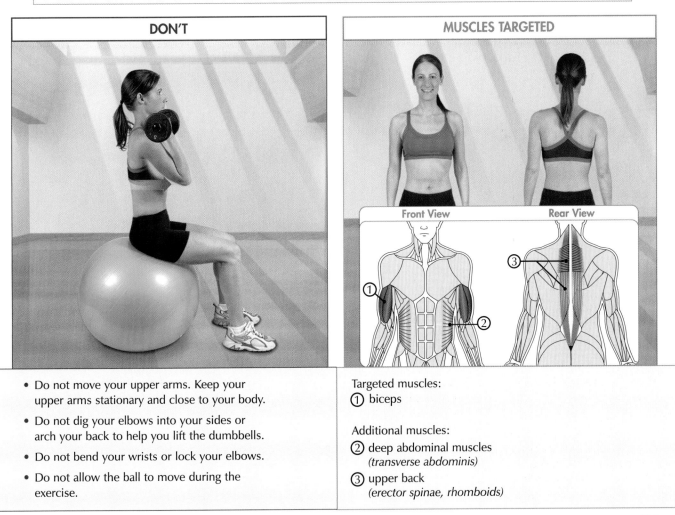

DON'T

MUSCLES TARGETED

Front View   Rear View

- Do not move your upper arms. Keep your upper arms stationary and close to your body.

- Do not dig your elbows into your sides or arch your back to help you lift the dumbbells.

- Do not bend your wrists or lock your elbows.

- Do not allow the ball to move during the exercise.

Targeted muscles:
① biceps

Additional muscles:
② deep abdominal muscles
   (transverse abdominis)
③ upper back
   (erector spinae, rhomboids)

abdominal crunch

The abdominal crunch focuses on flattening, toning and strengthening your front abdominal muscles, but also works your side and deep abdominal muscles and your lower back. This particular exercise is performed using an exercise ball. For more information on exercise balls, see page 168.

As you perform the abdominal crunch using an exercise ball, keep your abdominal muscles tight to prevent your lower back from overarching and to feel more tension in your abdominal muscles. You should

also avoid pulling your neck forward with your hands or letting your elbows draw in as you curl your head and shoulders up and forward.

To help maintain your balance, perform the exercise slowly and carefully. You should also keep your feet firmly on the floor for better support and balance.

Using an exercise ball to perform abdominal crunches is useful for people with lower back problems. However, people with neck problems should be careful performing this exercise.

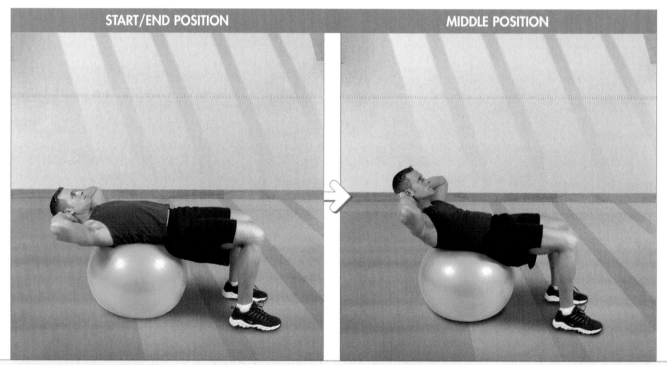

| START/END POSITION | MIDDLE POSITION |

1 Sit on the edge of a ball and position your feet flat on the floor with your feet roughly shoulder width apart.

2 Lean back on the ball so your hips and back are resting on the ball.

3 Place your hands behind your head and position your elbows out to the sides.

4 Push your lower back into the ball and tighten your abdominal muscles.

5 Slowly curl your head and shoulders a few inches up and forward so your upper back lifts off the ball. Keep your elbows out to the sides.

6 Pause for a moment and then slowly lower your head and shoulders back to the starting position.

Is there a way to make this exercise easier?

Yes. There are a couple of ways to make this exercise easier. You can place your feet against a wall for added support and stability. You can also position your arms across your chest to make this exercise easier. However, if you start feeling some neck strain, you can use one arm to help support your head.

How can I make this exercise harder?

To make this exercise harder, you can sit higher up on an exercise ball with only your hips and buttocks resting on the ball. Keep your upper back off the exercise ball. Curl up until your upper body is roughly perpendicular to your thighs. This variation allows a wider range of motion, which allows you to work your muscles more. You can also make this exercise harder by lifting one leg slightly off the floor to make you work harder to maintain balance.

DON'T

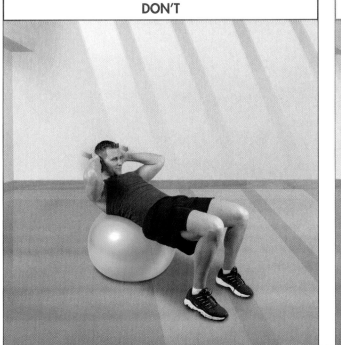

- Do not pull your neck forward with your hands. You should not bend your neck.
- Do not allow the ball to move during the exercise.
- Do not move your arms. Keep your elbows out to the sides.
- Do not interlock your fingers behind your head.

MUSCLES TARGETED

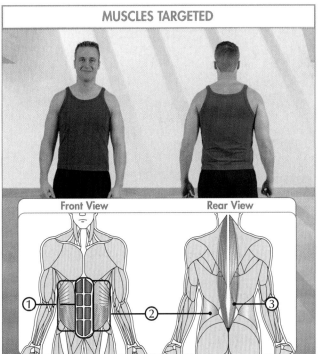

Front View　　　　Rear View

Targeted muscles:
① front abdominal muscles *(rectus abdominis)*

Additional muscles:
② side and deep abdominal muscles *(internal and external obliques, transverse abdominis)*
③ lower back *(erector spinae)*

side crunch

The side crunch focuses on strengthening and shaping your side abdominal muscles, but also works your deep abdominal muscles and your lower back. This exercise is performed using an exercise ball. For more information on exercise balls, see page 168.

When performing the side crunch using an exercise ball, focus on maintaining proper form and balance. Do not bend your neck as you raise your upper body. You should keep your head, neck and back in a straight line during the entire exercise. To help keep the ball steady

and maintain your balance, do not move your body forward or back.

At any point during the exercise, avoid quickly raising and lowering your upper body. As with other exercises, you should perform the side crunch in a slow, controlled manner to avoid injury and to get the full benefit of the exercise.

If you have neck problems, take extra care when performing the side crunch. You should not perform this exercise if you are suffering from back problems.

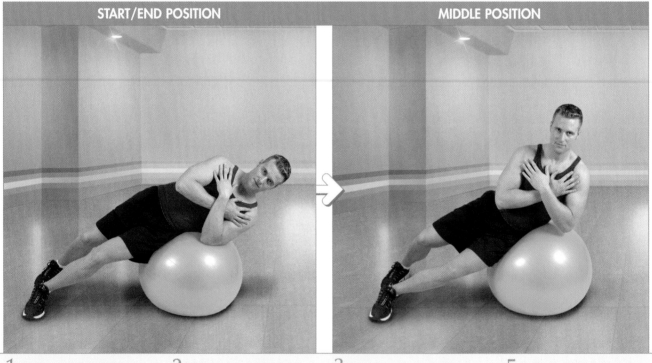

| START/END POSITION | MIDDLE POSITION |

1 Lie on your left side on a ball so your left hip is resting on the ball. Cross your arms over your chest. Tighten your abdominal muscles.

2 Position the edges of your feet on the floor with your left foot in front of your right foot, roughly shoulder width apart and your knees slightly bent.

3 Slowly curl your right shoulder toward your right hip.

4 Pause for a moment and then slowly lower your upper body back to the starting position.

5 After completing a set on your left side, repeat the exercise on your right side.

Are there ways to make the exercise easier?

Yes. There are a couple of ways to help make the exercise easier. For better stability, you can place your feet against a wall. You can also make the exercise easier by sitting lower on the exercise ball so that your left hip and upper left side are resting on the ball.

How can I make the exercise harder?

You can try a number of ways to make the exercise harder. You can place your hands behind your head with your elbows out or position your arms straight over your head. You can also make the exercise harder by holding a weight plate across your chest for added resistance. Another way to make the exercise harder is to hold a dumbbell with your arm closest to the floor, hanging the arm down with your elbow slightly bent and placing your other hand behind your head for support.

DON'T

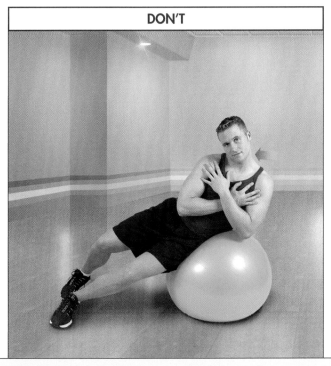

- Do not bend your neck. Keep your head, neck and back in a straight line.
- Do not move your body forward or back. Keep the ball stationary.
- Do not rapidly raise and lower your upper body. Keep the movement slow and controlled.

MUSCLES TARGETED

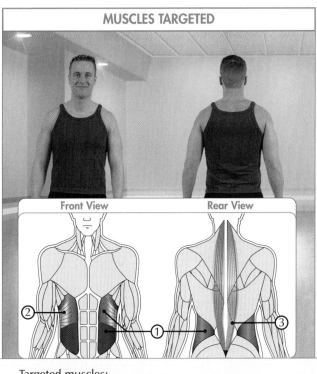

Front View   Rear View

Targeted muscles:
① side abdominal muscles
 (internal and external obliques)

Additional muscles:
② deep abdominal muscles *(transverse abdominis)*
③ lower back *(erector spinae)*

reverse crunch

The reverse crunch focuses on your front abdominal muscles, but also works your lower back and your side and deep abdominal muscles. This is a great exercise for flattening and toning the lower portion of your front abdominal muscles. To perform this exercise, you need to use an exercise ball. For more information on exercise balls, see page 168. The use of an exercise ball places you in a stable position, which makes it harder for you to cheat.

As you perform the reverse crunch using an exercise ball, focus on using your abdominal muscles to lift your buttocks off the ground. To keep the focus on your abdominal muscles, do not jerk your legs or thrust your hips to lift your buttocks. You should also avoid lifting your head or back off the ground and avoid arching your back as your lower your buttocks.

You should be careful performing this exercise if you are suffering from lower back problems.

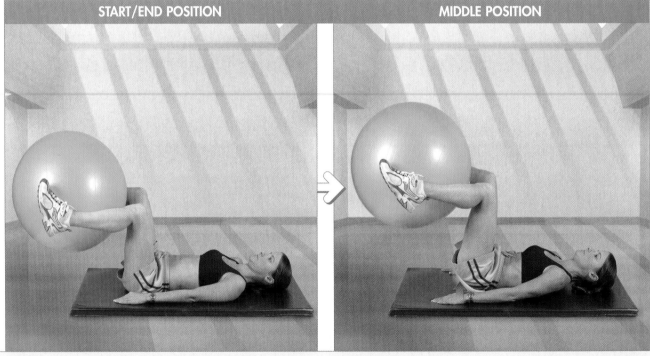

START/END POSITION   **MIDDLE POSITION**

1 Lie on your back on a mat and position a ball between your lower legs.

2 Bend your knees at roughly 90-degree angles and lift up your legs until your thighs are perpendicular to the floor.

3 Place your arms straight at your sides with your palms facing down. Rest your head on the mat and tighten your abdominal muscles.

4 While keeping your hips on the floor, slowly lift your buttocks a few inches off the floor so your knees lift up toward the ceiling.

5 Pause for a moment and then slowly lower your buttocks back to the starting position.

QUESTION & ANSWER
?

I have difficulty performing the reverse crunch. Is there an easier exercise I can perform?

Yes. You can perform the pelvic tilt by positioning yourself as described in the steps below and then tilting your hips toward your head. The pelvic tilt allows you to isolate your lower abdominal muscles but is easier to perform than the reverse crunch since you do not have to lift your buttocks off the ground.

How can I make the exercise harder?

You can try a couple of ways to make the exercise harder. You can perform the reverse crunch with your legs straight and perpendicular to the floor and the exercise ball positioned between your lower legs. You can also lie on your back with your legs straight, just off the floor, and the exercise ball placed between your lower legs. Raise your legs until they are perpendicular to the floor and then lower your legs back down. This last exercise also helps strengthen your hip flexors.

DON'T

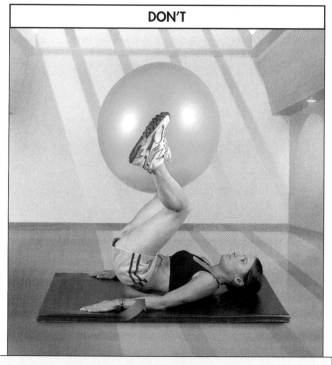

- Do not allow your back to lift off the mat.
- Do not swing your legs. Focus on just lifting your buttocks.
- Do not arch your back as you lower your buttocks.
- Do not lift your head off the mat.

MUSCLES TARGETED

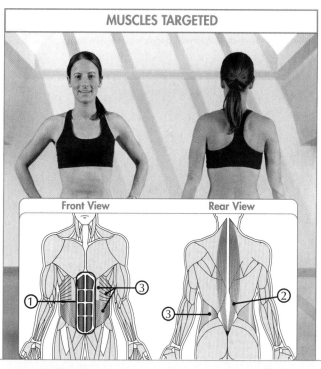

Targeted muscles:
① front abdominal muscles
   (rectus abdominis)

Additional muscles:
② lower back *(erector spinae)*
③ side and deep abdominal muscles
   (internal and external obliques and transverse abdominis)

back extension

The back extension focuses on strengthening your lower back. Performing this exercise can help give you the lower back support necessary for many daily activities. In addition to strengthening your lower back, the back extension also works your buttocks and your deep abdominal muscles. To perform this exercise, you need to use an exercise ball. For more information on exercise balls, see page 168.

When performing the back extension, try to keep the ball steady at all times. The effort of keeping yourself steady on the ball also helps to work your core

muscles, which includes your back and abdominal muscles.

As with other exercises, remember to perform the back extension in a slow, controlled manner and to maintain proper form throughout the entire exercise. Keep your knees slightly bent at all times and do not bend your neck as you raise and lower your upper body. You should try to always keep your head, neck and back in a straight line.

You should not perform this exercise if you are suffering from lower back problems.

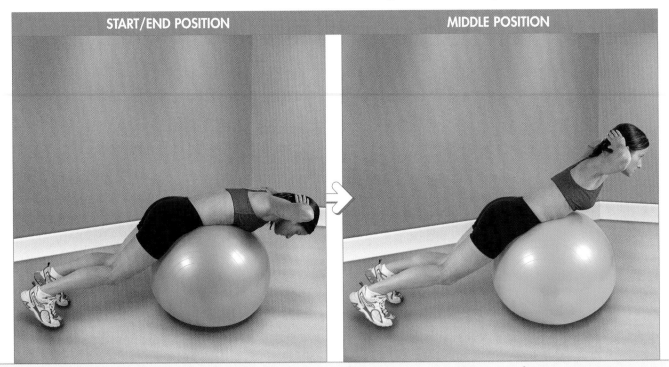

START/END POSITION　　　　　**MIDDLE POSITION**

1 Lie on your stomach on a ball with your feet roughly shoulder width apart, your knees slightly bent and the balls of your feet on the floor.

2 Place your hands behind your head and position your elbows out to the sides. Do not interlock your fingers.

3 Slowly raise your upper body until your hips and back are in a straight line.

4 Slowly lower your upper body back to the starting position.

Can I make the back extension easier?

Yes. You can make the back extension easier by placing your feet against a wall for better support. You can also place your arms across your chest or perform a shorter range of motion by not raising your upper body as high.

How can I make the back extension harder?

There are a few ways to make the back extension harder. You can hold a weight plate across your chest for added resistance or reposition yourself higher on the exercise ball so that you are lying on your hips instead of your stomach. For another variation, lie on your stomach on an exercise ball with your legs together and straight. With your hands on the floor, palms down and roughly shoulder width apart, slowly raise your legs until they are slightly above the level of your buttocks and then lower your legs back down.

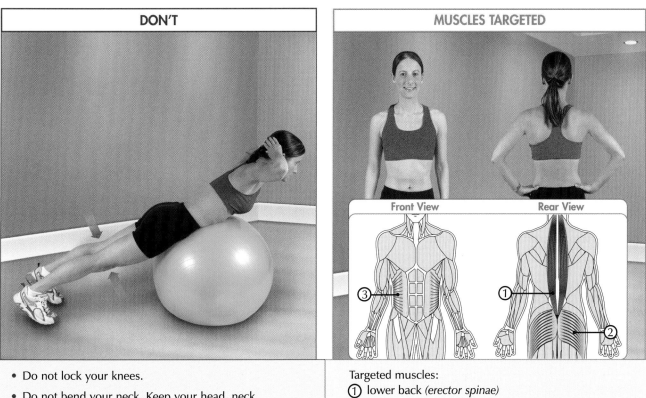

DON'T

MUSCLES TARGETED

Front View   Rear View

- Do not lock your knees.
- Do not bend your neck. Keep your head, neck and back in a straight line.
- Do not allow the ball to move during the exercise.
- Do not rapidly raise and lower your upper body. Keep the movement slow and controlled.

Targeted muscles:
① lower back *(erector spinae)*

Additional muscles:
② buttocks *(gluteus maximus)*
③ deep abdominal muscles *(transverse abdominis)*

introduction to exercise tubing

Exercise tubing is useful for strengthening, firming and toning your muscles. This piece of exercise equipment is handy when traveling or you can use it to vary your normal exercise routine.

Keep in mind that exercise tubing will not give you the same results as intense strength training or muscle building with weights, but using exercise tubing will help tone and define your muscles.

You can purchase exercise tubing at most sporting goods or exercise equipment stores.

You can also buy rubber strips called exercise bands, which are thin, flat strips that often do not have handles and can be used for exercises the same way as exercise tubing. If your tubing does not have handles and an exercise specifies that you should hold the handles of the tubing, wrap the ends of the tubing loosely around your palms.

BENEFITS OF EXERCISE TUBING

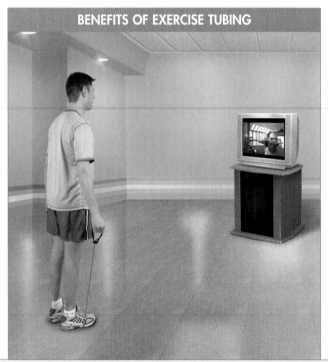

USE EXERCISE TUBING

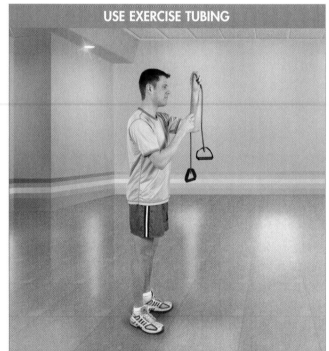

- You can use exercise tubing in almost any location for quick and easy workouts. Use exercise tubing while watching television, at a friend's house or when traveling.

- You can use exercise tubing to perform a variety of exercises. Exercise tubing is inexpensive, safe to use, lightweight and portable.

- Exercise tubing will wear over time. You should check your tubing frequently for holes and tears. If you find a hole or tear, you should replace the tubing immediately.

- Before starting an exercise using exercise tubing, make sure the tubing is securely in place to prevent injury.

- For the best results, perform 3 sets of each tubing exercise with 12 to 15 repetitions for each set.

Are there accessories I can buy to help enhance tubing exercises?

Yes. There are several tubing accessories that can enhance or vary your exercises. You can purchase accessories that make it easier to perform some exercises, such as door anchors or hooks that allow you to attach the tubing to a stable door or doorframe. If you will be using exercise tubing often, you may want to purchase an exercise tubing kit that has multiple attachments, such an ankle strap that will hold the tubing in place for some exercises.

What are the disadvantages of using exercise tubing?

Exercise tubing has some drawbacks, which include the limited amount of resistance they offer compared to weights. You may also have difficulty positioning yourself while holding the tubing or obtaining the desired tension in the tubing. Although they are relatively safe, exercise tubing can wear over time and may cause injury if it snaps while you are exercising. You should check your tubing regularly and replace the tubing at the first sign of wear.

CHANGE EXERCISE TUBING RESISTANCE

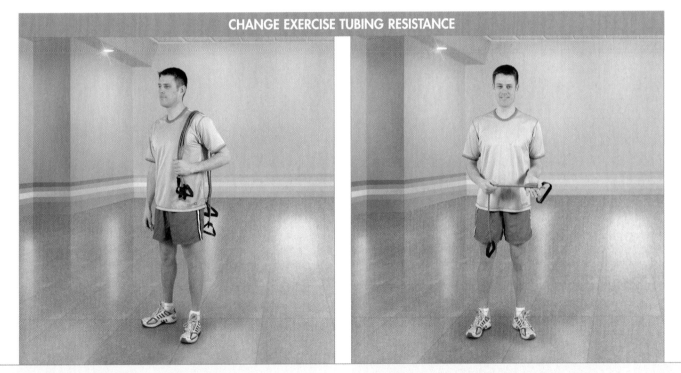

- Exercise tubing comes in various colors, which indicate the amount of resistance the tubing provides. The colors may vary between manufacturers, but darker colors usually indicate more resistance. In general, thicker tubing offers greater resistance.

- You can manually shorten or lengthen exercise tubing to quickly increase or decrease its resistance. For example, you can wrap the tubing around your hands or change where you stand on the tubing to change the resistance.

squat

The squat focuses on your quadriceps, hamstrings and buttocks, but also works your inner thighs and hip flexors. This is a great exercise for building strong legs, which can help make activities, such as walking and lifting objects off the floor, easier. Performing squats can also help give you more endurance when climbing stairs.

You need to use exercise tubing to perform this exercise. For more information on exercise tubing, see page 198. The use of exercise tubing gives you different resistance compared to using dumbbells or a barbell.

When performing squats, you should keep your head, neck and back in a straight line and also keep your abdominal muscles tight to help protect your back. You should bend your knees until your thighs are parallel to the floor, but you should not go lower than this point or let your knees pass your toes.

You should be careful performing this exercise if you have lower back, hip or knee problems.

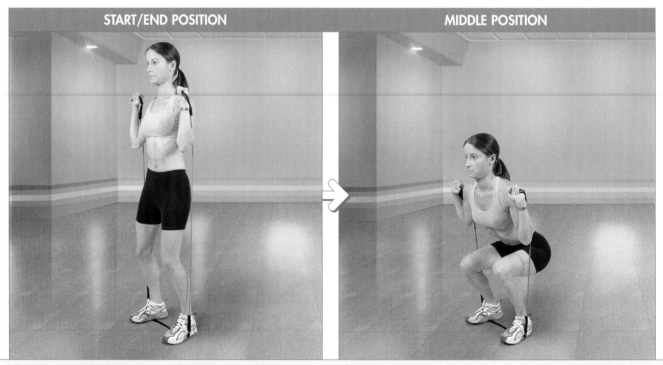

START/END POSITION   **MIDDLE POSITION**

1 Grasp a handle of the exercise tubing in each hand.

2 Stand on the middle of the tubing with both feet. Position your feet roughly shoulder width apart, knees slightly bent.

3 Position your upper arms at your sides and your hands in front of your shoulders with your palms facing forward. Tighten your abdominal muscles to help protect your back.

4 Slowly bend your knees until your thighs are parallel to the floor. Your knees should not pass your toes. Imagine you are sitting down in a chair.

• Make sure you keep your back straight, your head up and your feet flat on the floor.

5 Pushing through your heels, slowly lift yourself back to the starting position.

When performing squats, can I place my feet wider apart or closer together?

Yes. You can place your feet about one and a half shoulder width apart to work your inner thighs and buttocks more. You can also place your feet less than shoulder width apart to work your quadriceps and buttocks more.

How can I make this exercise harder?

You can slow down your movements to make the exercise harder and to help increase muscular and tendon strength. Take 2 seconds to perform the downward movement, pause momentarily and then take 4 to 6 seconds to rise back to the starting position. Slowing down your movements also maximizes the use of your muscles since you need to work harder against the resistance of the tubing to bring yourself back up to the starting position.

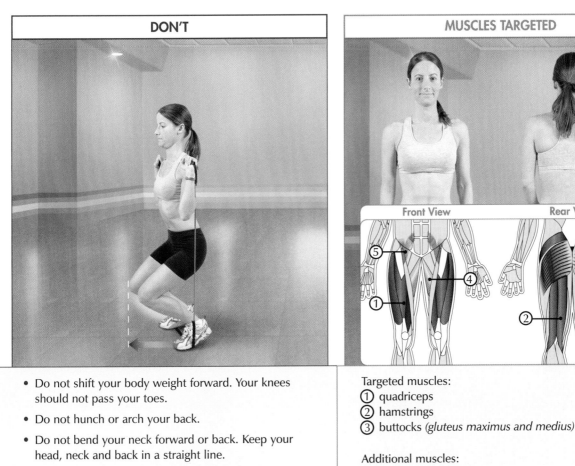

DON'T

MUSCLES TARGETED

Front View   Rear View

- Do not shift your body weight forward. Your knees should not pass your toes.

- Do not hunch or arch your back.

- Do not bend your neck forward or back. Keep your head, neck and back in a straight line.

- Do not lock your knees or lift your heels off the floor.

- Do not move your arms away from your body.

Targeted muscles:
① quadriceps
② hamstrings
③ buttocks (*gluteus maximus and medius*)

Additional muscles:
④ inner thighs (*adductors*)
⑤ hip flexors

standing leg curl

The standing leg curl focuses on your hamstrings and is a great exercise for toning the back of your legs. It is a convenient exercise to perform when you are away from the gym. In addition to working your hamstrings, this exercise also strengthens your calves.

You need exercise tubing to perform the standing leg curl shown in the steps below. For more information on exercise tubing, see page 198. When performing this exercise, you can change where you step on the tubing to adjust the tension. For example, placing the

foot of your supporting leg closer to the looped end of the tubing will increase the tension.

As you perform the standing leg curl, do not lean your body forward or backward. You should also avoid locking the knee of your supporting leg or moving the upper part of the leg you are working. As with other exercises, perform the standing leg curl in a slow, controlled manner.

If you have lower back problems, you should be careful performing the standing leg curl.

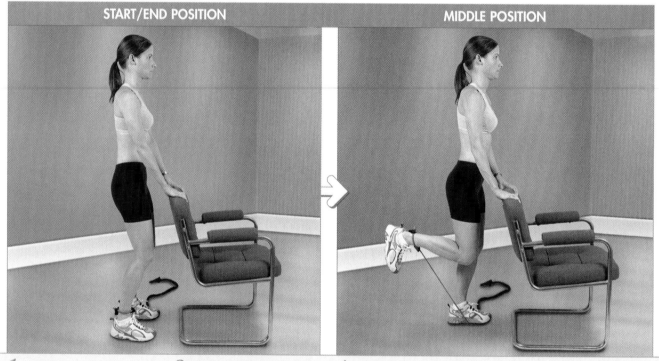

START/END POSITION   MIDDLE POSITION

1 Push one handle of the exercise tubing through the other handle to create a loop at one end of the tubing. Place the loop around your right ankle.

2 Stand roughly shoulder width apart with your left foot on the tubing. Slightly bend both knees.

3 Hold onto a chair or wall with both hands for support.

4 While keeping your upper right leg stationary, slowly lift your right foot towards your buttocks by bending your knee.

• Make sure you tighten your abdominal muscles to help protect your back.

5 Slowly lower your foot back to the starting position.

6 After completing a set with your right leg, repeat the exercise with your left leg.

In addition to working my hamstrings, how can I also work my buttocks, lower back and abdominal muscles?

To also work your buttocks, lower back and abdominal muscles, perform deadlifts using exercise tubing. Stand in the middle of the tubing with your feet shoulder width apart and your knees slightly bent. Bend from your hips and grasp a tubing handle in each hand with your arms straight, elbows

slightly bent and your palms facing back. To make sure the tubing is taut, you may need to wrap the tubing around your hands. Slowly raise your upper body until your body is straight and then bend at your hips to lower your body back down. Make sure your back remains completely straight.

DON'T

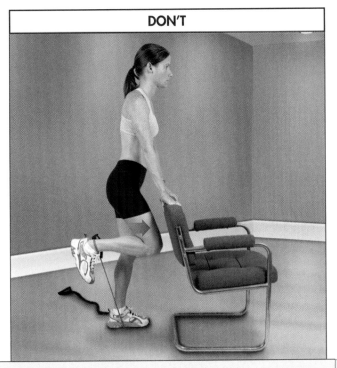

MUSCLES TARGETED

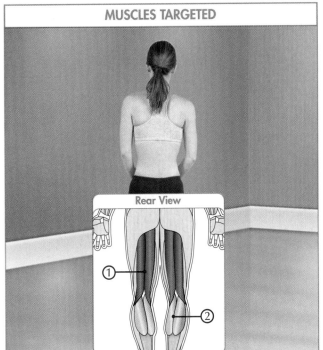

- Do not move the upper part of the leg you are strengthening forward or back.
- Do not lean your body forward or back.
- Do not raise or lower your leg too fast. Keep the movement slow and controlled.
- Do not lock the knee of your supporting leg.

Targeted muscles:
① hamstrings

Additional muscles:
② calves (*gastrocnemius*)

side-lying inner thigh lift

The side-lying inner thigh lift tones and firms your inner thighs. When positioning yourself for the exercise, you can stretch your right arm straight out on the mat and rest your head on your arm instead of supporting your head in your hand.

Your flexibility and muscle strength will determine how high you can lift your leg. However, you should not lift your leg higher than your bent knee. When you start to feel tension in your inner thigh muscles, stop lifting your leg, hold the position for a moment

and then lower your leg slowly.

Remember to maintain proper form as you perform the side-lying inner thigh lift. As with other exercises, perform the movements in a slow, controlled manner to avoid injury and to receive the full benefit of the exercise. Make sure the exercise tubing is taut before you begin. For more information on exercise tubing, see page 198.

You should be careful performing this exercise if you have lower back or hip problems.

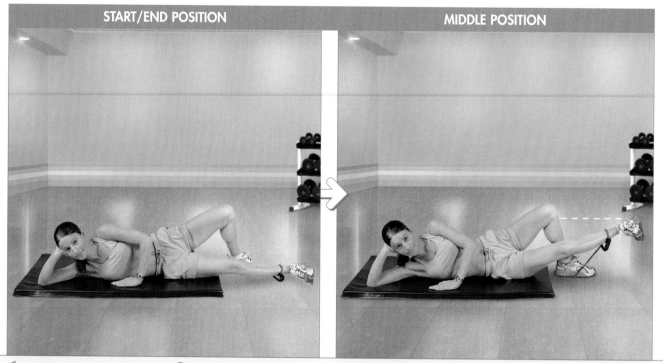

START/END POSITION   **MIDDLE POSITION**

1 Push one handle of the exercise tubing through the other handle and place the loop around your right ankle.

2 Lie on your right side with your right leg straight, left foot behind right knee.

3 Position the tubing under your left foot to hold it in place.

4 Rest your head in your right hand and place your left hand on the mat for support.

5 Keeping your right leg straight and your toes pulled toward your shin, slowly raise your right leg no higher than your left knee. Tighten your abdominal muscles to help protect your back.

6 Pause for a moment and then slowly lower your right leg back toward the floor.

7 After completing a set with your right leg, switch sides and repeat the exercise with your left leg.

How can I make the exercise easier?

To make the side-lying inner thigh lift easier, perform the exercise as described in the steps below, except keep the knee of the leg you are working slightly bent as you lift. Bending your leg will move the leg closer to the foot that is holding the tubing and help to reduce the tension in the tubing.

Is there a harder variation of the exercise I can perform?

Yes. You can make the exercise harder by positioning the leg you are working in a slightly different way. Lie on a mat as described in the steps below, except position your right leg in front of your body at about a 45-degree angle, bending at your hip. Keeping your right leg straight, slowly lift the leg and then slowly lower back to the starting position. After completing a set with your right leg, repeat the exercise with your left leg. This variation works your inner thigh more by adding more tension to the tubing.

DON'T	MUSCLES TARGETED

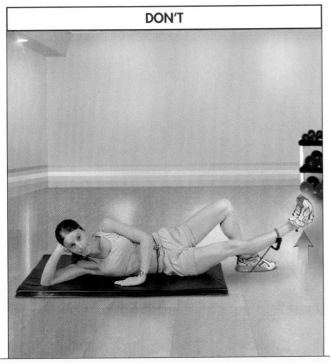

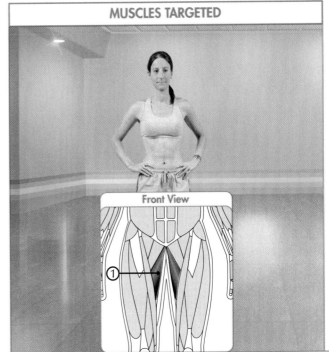

Front View

- Do not rotate the leg you are strengthening so your toes point to the ceiling. Keep your toes pointed to the side.

- Do not bend your neck. Keep your head, neck and back in a straight line.

- Do not lift your leg higher than your bent knee.

- Do not rapidly raise and lower your leg.

Targeted muscles:
① inner thighs (adductors)

kneeling kickback

The kneeling kickback is a good exercise for toning and tightening your buttocks as well as strengthening your hamstrings. Using exercise tubing when performing kneeling kickbacks provides extra resistance, making the exercise harder than without the tubing. For more information on exercise tubing, see page 198.

When you are in the starting position for the exercise, you should place your elbows directly under your shoulders and your knees directly under your buttocks.

As you perform kickbacks, keep your back straight and

your abdominal muscles tight to protect your back. You should also keep your head aligned with your back and your shoulders relaxed. Instead of jerking your leg up and letting it drop back to the starting position, focus on performing the movement in a slow, controlled manner. When you lift and lower your leg, try not to raise your knee higher than your hips or lean your body to the left or right.

You should be careful performing kneeling kickbacks if you have lower back, knee or shoulder problems.

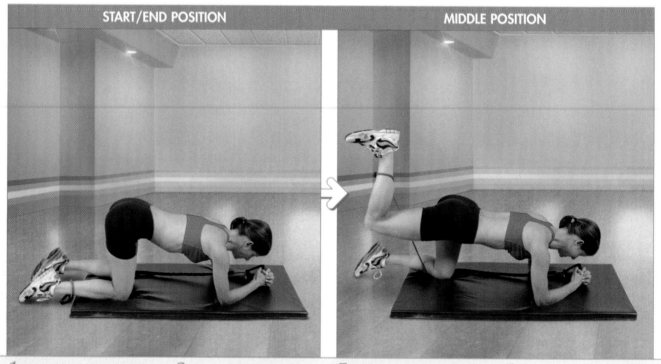

START/END POSITION | **MIDDLE POSITION**

1 Push one handle of the exercise tubing through the other handle to create a loop at one end of the tubing. Place the loop around your right ankle.

2 Kneel on a mat, resting your body weight on your knees and forearms.

3 Position your knees and elbows roughly shoulder width apart.

4 Place the tubing under your left knee and grasp the handle of the tubing with both hands, palms facing each other.

5 Keeping your right knee bent at a 90-degree angle, slowly lift your right leg until your thigh is parallel to the floor.

• Make sure you tighten your abdominal muscles to help protect your back.

6 Pause for a moment and then slowly lower your leg back toward the floor.

7 After completing a set with your right leg, repeat the exercise with your left leg.

How can I make the exercise harder?

To make the exercise harder, you can perform kneeling kickbacks with your leg straight instead of bent. Position yourself as described in the steps below, except stretch your right leg out behind you with the top of your toes touching the floor. Keeping your right leg straight, lift the right leg until it is parallel to the floor. Then lower your leg back to the starting position. Straightening your arms and resting your upper body weight on your hands instead of your forearms will also make the exercise harder.

Can I perform kickbacks while standing?

Yes. Create a loop at one end of the tubing and place the loop around your right ankle. Stand with your feet shoulder width apart with the tubing under your left foot and your knees slightly bent. Hold a chair or wall for support. Slowly push your right leg straight behind you as far as you can without moving the rest of your body. Then slowly return your leg to the starting position. After completing a set with your right leg, repeat the exercise with your left leg.

DON'T

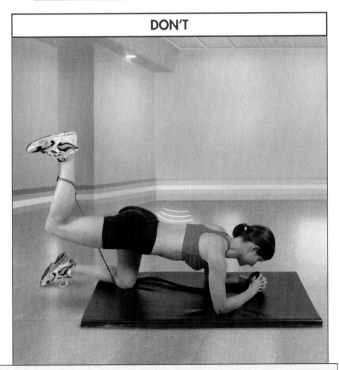

- Do not arch your back as you lift your leg.
- Do not shrug your shoulders.
- Do not bend your neck. Keep your head, neck and back in a straight line.
- Do not raise your thigh above parallel to the floor.
- Do not lean your body to the left or right.

MUSCLES TARGETED

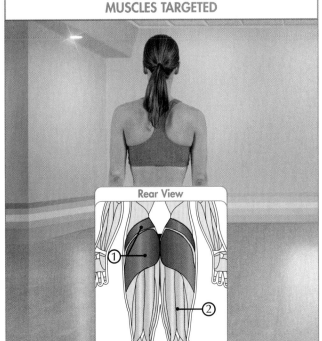

Rear View

Targeted muscles:
① buttocks (gluteus maximus and medius)

Additional muscles:
② hamstrings

lying leg abduction

The lying leg abduction focuses on your buttocks, but also works your outer hips. Performing this exercise helps give shape to your buttocks and tone your outer hip area. You need to use exercise tubing to perform this exercise. For more information on exercise tubing, see page 198.

When performing the lying leg abduction, make sure to keep your abdominal muscles tight to help protect your back. Avoid arching your back or lifting your head off the mat as you perform the exercise. You should also keep your arms stationary and your toes pointed toward your shins at all times.

As with other exercises, perform the lying leg abduction in a slow, controlled manner to help avoid injury and to receive the full benefit of the exercise. You should be careful performing the lying leg abduction if you have hip problems.

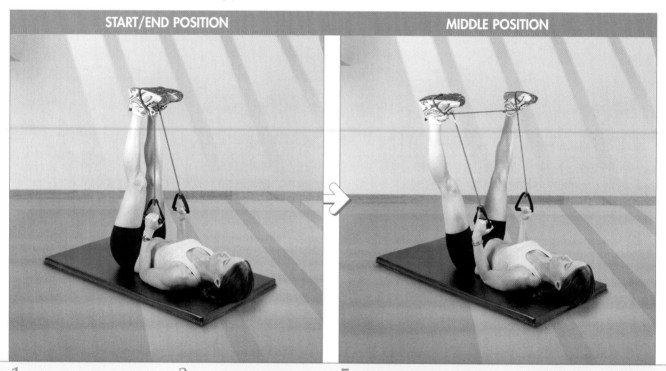

START/END POSITION   **MIDDLE POSITION**

1 Place the middle of the exercise tubing on the top of your feet. Wrap the tubing behind your feet and then between your feet so the tubing is wrapped around both feet.

2 Grasp a handle of the tubing in each hand.

3 Lie on your back on a mat and raise your legs perpendicular to the floor, keeping your legs together and straight.

4 Position your upper arms at your sides, elbows bent at 90-degree angles and palms facing each other over your stomach.

5 While pushing your elbows into the floor and keeping your toes pulled toward your shins, slowly move your legs as far apart as possible.

• Make sure you tighten your abdominal muscles to help protect your back.

6 Pause for a moment and then slowly bring your legs back together to return to the starting position.

How can I work one leg at a time?

Perform the lying leg abduction as described in the steps below, except keep one leg stationary while you work the other leg. Working one leg at a time allows you to focus on shaping and toning each side of your body separately.

Can I perform the exercise while standing?

Yes. After wrapping the tubing around your feet as described below, stand in front of a wall or chair with your feet slightly closer than shoulder width apart. Grasp both handles using your right hand with your palm facing back and your arm slightly in front of your body. Using your left hand, hold the wall or chair. Push your left leg to the side as far as you can without leaning your body over. Make sure to keep your supporting knee slightly bent. After completing a set, grasp the handles using your left hand and perform the exercise using your right leg.

DON'T

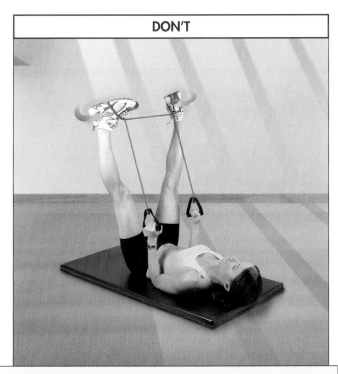

- Do not turn your feet in or out. Keep your toes pointed toward your shins.
- Do not move your arms. Keep your arms stationary.
- Do not lift your head off the mat.
- Do not arch your back.

MUSCLES TARGETED

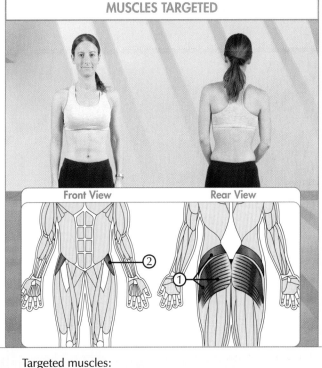

Front View | Rear View

Targeted muscles:
① buttocks (*gluteus maximus, medius and minimus*)
② outer hips

calf press

The calf press strengthens and tones your calf muscles. Performing the calf press can help make daily activities, such as walking, running and climbing stairs, easier. You need to use exercise tubing to perform this exercise. For more information on exercise tubing, see page 198. The use of exercise tubing to perform the calf press offers a variation from other exercises that work your calf muscles.

When performing the exercise, you can loop the tubing around the ball of your foot if you find the tubing easily slips off. To create a loop, push one handle of the tubing through the other handle and then place the loop around the ball of your foot. After the loop is in place, you can wrap the other end of the tubing around your hand to add tension. You hold the tubing using both hands.

As you perform the calf press, do not lock the knee of the leg you are strengthening. Keep this knee slightly bent throughout the entire exercise. You should also keep your back straight at all times.

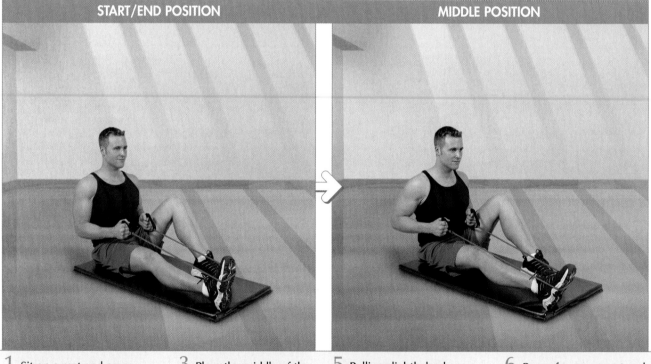

START/END POSITION	MIDDLE POSITION

1 Sit on a mat and grasp a handle of the exercise tubing in each hand.

2 Bend your left leg and position your left foot flat on the floor. Straighten your right leg with your knee slightly bent.

3 Place the middle of the tubing around the ball of your right foot.

4 Position your upper arms at your sides, elbows bent at roughly 90-degree angles and palms facing each other at stomach level.

5 Pulling slightly back on the tubing to add resistance, slowly point your toes forward.

6 Pause for a moment and then slowly pull your toes back to the starting position.

7 After completing a set with your right leg, repeat the exercise with your left leg.

How else can I position my supporting leg?

There are a couple of ways you can position your supporting leg for greater comfort. You can straighten your supporting leg or bend it so your knee points out and the bottom of your foot faces your other leg. No matter how you position your supporting leg, make sure to keep your back straight at all times.

Can I perform the exercise using both feet at the same time?

Yes. You can perform the exercise using both feet to work the calf muscles in both legs at the same time. Place the tubing around the balls of both your feet and then perform the exercise as described in the steps below. Make sure you keep your back straight.

DON'T

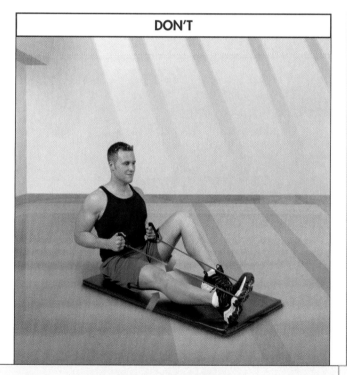

- Do not lock the knee of the leg you are strengthening. Keep the knee slightly bent.
- Do not hunch your back. Keep your back straight.

MUSCLES TARGETED

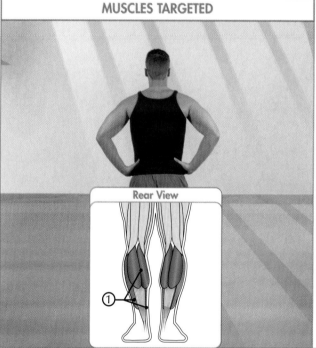

Rear View

Targeted muscles:
① calf muscles (*gastrocnemius and soleus*)

push-up

Push-ups work your chest as well as your shoulders and triceps. This is a great exercise for increasing your upper body strength and endurance, which can enhance your performance in sports that involve throwing, such as baseball or football.

Using exercise tubing when performing push-ups provides added resistance to make the exercise more challenging. For more information on exercise tubing, see page 198.

When you are in the starting position, you should make sure the exercise tubing is taut before you begin.

If the tubing is too loose, you can wrap the extra tubing around your palms to obtain the desired tension.

As you perform the exercise, keep your abdominal muscles tight and your back and legs in a straight line. Try to perform the full range of movement for the exercise, pushing your arms straight without locking your elbows and then lowering your chest close to the floor without touching.

You should be careful performing push-ups if have problems with your shoulders, elbows, wrists or lower back.

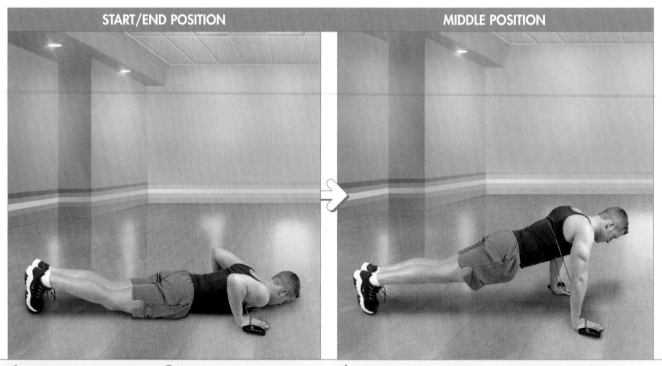

START/END POSITION | **MIDDLE POSITION**

1 Place the exercise tubing around your upper back and below your underarms. Wrap the ends of the tubing around your palms so that your hands are close to your underarms.

2 Lie on your stomach on the floor with your legs together and straight and the balls of your feet on the floor.

3 Bend your elbows and place your palms on the floor beside your shoulders, fingers pointing forward.

4 Slowly raise your body off the floor until your arms are straight. Keep your back and legs in a straight line.

• Make sure you tighten your abdominal muscles at all times to help protect your back.

5 Slowly lower your body until your chest almost touches the floor.

Is there an easier way to do push-ups?

Yes. You can perform modified push-ups. To do modified push-ups, perform the exercise as described in the steps below, except put your knees on the floor to help support your weight during the exercise. You can rest your lower legs together on the floor or keep them slightly raised, but do not cross your ankles. Your upper body should remain in a straight line as you perform push-ups.

Can I use the exercise tubing to perform a similar exercise while standing?

Yes. You can perform the chest press instead. Stand with your feet shoulder width apart. Wrap the exercise tubing across your upper back and below your underarms and grasp a handle of the tubing in each hand. Start with your arms bent with your elbows pointing back so your hands are near your shoulders and your palms are facing the floor. You may need to wrap the tubing around your hands to create enough tension. Straighten your arms in front of your chest so your hands almost touch and then bend your arms to return to the starting position.

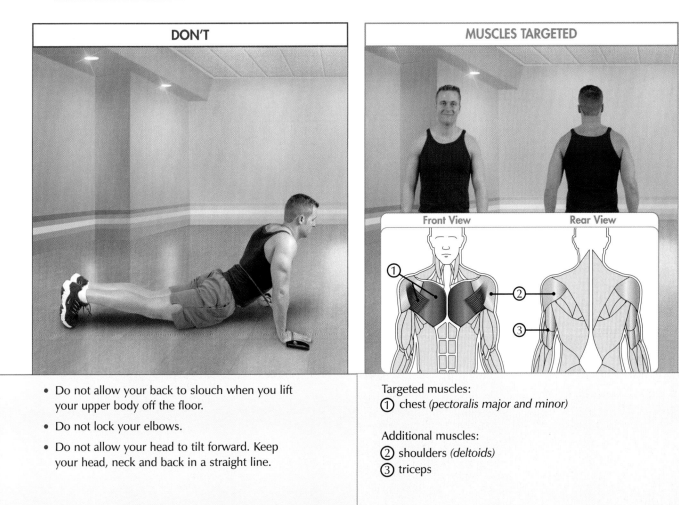

DON'T

MUSCLES TARGETED

Front View   Rear View

- Do not allow your back to slouch when you lift your upper body off the floor.

- Do not lock your elbows.

- Do not allow your head to tilt forward. Keep your head, neck and back in a straight line.

Targeted muscles:
① chest (*pectoralis major and minor*)

Additional muscles:
② shoulders (*deltoids*)
③ triceps

bent
over row

The bent over row focuses on your upper back, but also works your rear shoulders. In addition to adding definition to the muscles in your upper back, this exercise helps to improve your posture. You need to use exercise tubing to perform this exercise. For more information on exercise tubing, see page 198. You may need to wrap the tubing around your hands to get enough tension to perform the exercise properly.

During the exercise, remember to keep your back straight and your abdominal muscles tight to help protect your back. Do not hunch your back as you raise your elbows. You should also keep your knees slightly bent and your wrist and neck straight throughout the exercise.

Be careful performing the bent over row if you have lower back, shoulder or neck problems.

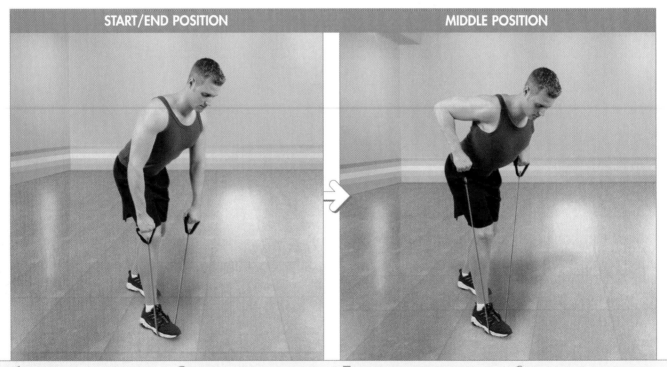

START/END POSITION	MIDDLE POSITION

1 Grasp a handle of the exercise tubing in each hand.

2 Stand with your feet roughly shoulder width apart, your right foot one step forward, knees slightly bent and feet flat on the floor.

3 Position the middle of the tubing under your right foot. Bend forward at your hips at a 45-degree angle.

4 Start with your arms hanging down, elbows slightly bent and your palms facing back.

5 Slowly bend your arms to raise your elbows back as far as you can, squeezing your shoulder blades together.

• Make sure you keep your back straight and tighten your abdominal muscles during the exercise.

6 Pause for a moment and then slowly straighten your arms to return to the starting position.

I have back problems. Is there an easier way to perform the exercise?

Yes. Position a bench with back support in front of a stable object, such as a column or railing, and wrap the tubing around the object. Grasp a handle in each hand and then sit on the bench. To ensure the tubing is taut, move the bench farther away from the object. Place the tubing at shoulder height and straighten your arms in front of you with your elbows slightly bent and your palms facing down. Slowly bring your elbows back as far as you can before returning to the starting position.

How can I focus more on my rear shoulders?

You can perform the bent over lateral raise to focus more on your rear shoulders. Position yourself as described in the steps below, except grasp the handles of the tubing with your palms facing each other. While keeping your elbows slightly bent, slowly raise your arms out to your sides until they are at shoulder height. Squeeze your shoulder blades together at the top of the movement. Then lower your arms back to the starting position.

DON'T

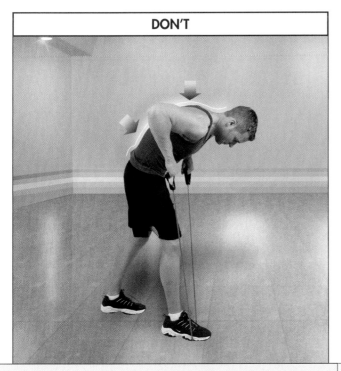

- Do not hunch your back or shrug your shoulders.
- Do not lock your knees. Keep your knees slightly bent at all times.
- Do not lock your elbows when you straighten your arms.
- Do not bend your wrists or neck.

MUSCLES TARGETED

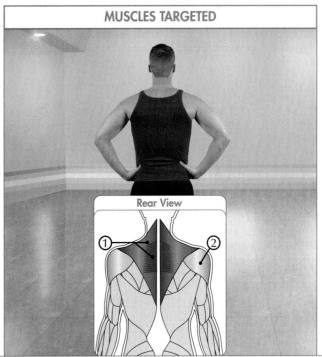

Rear View

Targeted muscles:
① upper back (*rhomboids* and *upper trapezius*)

Additional muscles:
② rear shoulders (*posterior deltoids*)

lateral raise

The lateral raise works your shoulders as well as your upper back. This is a good exercise for shaping and defining your shoulders. Using exercise tubing to perform lateral raises gives you a different resistance compared to using free weights. For more information on exercise tubing, see page 198.

You should perform the exercise slowly, without raising your arms too high or arching your back to help lift your arms. Also remember to keep your wrists straight

and your elbows and knees slightly bent throughout the exercise.

You should be careful performing lateral raises if you have neck or lower back problems. You should not perform this exercise if you have shoulder problems.

If you have back problems, you can help protect your back by performing the exercise while sitting on a bench or chair with back support. If the tubing is too loose when you are sitting, you can wrap the extra tubing around your hands to increase the tension.

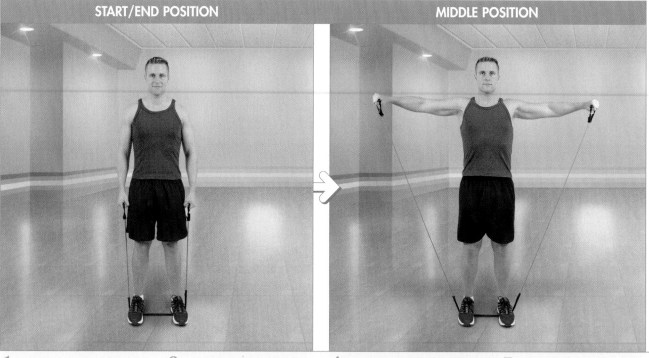

START/END POSITION

MIDDLE POSITION

1 Grasp a handle of the exercise tubing in each hand.

2 Stand straight on the middle of the tubing with both feet. Position your feet roughly shoulder width apart, knees slightly bent.

3 Start with your arms at your sides, your elbows slightly bent and both palms facing each other. Tighten your abdominal muscles to help protect your back.

4 Slowly raise your arms out to your sides until they are at shoulder height. Keep your elbows slightly bent and your palms facing down as you lift your arms.

5 Pause for a moment and then slowly lower your arms back to your sides.

Can I work only one arm at a time?

Yes. Perform the exercise as described in the steps below, except raise only one arm at a time, keeping your other arm at your side. You can change the resistance for each arm by repositioning yourself on the tubing. Standing closer to the handle of the arm you are working increases the resistance and standing farther away from the handle decreases the resistance. Working one arm at a time allows you to focus on strengthening each arm separately. This is useful when one arm is stronger than the other and you want to balance the strength in your arms.

How can I work the front of my shoulders more?

To work the front of your shoulders more, you can perform front raises instead of lateral raises. Perform the exercise as described in the steps below, except start with your palms facing the front of your thighs. Keeping your elbows slightly bent, raise your arms straight out in front of you until your hands are at shoulder height. Then lower your arms and repeat the exercise.

DON'T

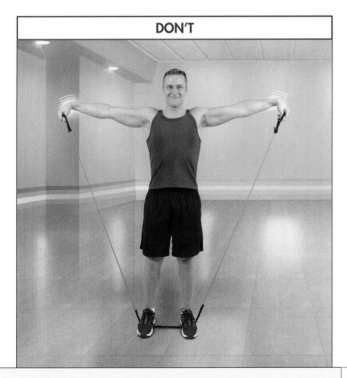

- Do not bend your wrists.
- Do not lock your elbows or knees. Keep your elbows and knees slightly bent.
- Do not raise your arms above your shoulders.
- Do not arch your back or swing your body back and forth to help lift your arms. Keep your back straight at all times.

MUSCLES TARGETED

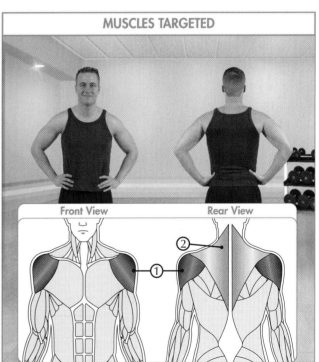

Front View   Rear View

Targeted muscles:
① middle shoulders (*middle deltoids*)

Additional muscles:
② upper back (*upper trapezius*)

external rotation

The external rotation works your rotator cuff muscles, which are located deep in your shoulders. Strengthening your rotator cuff muscles can help you perform better in racquet sports and in sports that involve throwing objects. This exercise can also help maintain stability within your shoulder joints.

You need to use exercise tubing to perform the external rotation shown in the steps below. For more information on exercise tubing, see page 198. To perform this exercise, you will need to wrap the tubing around a stable object, such as a stair banister at home, a door handle or a weight machine at a gym. You may need to take a few steps away from the object to help create tension in the tubing.

Performing the external rotation can help prevent shoulder injuries and is also beneficial for people who are recovering from shoulder injuries. However, you should be careful performing the external rotation if you have a recent injury to your rotator cuff muscles.

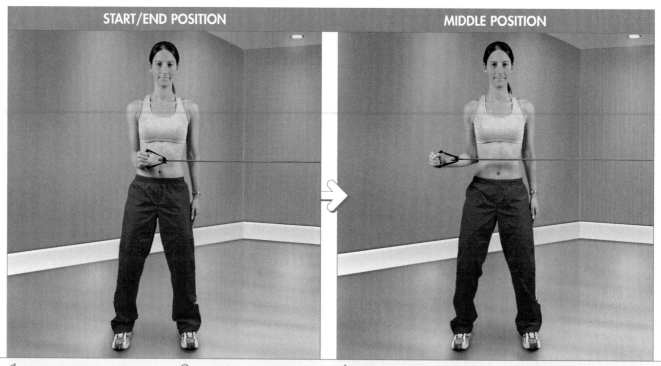

START/END POSITION

MIDDLE POSITION

1 Wrap the exercise tubing around a stable object and push one handle of the tubing through the other handle so the end of the tubing is looped around the object. Position the tubing at waist level. Grasp the handle of the tubing with your right hand.

2 Stand with your left side facing the object, feet roughly shoulder width apart and knees slightly bent.

3 Position your right elbow at your side, arm bent at a 90-degree angle and palm facing your body.

4 While keeping your upper right arm stationary, slowly move your hand away from your body as far as you can without moving your upper arm. Tighten your abdominal muscles to help protect your back.

5 Pause for a moment and then slowly return your hand to the starting position.

6 After completing a set with your right arm, switch sides and repeat the exercise with your left arm.

What other rotator cuff exercise can I perform using tubing?

You can perform the internal rotation. With the tubing wrapped around a stable object, grasp the tubing handle with your right hand and stand with your right side facing the object and your feet shoulder width apart. Position your right elbow at your side, bent at a 90-degree angle, with your hand out to the side and your palm facing forward. Without moving your upper arm, bring your right hand toward your stomach. Pause for a moment and then bring your hand back to the starting position. This exercise works a different part of your rotator cuff muscles.

How can I make this exercise harder?

To make the exercise harder, step on one end of the tubing with your right foot and stand with your feet shoulder width apart. Grasp the handle on the other end of the tubing with your right hand. Keep your right upper arm parallel to the floor and your elbow pointing to the side, bent at a 90-degree angle. Starting with your palm facing the floor, raise your right forearm until your palm is facing forward and then bring your forearm back to the starting position.

DON'T

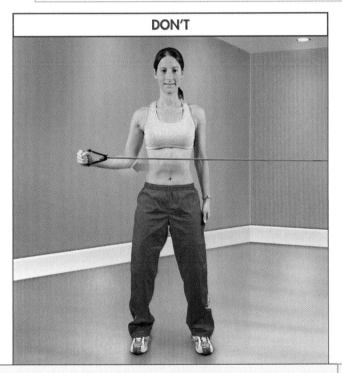

- Do not lift your elbow off your side.
- Do not bend your wrist.
- Do not twist your body as you move your hand. Keep your body stationary.

MUSCLES TARGETED

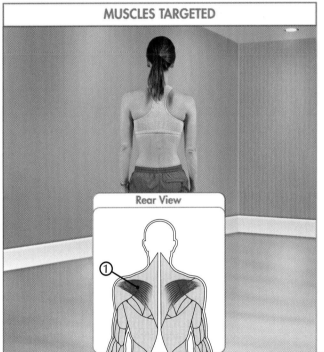

Rear View

Targeted muscles:
① deep shoulder muscles (*rotator cuff*)

tricep extension

The tricep extension focuses on toning and strengthening your triceps. This exercise allows you to focus on working one arm at a time. You need to use exercise tubing to perform the tricep extension shown in the steps below. For more information on exercise tubing, see page 198.

As you perform the tricep extension, try to keep your back straight and your abdominal muscles tight to help protect your back. You should also try to keep your upper arm stationary and your knees slightly

bent at all times. Do not bend your wrist or lock your elbow as you straighten your arm.

As with any other exercise, perform the tricep extension in a slow, controlled manner to get the most out of the exercise and to avoid injury.

If you have neck or wrist problems, you should be careful when performing the tricep extension. Do not perform this exercise if you have shoulder or elbow problems.

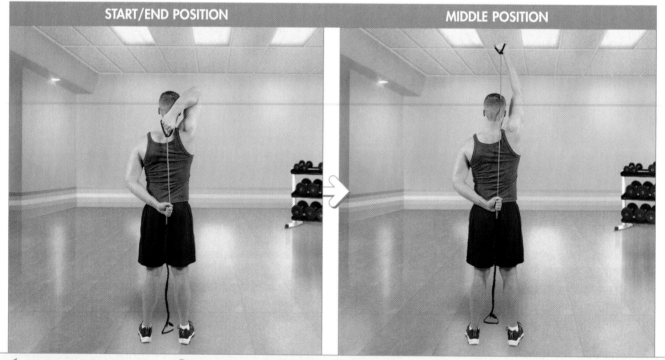

| START/END POSITION | MIDDLE POSITION |

1 Grasp a handle of the exercise tubing in your right hand.

2 Stand straight with your feet roughly shoulder width apart and your knees slightly bent. Tighten your abdominal muscles to help protect your back.

3 Bend your right arm and point your elbow toward the ceiling with your palm facing the back of your head.

4 Bend your left arm and grasp the tubing behind your back, palm facing backward.

5 Slowly straighten your arm to raise your hand above your head.

6 Pause for a moment and then slowly bend your arm to lower your hand back to the starting position.

7 After completing a set with your right arm, repeat the exercise with your left arm.

I have neck problems. Is there an easier tricep exercise I can perform?

Yes. Stand in the middle of the tubing with your feet shoulder width apart and knees slightly bent. With your palm facing your body, grasp a handle in your right hand and bend forward from your hips at a 45-degree angle. Keep your right upper arm against your side with your arm bent at 90 degrees and place your left hand on your left thigh. Keeping your upper arm stationary, straighten your right arm and then bend your arm back to the starting position.

How can I work both arms at the same time?

To work both arms at the same time, stand with your feet a few inches apart and your knees slightly bent. Step on one end of the tubing and then bring the tubing up along your back. Using both hands, grasp the handle of the tubing with your palms facing back and your elbows bent and pointing toward the ceiling. Straighten your arms until your hands are above your head and then bend your arms to lower your hands back to the starting position.

DON'T

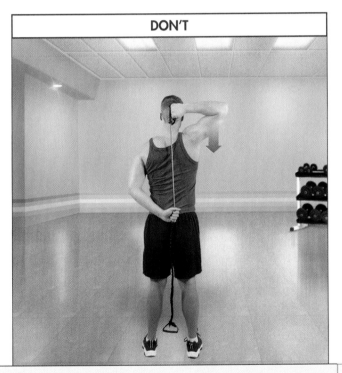

- Do not move your upper arm when you raise and lower your hand.
- Do not lock your elbow when you straighten your arm.
- Do not bend your wrist.
- Do not lock your knees. Keep your knees slightly bent.
- Do not arch your back.

MUSCLES TARGETED

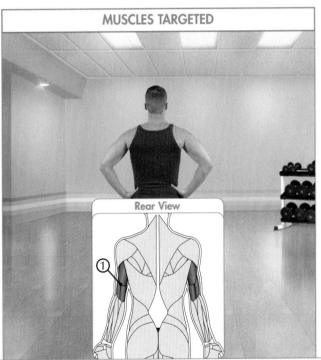

Rear View

Targeted muscles:
① triceps

biceps curl

The biceps curl strengthens and tones your biceps, as well as your forearms. You should be careful performing this exercise if you have elbow or wrist problems. Strong biceps help you lift heavy objects more easily.

Using exercise tubing to perform curls gives you a different resistance compared to using weights and is a good way to vary your routine. For more information on exercise tubing, see page 198.

Before you start the exercise, you should make sure

you stand in the middle of the exercise tubing to ensure you have equal resistance for both arms. As you perform the curls, keep your upper arms stable and hold your elbows close to your sides, without digging them into your body for support. As with all exercises, concentrate on keeping your movements slow and controlled as you lift and lower your arms. Try to perform the full range of movement for each repetition, lifting all the way up until the tubing is taut and lowering all the way down without locking your elbows.

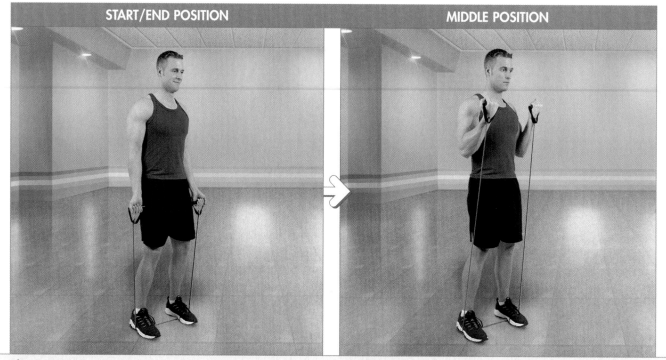

START/END POSITION

MIDDLE POSITION

1 Grasp a handle of the exercise tubing in each hand.

2 Stand on the middle of the tubing with both feet. Position your feet roughly shoulder width apart, knees slightly bent.

3 Start with your arms at your sides, your elbows slightly bent and both palms facing forward. Tighten your abdominal muscles to help protect your back.

4 Keeping your elbows close to your sides, slowly bend your arms to raise your hands toward your shoulders.

• Make sure you keep your back straight and your head up.

5 Slowly straighten your arms to lower your hands back to the starting position.

QUESTION & ANSWER

How can I work only one arm at a time?

Perform the exercise as described in the steps below, except alternate between lifting your left arm and your right arm. You can also hold only one handle of the exercise tubing and perform curls while your other arm is resting at your side. When performing this last variation, you can increase the resistance for each arm by standing closer to the handle of the arm you are working, or standing farther away from the handle for less resistance.

Is there a harder variation of the exercise that I can perform?

Yes. Perform the exercise as described in the steps below, except hold both handles of the exercise tubing in your left hand. Standing on the tubing with your feet slightly closer than shoulder width apart, slowly raise and lower your left hand to perform the exercise. After completing a set with your left arm, switch arms and then repeat the exercise with your right arm.

DON'T

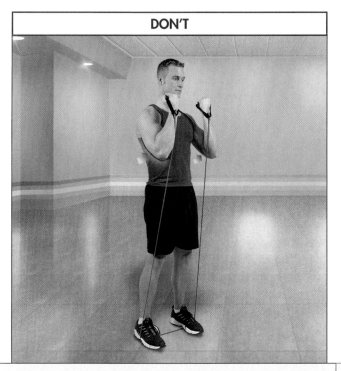

- Do not move your upper arms. Keep your upper arms stationary and close to your body.

- Do not dig your elbows into your sides or arch your back to help you raise your hands.

- Do not shrug your shoulders or bend your wrists.

- Do not lock your knees or lock your elbows when you straighten your arms.

MUSCLES TARGETED

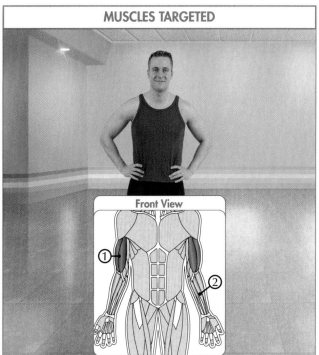

Front View

Targeted muscles:
① biceps

Additional muscles:
② forearm flexors

abdominal crunch

The abdominal crunch focuses on tightening, toning and strengthening your front abdominal muscles, but also works your side abdominal muscles. You need to use exercise tubing to perform this exercise. For more information on exercise tubing, see page 198.

Remember to maintain proper form when performing the exercise. Keep your elbows out to your sides and your feet on the mat. As you curl your head and shoulders off the mat, you should avoid bending your neck forward.

As your abdominal muscles become stronger, you can try lifting your shoulders higher off the ground. You can also grasp the tubing rather than the handles if you want to increase the tension in the tubing.

If you have neck problems, you should be careful when performing this exercise.

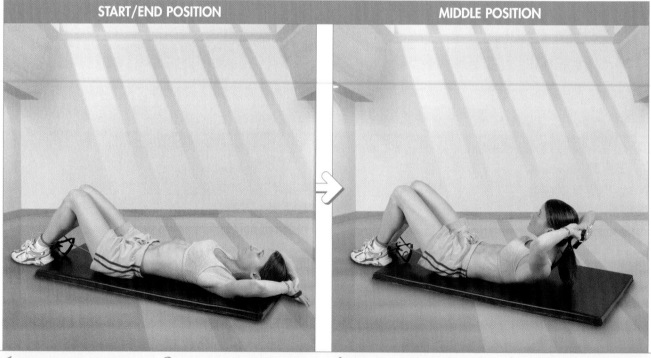

START/END POSITION → **MIDDLE POSITION**

1 Push one handle of the exercise tubing through the other handle to create a loop at one end of the tubing. Place the loop around both ankles.

2 Lie on your back on a mat, with your knees bent and your feet together.

3 Position the tubing under your back and grasp the handle of the tubing behind your head with both hands, palms facing up.

4 Push your lower back into the mat and tighten your abdominal muscles.

5 While keeping your elbows out to the sides, slowly curl your head and shoulders a few inches off the mat.

6 Pause for a moment and then slowly lower your head and shoulders back to the starting position.

Is there a way to make this exercise harder?

Yes. To make this exercise harder, you can perform the exercise with your legs lifted off the floor and your knees bent at 90-degree angles. Make sure to keep your thighs perpendicular to the floor as you perform the exercise. Lifting your legs off the floor makes your muscles work harder by increasing the tension in the tubing and engaging the lower part of your front abdominal muscles to work.

How can I put more focus on my side abdominal muscles?

You can perform the twist crunch to put more focus on your side abdominal muscles. Position yourself in the same starting position as described in the steps below and then slowly curl your head and shoulders a few inches off the mat toward your right knee. Pause for a moment and then slowly lower your head and shoulders back to the starting position. After completing a set toward your right knee, repeat the exercise toward your left knee.

DON'T

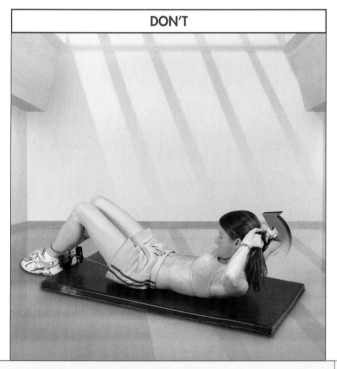

- Do not bend your neck forward as you curl your head and shoulders off the mat.

- Do not move your arms. Keep your elbows out to the sides.

- Do not lift your feet off the mat.

MUSCLES TARGETED

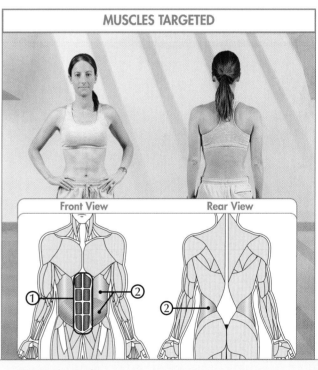

Front View   Rear View

Targeted muscles:
① front abdominal muscles *(rectus abdominis)*

Additional muscles:
② side abdominal muscles *(internal and external obliques)*

Section 5

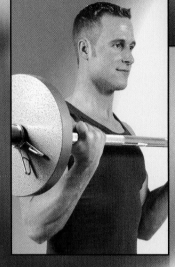

Now that you know how to perform weight training exercises, you can set up a weight routine that will help meet your fitness goals. Section 5 provides the information you need to set up a routine to ensure you weight train effectively. For example, you will learn how many times to lift a weight, how long you should rest between exercises and how to prevent and treat injuries. This section also provides sample routines to get you started.

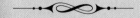

Design a Weight Routine

In this Section...

Design a Weight Routine

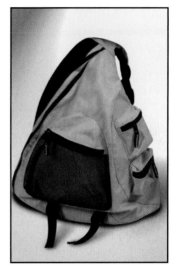

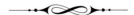

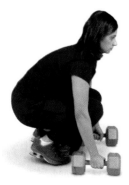

weight routine basics

Repetitions

A repetition, or rep, is the basic element used in weight training. One repetition of a weight training exercise usually consists of an up movement and a down movement. For example, when performing the dumbbell curl, lifting the dumbbell up to your shoulders and then lowering it back to the starting position counts as one repetition. You should be careful not to perform repetitions too quickly, as this can result in joint injury. As a general rule, a complete repetition should take about 4 to 6 seconds. You should take 2 to 3 seconds to raise the weight, pause for a moment, and then take 2 to 3 seconds to lower the weight.

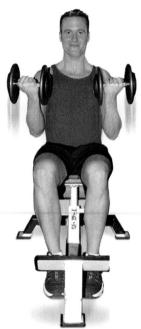

Sets

A series of consecutive repetitions is called a set. The number of sets and repetitions you should perform depends on your goals.

If you are new to weight training, start by doing 1 or 2 sets of 12 to 15 repetitions and then increase to about 3 sets in a month or two. If you are already in shape, performing 1 to 2 sets is enough to maintain your strength.

As you perform an exercise, you should try to move smoothly from one repetition to the next until you complete a set.

Rest Between Sets

After completing a set, you should give your muscles time to recover before performing another set. To determine the amount of rest to take between sets, consider your goals. If you are lifting heavy weights to develop strength and power, you should rest for about 2 to 5 minutes between sets. If you are using moderate weights for building muscle size, rest for 1 to 2 minutes. If you are using lighter weights for building muscle tone and endurance, rest for 30 seconds to 1 minute.

For most people, 60 to 90 seconds is usually enough recuperation time between sets. Resting for too long will allow your muscles to cool down, which can result in injury when you resume your workout. For variety, you can vary the amount of rest between sets, but keep in mind that the less rest you take, the less weight you will be able to lift in the next set.

Amount of Weight

It is important to use the correct amount of weight for each exercise to prevent injury and maximize results. You should choose a weight that allows you to complete the desired number of repetitions with proper form, while fatiguing the muscles enough to make the last 2 to 3 repetitions of a set challenging. When you lift weights that are too heavy, you risk muscle injury or losing control of the weight and dropping it. Larger muscles, such as those in your legs, can generally lift more weight than smaller muscles, such as the muscles in your arms.

You may need to try a number of different weights with an exercise before finding the right one. Do not feel forced to complete a set with weights that are too light or too heavy. If necessary, you can add or remove weight during a set. Start an exercise with a light weight and then gradually increase to a more challenging weight. When you can complete each set without feeling tired for the last 2 or 3 reps, you can increase the weight.

Proper Form

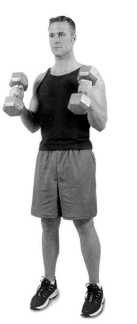

Using proper form for each repetition is crucial to getting the maximum benefit from an exercise and avoiding injury. To help maintain proper form throughout an exercise, you can perform the exercise in front of a mirror. Keep in mind that how well you lift the weight is more important than the amount of weight you lift.

Work Every Major Muscle Group

Although you do not need to work all your muscles on the same day, you should make sure your weight training routine includes at least one exercise for each major muscle group, 2 to 3 times per week. Omitting a major muscle group can lead to injury or make your body look out of proportion. Your weight training program should focus on all of the following major muscle groups:

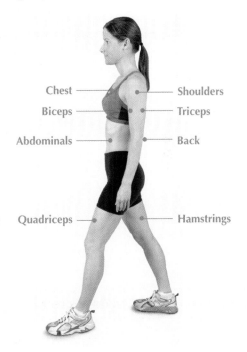

Chest — Shoulders
Biceps — Triceps
Abdominals — Back
Quadriceps — Hamstrings

Proper Breathing

Breathing properly helps you lift weights more efficiently and contributes to regulating your blood pressure as you weight train. You should exhale deeply through your mouth during the hardest part of an exercise and inhale normally through your nose during the least difficult part.

weight routine basics

Warm Up

Warming up before weight training increases blood flow to your muscles, making them more flexible so you can perform exercises with greater ease and avoid injury. About 5 minutes of cardiovascular exercise, such as running at an easy pace, is sufficient to warm up. If you will be working a specific muscle especially hard, you may want to use a light weight for the first set to further warm up the muscle.

Perform Exercises in the Right Order

To work your muscles efficiently, consider the order in which you perform exercises. It is generally best to work larger muscles before smaller ones.

Think of your body as divided into an upper, middle and lower section. If you are performing a full body workout, you should work your lower section, then your upper section and then your midsection. Work the muscles within each section in the following order:

LOWER BODY
1 Quadriceps and hamstrings
2 Inner thighs
3 Buttocks
4 Hip flexors and outer hips
5 Calves and shins

UPPER BODY
1 Chest, upper and middle back
2 Shoulders
3 Biceps and triceps
4 Forearms

MIDDLE BODY
1 Abdominals and lower back

Rest Muscles for at least 48 Hours

To become stronger, your muscles need time to recuperate after a workout. It is actually during the rest period, rather than during the workout, that muscles gain strength, so overworking your muscles is counter-productive. You should never work the same muscle two days in a row, since working your muscles before they have adequately recovered can result in injury. Instead, allow your muscles at least 48 hours rest between workouts.

Cool Down

Cooling down helps to release the tension in your muscles and flush out waste products that build up during your workout. Generally, if your workout was slow with lots of rest between sets, you can stretch for a few minutes to cool down. However, after a fast-paced weight training workout, perform about 5 minutes of light cardiovascular exercise to get rid of built-up lactic acid in your muscles to help prevent soreness after your workout. You should then stretch for a few minutes.

Schedule

How you structure your weight training schedule depends on many factors, including your time, goals and how hard you train. The harder you train, the more recovery time you will need between workouts. For best results, try to work out between 3 to 4 days a week. Beginners should aim for 3 sessions per week, performing a full-body workout at each session. If you can manage only 2 days per week, this can be enough to maintain your current strength levels. Keep in mind that if you wait too long between sessions, you risk losing gains you made in previous workouts.

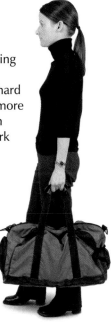

Weight Training Routine

A weight training routine, or program, consists of all the elements of a weight training session, including the equipment used, rest periods, exercise order and the exercises you perform. Your routine should be customized for your specific needs, taking into account your goals and the amount of time you can allot to each session. A good routine should include a variety of exercises and should be adaptable as you progress.

TRADITIONAL VERSUS FUNCTIONAL WEIGHT TRAINING

Your routine should incorporate both traditional and functional weight training. Traditional weight training exercises isolate individual muscles to build size and strength. Functional weight training exercises work multiple muscle groups at once. Including both types of exercises balances your weight training program.

Weight Training Progression

To increase your strength, you need to increase the intensity of your exercises periodically. You would generally start by weight training about 2 or 3 times a week, working all the major muscle groups by performing 1 to 2 sets of 12 to 15 repetitions for each exercise. After a month or two, when the exercises become less challenging and you fail to achieve muscle fatigue during the last 1 or 2 repetitions in a set, you can increase to 3 sets for each exercise. In a few more weeks, you can increase the amount of weight for each exercise. When you first start weight training, it is generally better to start with weight machines and add free weight exercises as you progress. Also, consider changing the exercises in your routine every 4 to 6 weeks. This is a good way to keep challenging your muscles so they do not get used to the same movements. To progress further, you can explore more advanced types of weight training, such as split training.

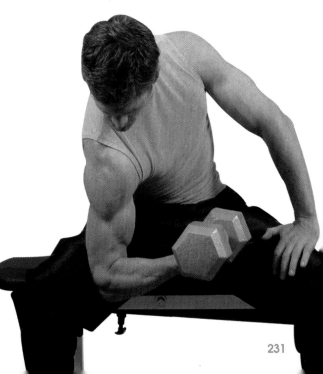

sample weight routines

The routines shown here are samples you can use to structure a customized routine. When you first start weight training, it is generally better to start with weight machines (if you have access to them) and then add free weight exercises as you progress. Beginners can start by training 2 to 3 times a week. The entire workout should take about 20 to 30 minutes to complete.

Sample Beginner Routine 1

1
leg press
Quadriceps and Hamstrings
Page 132

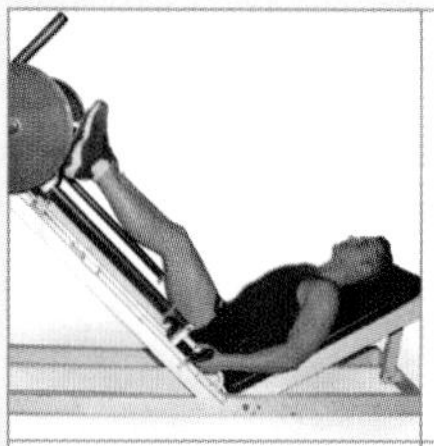

2
leg curl
Hamstrings
Page 136

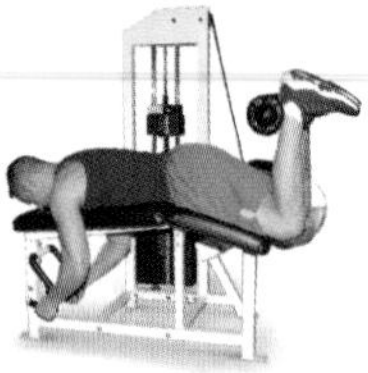

3
leg extension
Quadriceps
Page 134

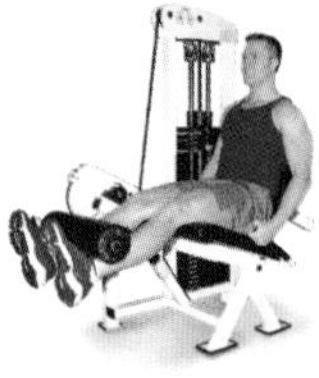

4
seated calf raise machine
Calves
Page 160

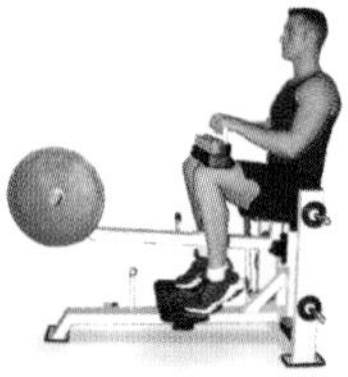

5
lat pulldown
Back
Page 62

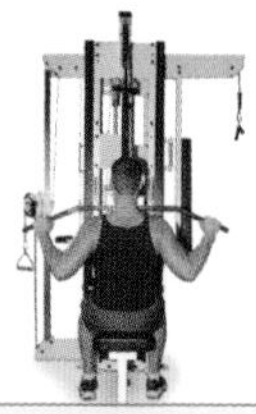

6
chest press machine
Chest
Page 40

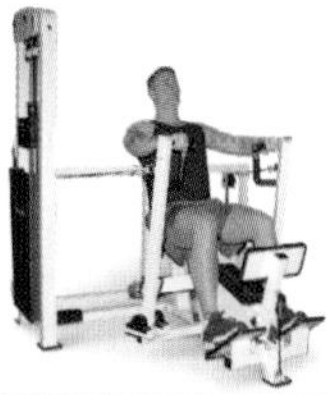

7
shoulder press machine
Shoulders
Page 56

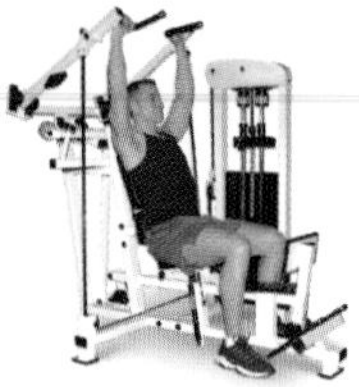

8
triceps extension machine
Triceps
Page 90

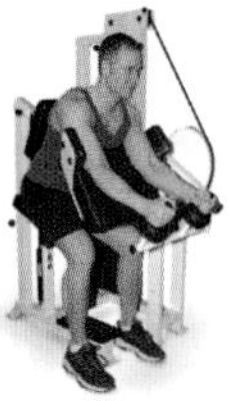

9
arm curl machine
Biceps
Page 104

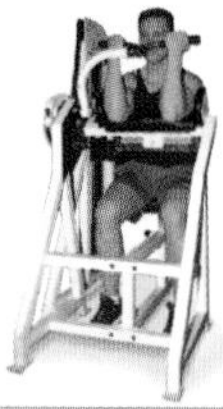

10
abdominal machine
Abdominals
Page 114

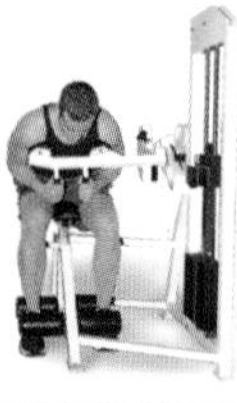

How do I know if I'm using the correct amount of weight?

You should feel a burning sensation in your muscles at the end of each set. This sensation, called the "burn," is caused by an accumulation of lactic acid in your muscles when they are exerted. The burn is harmless and the sensation usually disappears a few seconds after you finish the exercise.

Sample Beginner Routine 2

1 wall squat
(with exercise ball)

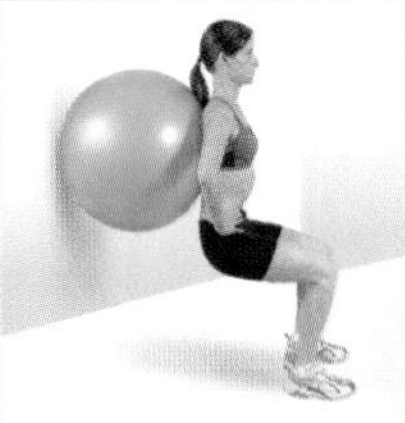

Quadriceps
Page 170

2 lunge

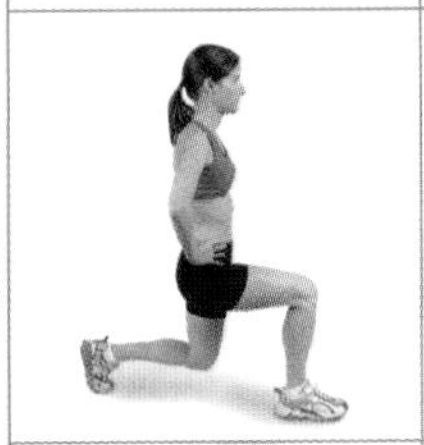

Quadriceps and Hamstrings
Page 138

3 single-leg
calf raise

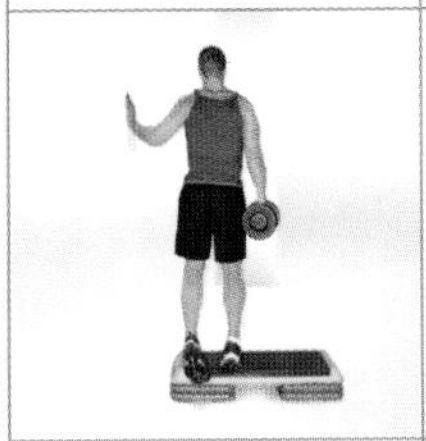

Calves
Page 162

4 push-up

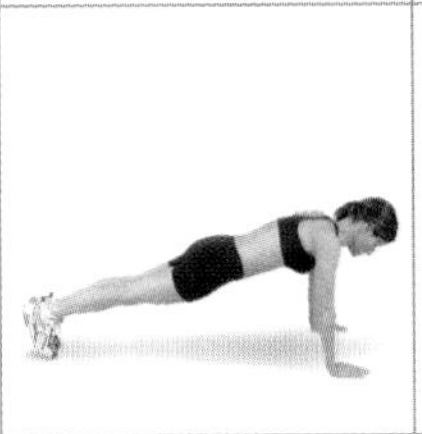

Chest and Triceps
Page 36

5 bent over row
(with exercise tubing)

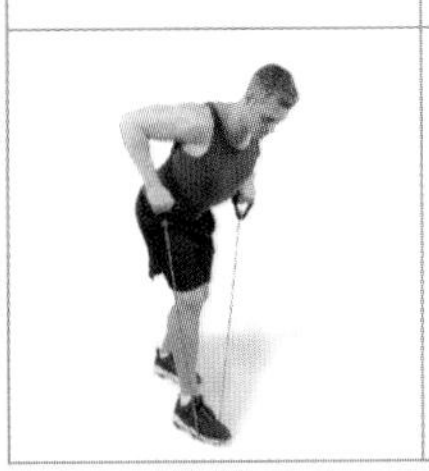

Upper Back
Page 214

6 bench dip

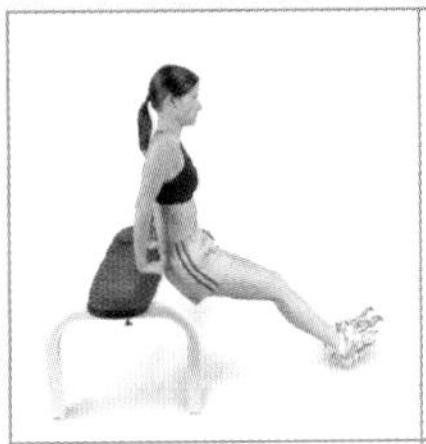

Triceps
Page 78

7 lateral raise

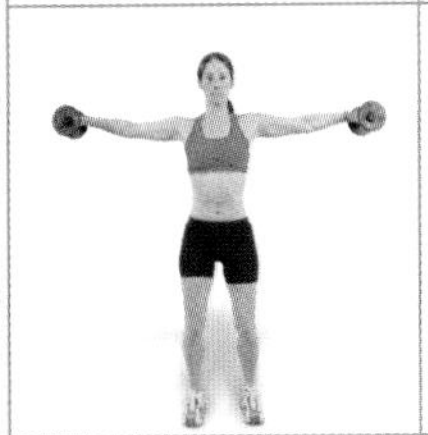

Shoulders
Page 48

8 seated
dumbbell curl

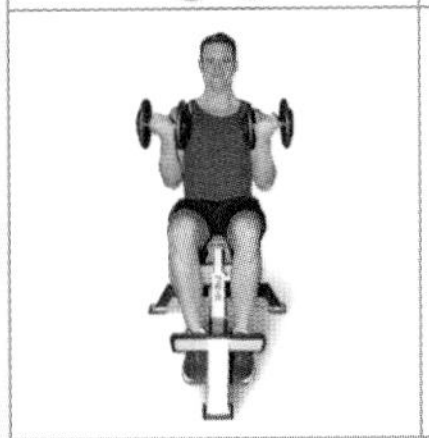

Biceps
Page 92

9 back extension
(with exercise ball)

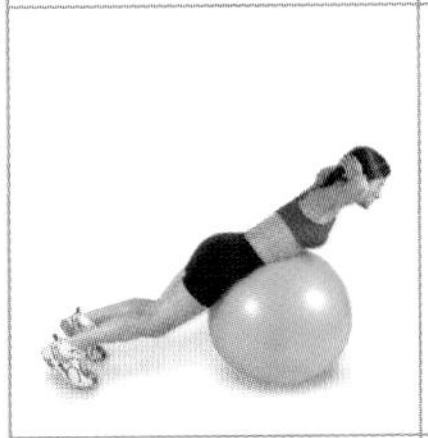

Lower Back
Page 196

10 abdominal crunch

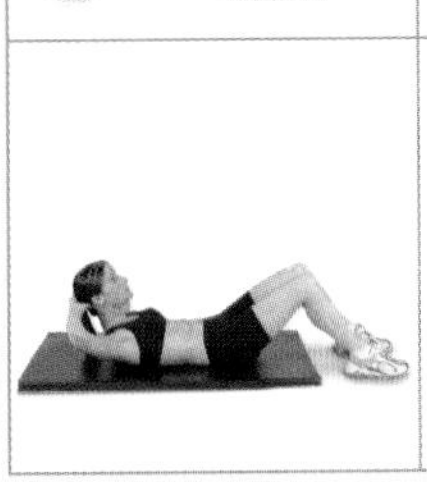

Abdominals
Page 108

sample weight routines

Once you are comfortable performing the beginner routines, you may feel you are ready to perform one of the intermediate routines shown here. For an intermediate routine, the number of sets, repetitions and workouts you should perform each week depends on your goals.

Sample Intermediate Routine 1

1

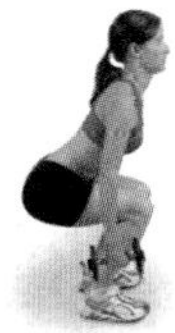

dumbbell squat
Quadriceps and Hamstrings
Page 126

2

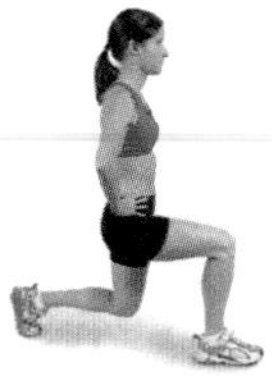

lunge
Quadriceps and Hamstrings
Page 138

3

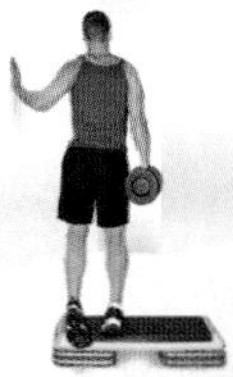

single-leg calf raise
Calves
Page 162

4

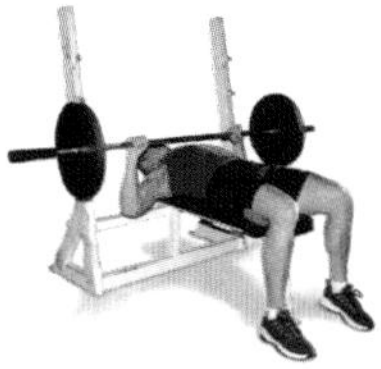

barbell bench press
Chest
Page 32

5

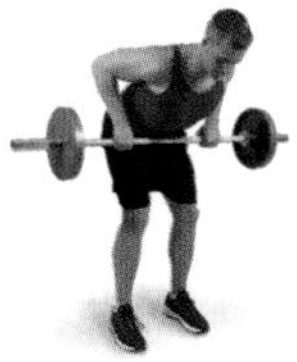

bent over barbell row
Back
Page 66

6

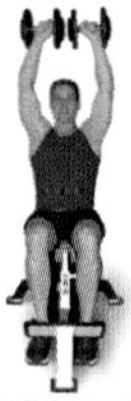

dumbbell shoulder press
Shoulders and Upper Back
Page 46

7

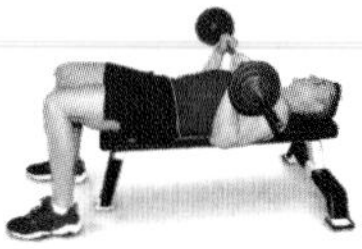

barbell triceps press
Triceps
Page 84

8

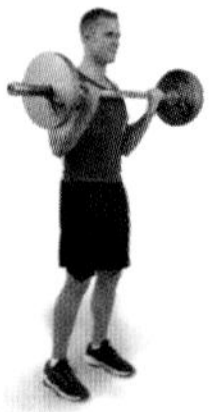

barbell curl
Biceps
Page 94

9

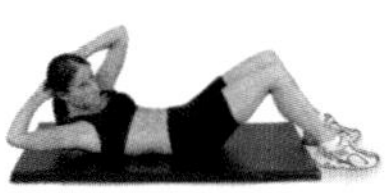

twist crunch
Side and Front Abdominals
Page 110

10

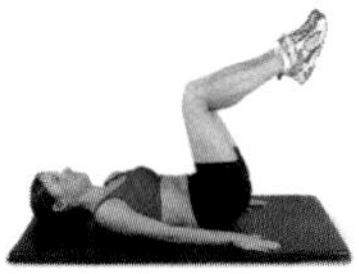

reverse crunch
Front Abdominals
Page 112

Sample Intermediate Routine 2

1
barbell squat
Quadriceps and Hamstrings
Page 128

2
barbell deadlift
Hamstrings and Buttocks
Page 142

3
calf press
Calves
Page 164

4
one-arm dumbbell row
Back
Page 64

5
dumbbell fly
Chest
Page 34

6
lateral raise
Shoulders
Page 48

7
dumbbell overhead triceps extension
Triceps
Page 86

8
concentration curl
Biceps
Page 96

9
plank
Abdominals and Lower Back
Page 118

10
leg raise
Front Abdominals
Page 116

super slow, negatives, drop sets and pyramids

There are several effective techniques you can use to enhance your weight training workouts.

Super Slow

The super slow technique is based on slowing down your movements to prevent momentum and achieve the maximum contraction from your muscles. When using this technique, you take a minimum of 4 seconds to lift the weight (positive phase) and a minimum of 4 seconds to return the weight to the starting position (negative phase). Increasing the amount of time you take to lift and lower the weight makes the exercise more difficult, especially when you increase the time for the lowering phase. The time taken for the negative and the positive phases does not need to be the same. For example, you can take 5 seconds to lift and 10 seconds to lower. You can perform 4 to 8 repetitions per set.

Using the super slow technique helps prevent injury to your joints, makes it easier for you to maintain proper form and results in faster strength gains. However, you will not be able to lift heavy weight.

You can perform a super slow set once a week for each muscle. For each exercise, you would perform one set using the super slow technique and then perform all other sets normally.

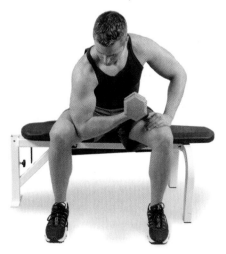

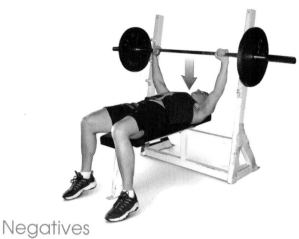

Negatives

When you perform negatives, you emphasize the negative phase of a weight training exercise. In weight training, the lifting movement is called the positive phase and the lowering movement to return the weight to the starting position is called the negative phase.

Since you can generally lower more weight than you can lift, this technique allows you to use heavier weight than usual, using a spotter to help you lift the weight. After the spotter helps you lift the weight, you are then left on your own to concentrate on lowering the weight to the starting position in a slow, controlled motion. Take about 4 to 10 seconds to lower and then repeat until you complete a set.

Performing negatives helps to increase your strength and is a good way to get familiar with handling heavier weight. You can do negatives once every week or two to increase your strength gains.

You need to be particularly careful when performing this technique with free weights, since heavier weights increase your risk of injury from dropping the weight or using incorrect form. Using a machine to perform negatives reduces the risk of injury. Keep in mind that concentrating on the negative phase also places a lot of stress on your muscles, which increases the amount of muscle soreness that can occur after your workout.

Drop Sets

When you perform drop sets, you start with heavy weight and reduce the weight each time your muscles reach failure so you can perform additional repetitions. To perform one drop set, you start by completing as many repetitions as possible with heavy weight and you continue to reduce the weight until you reach a weight that allows you to perform about 15 repetitions.

You would usually reduce the weight a minimum of three times during each drop set. For example, you can perform 6 to 8 repetitions with heavy weight, reduce the weight and perform 10 repetitions, reduce the weight again and perform 12 repetitions, and then reduce the weight and perform 15 repetitions. You should aim for 2 to 3 drop sets for each exercise, resting for at least 2 minutes between drop sets.

Drop sets are useful when you want to vary your routine so your muscles do not get used to being worked the same way. You can perform drop sets as the last exercise for a muscle group to help tone and define the muscles worked. For example, you can perform drop sets for your last tricep exercise.

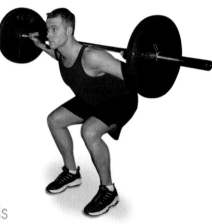

Pyramids

To exercise using pyramids, you start with light weight for the first set of an exercise and then gradually move to heavier weight for each successive set. Then you work backwards, decreasing the weight so that you perform the last set of the exercise with the same amount of weight you used for the first set.

You can perform about 12 to 15 repetitions when using light weight and about 4 to 6 repetitions when using heavy weight. Aim to perform 6 to 10 sets to complete a pyramid, resting 1 to 2 minutes between pyramids. If you are using a machine, you can increase or decrease the weight by roughly one plate each time. When using free weights, you can use increments of about 5 pounds.

There are two main types of pyramids: ascending and descending. Ascending pyramids involve using light weight for the first set of an exercise and gradually increasing the weight with each successive set until you reach about 4 to 6 repetitions for the last set. This is the most common type of pyramid. Descending pyramids involve starting with heavy weight and then moving to lighter weight for each successive set until you reach about 12 to 15 repetitions for the last set. Before starting descending pyramids, make sure you warm up your muscles properly. Descending pyramids are more difficult than ascending pyramids, but will result in greater strength gains.

Performing pyramids is great for building muscle strength and mass. You can perform pyramids for every weight training exercise and at every session.

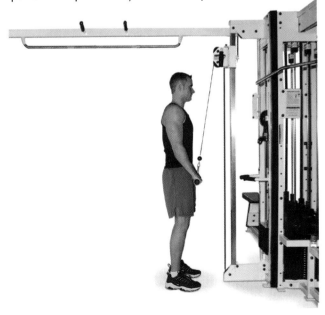

circuit training

Circuit training involves performing a series of exercises one after the other without taking a break between exercises. One weight training circuit normally includes 8 to 12 exercises. You perform 1 set of 10 to 15 repetitions for each exercise. After performing 1 circuit, you can rest for about 2 minutes and then move on to the next circuit until you complete 2 to 4 circuits.

You can include free weight or machine exercises, or a combination of both. For full-body circuits, make sure you include an exercise for every major muscle group. You can complete 1 circuit training workout a week as part of your routine.

Circuit training can allow you to work out more efficiently in a shorter time and is a great way to change your routine. This is also a good way to build muscular endurance and achieve weight loss. You may find it difficult to circuit train effectively at a gym, since the machines or weights may not be readily available and changing settings on machines can take time.

Circuit Training Considerations

To ensure that one muscle group will not fatigue too quickly, you should structure your circuit training workout so you do not perform 2 exercises in a row that work the same muscle group. You can alternate between your upper and lower body or you can work opposing muscle groups in the same section of the body, such as back and chest or hamstrings and quadriceps. Also try to work larger muscle groups, such as quadriceps, hamstrings, back and chest, before smaller muscle groups, such as triceps, biceps, shoulders and calves.

When switching between exercises in different positions, such as lying and standing, be cautious about moving too quickly, since this can cause dizziness.

Keep in mind that the fast pace of circuit training is based on skipping the rest between sets, not on speeding up repetitions. Perform each repetition in a slow, controlled manner, as you would during regular workouts. You will also need to use less weight when circuit training.

Circuit Training Variations

You can vary your circuit training workout by split training, which involves working different sections of your body on different days. For example, you can perform a circuit that works your upper body on Monday and Wednesday and then perform a lower body circuit on Tuesday and Thursday.

You can also incorporate cardiovascular training into your strength training circuit to burn fat. After every 1 or 2 weight training exercises, you can perform 2 to 4 minutes of a high-intensity cardiovascular exercise, such as cycling, jumping rope, jumping jacks, running or using a cardio machine.

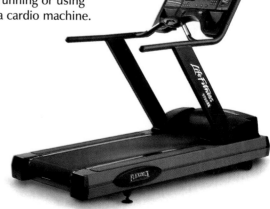

Sample Circuit Training Routine

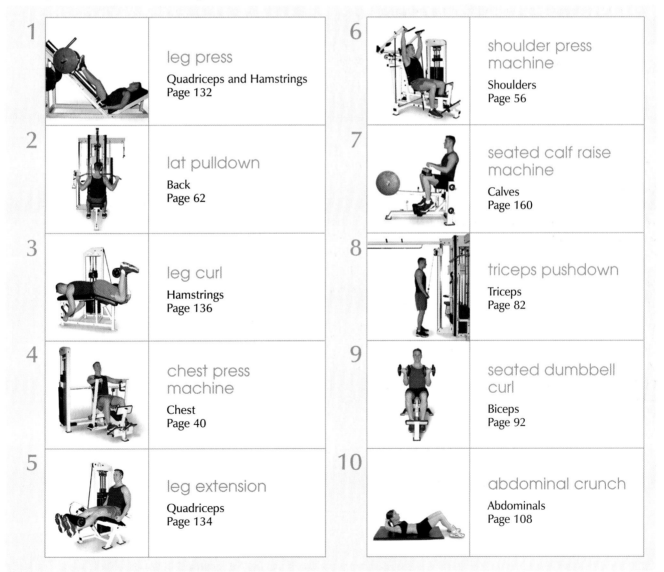

1 leg press

Quadriceps and Hamstrings
Page 132

2 lat pulldown

Back
Page 62

3 leg curl

Hamstrings
Page 136

4 chest press machine

Chest
Page 40

5 leg extension

Quadriceps
Page 134

6 shoulder press machine

Shoulders
Page 56

7 seated calf raise machine

Calves
Page 160

8 triceps pushdown

Triceps
Page 82

9 seated dumbbell curl

Biceps
Page 92

10 abdominal crunch

Abdominals
Page 108

split routines

A split routine is a training program you can use to work different body parts or muscle groups on separate days. You can divide your body into different parts, such as upper and lower body, or into different types of muscles, such as pushing and pulling muscles. You exercise only one part or group of muscles at each workout, making sure you do not work the same muscles two days in a row.

Split routines allow you to take two or more days to complete a total body workout, which is helpful if you

want to perform multiple exercises for each body part or muscle group at each session. This type of routine can help you gain strength faster and may work well for people who can work out several days a week, but for only a short time each day. Shorter and more frequent workouts can also help prevent fatigue or boredom and keep you motivated.

You should make sure you work each muscle group or body part at least 2 to 3 times a week.

Upper and Lower Body Split

An upper and lower body split routine is based on working your upper body and lower body on alternate days. This allows you to rest your muscles between workouts. For example, you can

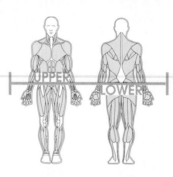

work your upper body on Monday and Thursday and your lower body on Tuesday and Friday. You can work your abdominals during either the upper or lower body workout.

SAMPLE EXERCISES

	MUSCLES TARGETED	EXERCISES
UPPER BODY	Back	Lat Pulldown, Bent Over Barbell Row
	Chest	Barbell Bench Press, Dumbbell Fly
	Shoulders	Dumbbell Shoulder Press, Reverse Fly
	Biceps	Standing Barbell Curl
	Triceps	Dumbbell Overhead Triceps Extension
	Lower Back	Back Extension on a Roman Chair
LOWER BODY	Quadriceps and Hamstrings	Leg Press, Lunge
	Quadriceps	Leg Extension
	Hamstrings	Leg Curl
	Buttocks and Outer Hips	Hip Abduction Machine
	Inner Thighs	Hip Adduction Machine
	Calves	Standing Calf Raise Machine
	Abdominals	Abdominal Machine, Reverse Crunch

SAMPLE OF A WEEKLY ROUTINE

DAY 1	Upper Body
DAY 2	Rest
DAY 3	Lower Body
DAY 4	Rest
DAY 5	Upper Body
DAY 6	Rest
DAY 7	Lower Body

Push and Pull Split

This routine separates your upper body muscles into two groups: muscles that push and muscles that pull. You work pushing muscles one day and pulling muscles the next. Make sure you do not work the same muscle group two days in a row.

Pushing muscles are used in exercises that move the weight away from you, such as bench press, while pulling muscles work in exercises that bring the weight toward you, such as lat pulldown.

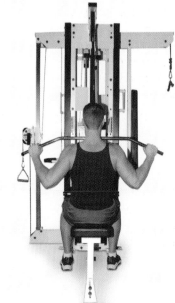

Pushing exercises work your chest and triceps and pulling exercises work your back and biceps. The shoulder muscles fit into both categories.

You can perform shoulder, lower body and abdominal exercises on a separate day or on a day when you work either of the pushing or pulling muscle groups.

SAMPLE EXERCISES

MUSCLES TARGETED	EXERCISES
Chest	Assisted Dip, Dumbbell Bench Press, Pec Fly Machine, Cable Crossover
Triceps	Lying Barbell Triceps Extension, Dumbbell Overhead Triceps Extension, Triceps Pushdown
Back	Assisted Chin-Up, One-Arm Dumbbell Row, Upright Row, Dumbbell Shrug
Biceps	Preacher Curl, Seated Dumbbell Curl, Concentration Curl
Quadriceps and Hamstrings	Hack Squat, Lunge
Quadriceps	Leg Extension
Hamstrings	Leg Curl, Barbell Deadlift
Shoulders	Dumbbell Shoulder Press, Front Raise, Bent Over Lateral Raise
Abdominals	Leg Raise, Twist Crunch

SAMPLE OF A WEEKLY ROUTINE

DAY 1	Chest and Triceps
DAY 2	Rest
DAY 3	Back and Biceps
DAY 4	Quadriceps and Hamstrings
DAY 5	Rest
DAY 6	Shoulders and Abdominals
DAY 7	Rest

super
sets

Super sets involve performing two exercises one after another without rest. Performing super sets can create more efficient workouts, especially if you have limited time, but may not be ideal if you work out in a busy gym since the equipment you need may not always be readily available. There are two types of super sets—those that work opposing muscle groups and those that work the same muscle group.

When performing super sets, make sure to go from one exercise to another as efficiently as possible. Any time lost between exercises can decrease the effectiveness of the super set. Since performing super sets can lead to injuries, you should perform super sets about once a week for each muscle group. Also make sure to rest for about 1 to 2 minutes between super sets.

For a greater challenge and a more efficient workout, you can try performing three exercises one after another without rest. For example, if you want an intense abdominal workout, perform three different abdominal exercises one after another.

Opposing Muscles Super Sets

Performing super sets on opposing muscle groups, such as your chest and back, helps create good muscle balance. For example, to work your chest and back, you can perform the barbell bench press immediately followed by the lat pulldown. Remember to rest for about 1 to 2 minutes before performing another super set.

Examples

MUSCLES TARGETED	EXERCISES
Chest and Back	Barbell Bench Press + Lat Pulldown
Biceps and Triceps	Seated Dumbbell Curl + Dumbbell Overhead Triceps Extension
Abdominals and Lower Back	Abdominal Crunch + Back Extension on a Roman Chair
Quadriceps and Hamstrings	Leg Extension + Leg Curl

Same Muscle Super Sets

Performing super sets on the same muscle group gives the muscles an intense workout. For example, to thoroughly work your back, you can perform the lat pulldown immediately followed by the seated cable row. You may need to use less weight when performing the second exercise since your muscles will be fatigued after the first exercise.

Examples

MUSCLES TARGETED	EXERCISES
Chest	Barbell Bench Press + Dumbbell Fly
Back	Lat Pulldown + Seated Cable Row
Triceps	Lying Barbell Triceps Extension + Bench Dip
Biceps	Barbell Curl + Hammer Curl
Abdominals	Plank + Abdominal Crunch
Quadriceps	Dumbbell Squat + Leg Extension
Hamstrings	Leg Press + Leg Curl

free weights safety tips

Keep the following safety tips in mind when using free weights during your workouts.

Use Proper Form

How you lift weight is more important than how much weight you are lifting. When performing exercises using free weights, maintaining proper form helps prevent injury and ensures you get the most out of your workouts. Placing your body in incorrect positions puts unnecessary stress on your muscles, tendons and joints, which can lead to injury. To avoid injury, many exercises require that you keep your back straight, your knees or elbows slightly bent and your abdominal muscles tight to help protect your back.

Use a Spotter

When performing exercises, you should ask someone to act as a spotter, especially if the weight is heavy. A spotter is a person who stands close by and is ready to offer assistance if needed. You should tell the spotter how many repetitions you plan to perform, so he or she can be ready to assist when you perform the last few repetitions.

Safely Pick Up and Return Weight

At the start and end of an exercise, make sure to safely pick up and lower the weight. When lifting dumbbells off a rack, make sure to always bend at the knees and not at the hips. If you are picking weight off the floor, you should lift with your legs and not with your back. When performing exercises that require you to lie on a bench, you should first sit on the bench and place the weight on your thighs. As you lie down, use your legs to assist in moving the weight into position.

Use Collars

Collars are metal screws or clamps placed on a barbell to prevent the weight plates from rattling or falling off. You should use collars to secure the weight plates to a bar so you do not injure yourself or someone else.

track your progress

Keeping a record of your workouts is an important part of your weight training routine. Recording your workout information in a daily log allows you to track your progress over time and can help keep you motivated to continue exercising.

In addition to showing your progress, a daily workout log can help you pinpoint areas where you can adjust your training to achieve better results.

You can use the sample log on page 245 to record your workout information.

Information to Record in Your Workout Log

You should record the details of each weight training session in your log. The information should include the date and time of your workout and the name of each exercise you completed. For each exercise, record the number of repetitions and sets and how much weight you used. It is also useful to make notes about additional items, such as specific adjustments you made to the machine or how you plan to modify the exercise next time.

You can also record information about cardiovascular exercise. For example, if you used a treadmill, you can note the length, intensity, heart rate and distance traveled during the exercise.

General comments about the exercise session, such as whether you felt tired or energized, can also be useful.

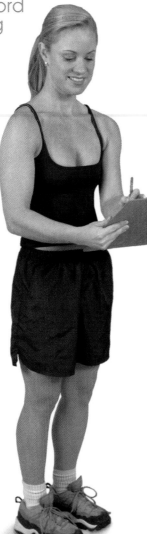

Review Your Workout Logs

You should review your workout logs every few weeks to check your progress. When reviewing your logs, look for increases in the amount of weight you used for an exercise. This helps show which muscles are getting stronger and whether there are any muscle imbalances. For example, if your hamstrings are getting stronger and your quadriceps are not, you may want to focus on strengthening your quadriceps.

If you notice that you have not increased the amount of weight for 3 to 4 weeks or that you have not changed the number of sets and repetitions over the past 2 months, consider changing your routine. You will need to make changes to your routine periodically in order to continue gaining strength.

Make sure you are not constantly skipping specific exercises in your routine. If you often skip an exercise, you should replace it with a similar exercise you will perform regularly. Also, check the consistency of your workouts to ensure you are weight training at least 3 days a week.

Examining your cardiovascular exercise is also important. Note changes in the intensity of your workouts and in your heart rate. You should notice a gradual drop in heart rate at the same intensity level over time, which indicates you can increase the intensity or the length of the exercise to push yourself a bit harder.

DAILY WORKOUT LOG

Date:				Time:			

EXERCISE		SET 1	SET 2	SET 3	SET 4	SET 5	SET 6	NOTES
	WT							
	REP							
	WT							
	REP							
	WT							
	REP							
	WT							
	REP							
	WT							
	REP							
	WT							
	REP							
	WT							
	REP							
	WT							
	REP							
	WT							
	REP							
	WT							
	REP							
	WT							
	REP							

CARDIOVASCULAR TRAINING

COMMENTS

REP(REPETITIONS) WT(WEIGHT)

common weight training injuries

Injuries, such as sprains and strains, can happen to anyone, even to careful weight lifters. Depending on how severe your injury is, the time of recovery can range from a couple of days to a few months. You should see your doctor if an injury persists for more than a few days or if the pain is excruciating and troublesome. You can limit the severity of an injury and speed up your recovery time by stopping an exercise as soon as you feel pain. Continuing to work out can cause further damage to the area, making the injury worse and prolonging the recovery period.

Strain

A strain is a tear of a muscle or tendon. Strains can be caused by lifting extremely heavy weight, by not warming up before exercising or by stretching beyond your limits. If you suffer from a strain, you will feel an immediate, sharp pain in your muscles. The affected area may become swollen, red and painful to move.

Sprain

A sprain is a tear in your ligaments, which are strong bands of connective tissue found around joints, such as your wrists, elbows and knees. Although typically avoidable, sprains are caused mainly by trauma. If you suffer from a sprain, you will feel immediate pain in the affected joint, which may appear red, swollen and bruised. You will also experience limited movement in the injured joint.

Overuse Injuries

An overuse injury usually starts as a slight pain felt after exercising, but the pain gradually becomes worse over time until the affected area hurts all the time. This type of injury is most commonly an inflammation of a tendon or bursa, caused by the overuse of a muscle group or a certain repetitive movement.

Delayed Onset Muscle Soreness (DOMS)

About 24 to 48 hours after your workout, you may feel tightness or soreness in your muscles. This muscle pain is referred to as Delayed Onset Muscle Soreness (DOMS) and is common after a hard workout, especially if you are a beginner or if you haven't exercised in a while. DOMS is not an injury, but is a result of microscopic tears that occur in the muscles when they are exerted, allowing the muscles to regenerate and grow larger and stronger. The soreness normally peaks about 48 hours after exercising and dissipates within a few days. If the soreness lasts more than a few days or becomes worse, you should see a doctor.

Preventing Injuries

To help prevent injuries:

1 You should perform about 5 minutes of cardiovascular exercise before each workout to warm up your muscles and to increase blood circulation.

2 Remember to train gradually. You should take note of the weight you are lifting, increase the weight gradually and avoid using more weight than your body is capable of handling.

3 Try to always maintain proper form. You can place excessive stress on your joints by placing your body in incorrect positions.

4 Work all major muscle groups to prevent muscle imbalances.

5 Remember to stretch between sets and at the end of your workout.

6 Do not work the same muscle two days in a row. You should give your muscles time to recover.

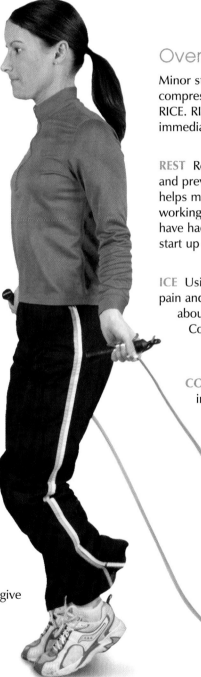

Overcoming Injuries

Minor strains and sprains can be treated with rest, ice, compression and elevation, commonly referred to as RICE. RICE is most effective when you start treatment immediately after suffering an injury.

REST Resting reduces the stress on the affected area and prevents further aggravation of the injury. It also helps minimize internal bleeding or swelling. Before working the affected area, you should wait until you have had at least two pain-free days. Make sure you start up slowly when you begin exercising again.

ICE Using ice on the affected area helps reduce the pain and swelling. You can ice the injured area for about 15 to 20 minutes, 3 to 4 times a day. Continue to apply ice on the affected area for as long as pain and swelling are present.

COMPRESSION Placing pressure on the injured area can help keep the swelling to a minimum. You can use an elastic bandage or purchase a special brace or wrap for your wrist, knee or elbow. Wrap the bandage tight enough to feel tension, but not too firmly that you cut off blood circulation.

ELEVATION You should keep the injured area elevated. Elevating the area reduces the blood flow and drains fluids and waste products away, which helps reduce the swelling of the injured area.

weight training
when traveling

When you are away from home on vacation or business, it is important that you continue weight training so you do not lose all the benefits you previously gained. Even a short weight training session once a week can help keep you in shape and make it easier for you to get back to your regular routine after your trip.

It may require a bit of planning and discipline to continue exercising while traveling, but the benefits are worth the effort. Exercising when traveling can reduce stress, minimize the effects of jet lag and help maintain your regular sleep pattern. You may tend to eat more on your trip than you would normally eat at home, especially if you eat at restaurants regularly. Exercise can help keep your metabolism up and burn the extra calories you consume.

If you did not exercise at least once a week while on your trip, when you return home, you may want to gradually ease back into your normal exercise routine by performing your workouts at a lower intensity until you return to your previous fitness level.

STAY AT A HOTEL WITH A GYM

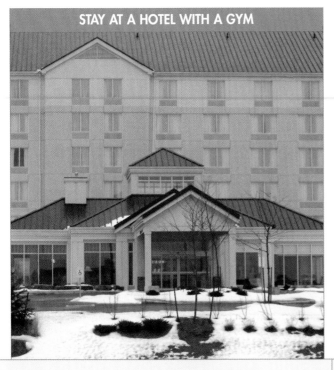

- When traveling, stay at a hotel that has a gym where you can continue your weight training routine. Many hotels offer weight-training facilities that guests can use for free or for a minimal cost.

FIND A GYM NEARBY

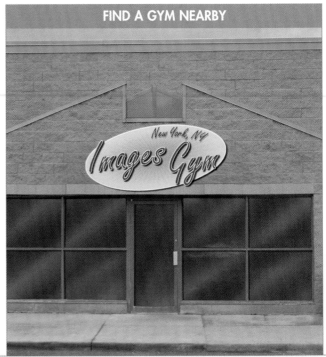

- If your hotel does not have a gym, try to find a gym nearby that you can use. You can ask hotel employees at the front desk or look in the yellow pages for a nearby gym.
- A gym near your hotel that is affiliated with your gym at home may allow you to use their facilities for free or for a discounted rate.

What cardiovascular exercises can I perform when traveling?

You can use the cardiovascular equipment at a gym or the hotel's swimming pool if these are available. If there are no facilities available, you can exercise in your room by jogging on the spot, jumping rope or performing jumping jacks. You can also take the stairs to and from your room or go outside for a walk or jog around the neighborhood. You should aim to perform 15 to 20 minutes of cardiovascular exercise every other day while traveling.

How can I maintain a healthy diet when traveling?

While you are away, you should continue to eat foods from all the food groups, especially fruits and vegetables. To prevent hunger and overeating at restaurants, take along lightweight, nutritious snacks, such as dried fruit and nuts, to eat during the day. At restaurants, ask for sauces, such as salad dressing, on the side and order grilled, broiled or baked foods instead of fried foods. Pay attention to portion sizes, since restaurants usually serve larger portions than you would normally eat at home. Also, remember to keep your body hydrated by drinking lots of water.

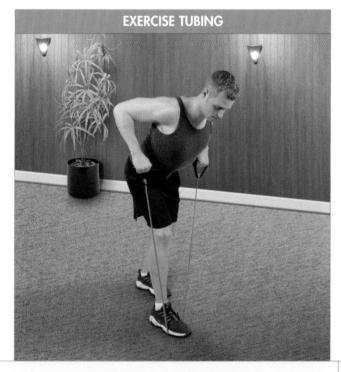

EXERCISE TUBING

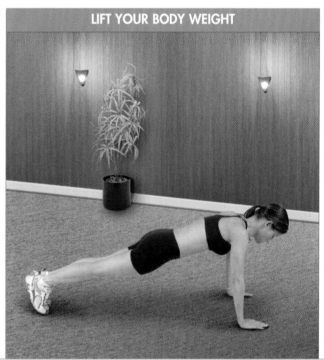

LIFT YOUR BODY WEIGHT

- If you will not have access to weight training equipment while traveling, you can bring exercise tubing with you. Exercise tubing is lightweight and can easily fit in a suitcase. You can use exercise tubing to perform various exercises in the comfort of your hotel room. For more information on exercise tubing, see pages 198 to 225.

- You can always maintain your workout routine without exercise equipment by lifting your own body weight. In your hotel room, perform exercises such as push-ups, abdominal crunches, dips and lunges, to keep in shape while traveling. For more information on exercises you can perform, see page 250.

exercises to perform
when traveling

Continuing your weight training program when traveling can be difficult if you do not have access to a gym, but there are several exercises you can perform to work the main muscle groups in your body and keep in shape without equipment.

Before you perform the exercises below, you should warm up for about 5 minutes with a light cardio exercise, such as jogging, doing jumping jacks or climbing stairs, and then stretch for 10 minutes after you finish the resistance training exercises. For each exercise, perform 3 sets of 15 repetitions. The entire workout takes about 20 minutes to complete.

You can use ankle weights or exercise tubing to make some of the exercises harder. For information on exercise tubing, see page 198.

EXERCISES TO PERFORM WHEN TRAVELING

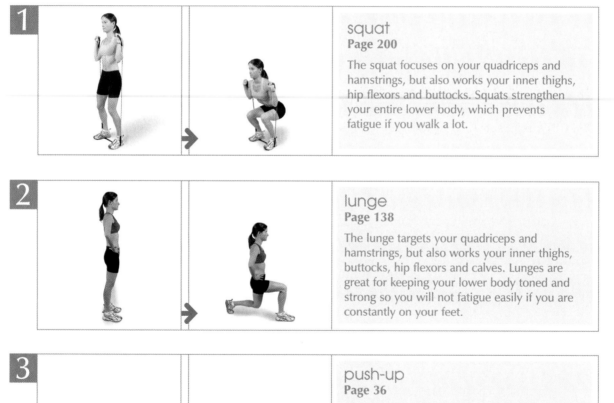

1

squat
Page 200

The squat focuses on your quadriceps and hamstrings, but also works your inner thighs, hip flexors and buttocks. Squats strengthen your entire lower body, which prevents fatigue if you walk a lot.

2

lunge
Page 138

The lunge targets your quadriceps and hamstrings, but also works your inner thighs, buttocks, hip flexors and calves. Lunges are great for keeping your lower body toned and strong so you will not fatigue easily if you are constantly on your feet.

3

push-up
Page 36

The push-up targets your chest, but also works your shoulders and triceps. Push-ups help maintain your upper body strength, which helps you more easily perform tasks when traveling, such as carrying heavy bags.

EXERCISES TO PERFORM WHEN TRAVELING (CONTINUED)

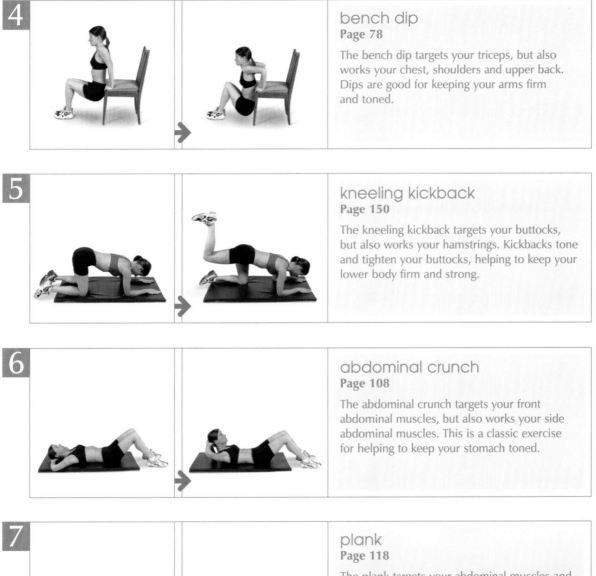

4

bench dip
Page 78

The bench dip targets your triceps, but also works your chest, shoulders and upper back. Dips are good for keeping your arms firm and toned.

5

kneeling kickback
Page 150

The kneeling kickback targets your buttocks, but also works your hamstrings. Kickbacks tone and tighten your buttocks, helping to keep your lower body firm and strong.

6

abdominal crunch
Page 108

The abdominal crunch targets your front abdominal muscles, but also works your side abdominal muscles. This is a classic exercise for helping to keep your stomach toned.

7

plank
Page 118

The plank targets your abdominal muscles and lower back, but also works your shoulders and middle back. This exercise strengthens your core, which includes your back and abdominal muscles. Strong core muscles help improve posture and prevent lower back pain.

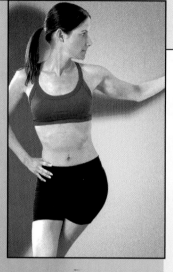

Section 6

S tretching is an important part of your weight training routine, since regular stretching can help prevent injury and reduce muscle soreness after workouts. Stretching is also important for increasing your flexibility, which can make it easier for you to perform everyday tasks. Section 6 shows you how to stretch the major muscles in your body properly.

Stretching

In this Section...

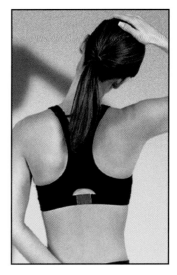

introduction to stretching

Stretching helps prevent injuries, keeps your muscles relaxed and your body flexible. Stretching can also help make daily activities easier to perform, improve your posture, reduce muscle soreness after workouts and make your muscles look leaner and longer.

Age and lack of exercise tend to shorten the length of our muscles. Stretching helps to lengthen the muscles and loosen up the joints. As a result, the body becomes more flexible and we are able to feel and perform better.

You should avoid comparing your flexibility with other people. Your flexibility will improve as you perform stretches on a regular basis. If you perform stretches at least 3 times a week, you will notice a marked increase in your flexibility after just a few weeks.

When performing stretches, you can concentrate on muscles that you use on a daily basis and when you workout. However, you should not neglect any major muscle group.

HOW TO STRETCH

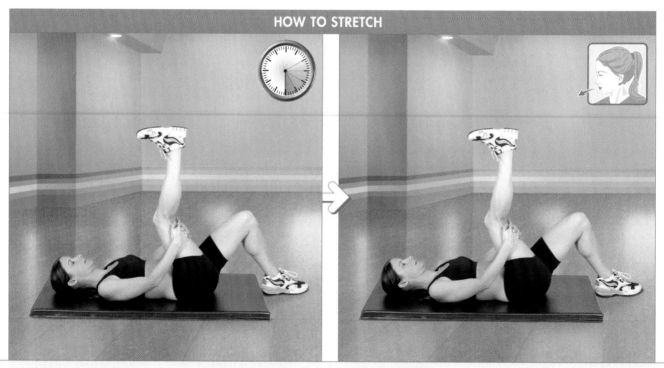

- Hold each stretch for 10 to 30 seconds.
- Stretch to the point where you feel mild tension in your muscles.
- Stretch slowly and smoothly.

- Perform at least one stretch for every major muscle group.
- Inhale deeply through your nose before each stretch and exhale through your mouth as you move into a stretch.

- Continue to breathe deeply as you hold a stretch. Deep breathing increases your flexibility by helping you to relax and by sending fresh blood to your muscles.

- When you feel the muscle loosen after holding a stretch, slowly stretch a little further.
- If you feel a muscle needs further stretching, wait about 15 seconds and then perform the stretch once or twice more.

Question & Answer

What is assisted stretching?

Assisted stretching typically involves the use of a partner to achieve a better stretch. However, if a partner is not available, you can use an object, such as a wall, chair or bench. Make sure your partner helps you ease into a stretch slowly. You should give your partner constant feedback as to how the stretch feels so you avoid injuries caused by your partner overstretching you. A personal trainer can teach you how to properly perform assisted stretches.

What is PNF?

PNF, which stands for Proprioceptive Neuromuscular Facilitation, is another method of stretching that can greatly improve flexibility compared to regular stretching. For safety reasons, PNF is best performed with the help of a trainer. PNF involves the application of resistance to the muscle being stretched for 6 to 10 seconds. This is then followed by a period of relaxation for about 20 seconds. The process of applying resistance and then allowing the muscle to relax is repeated 3 to 6 times. With each repetition, the muscle is stretched a bit further. Make sure not to push beyond your muscle's capacity to prevent injury and to make sure you get a good stretch.

WHEN TO STRETCH

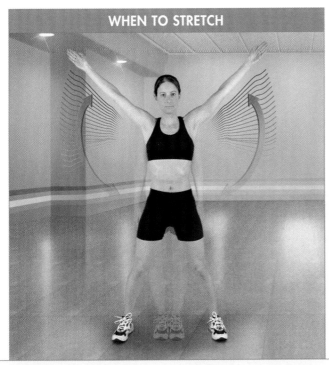

DON'T

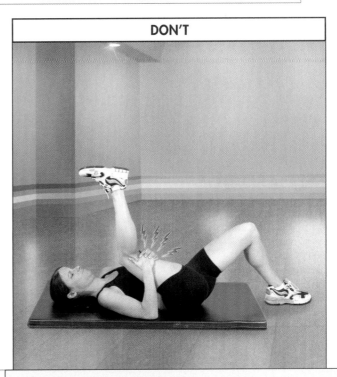

- Before stretching, warm up your muscles to prevent injury. You should perform at least 5 minutes of aerobic exercise such as jumping jacks or cycling before stretching.

- When performing weight training exercises, you can stretch the muscle targeted after each set. You should stretch all your muscles at the end of your workout.

- You should stretch at least 3 times a week. If possible, stretch every day.

- You should not feel pain when you stretch.

- Do not bounce when stretching.

- Do not hold your breath while you stretch.

- Do not stretch before you warm up or exercise.

chest stretches

Chest stretches focus on your pectoral muscles, which are the muscles used to pull your arms forward. You can perform chest stretches in between sets or at the end of your workout.

If you spend a lot of time sitting at your desk and find yourself slumping, you can perform chest stretches to help improve your posture. For more information on the benefits of stretching, see page 254.

When performing chest stretches, you should hold each stretch for about 15 to 30 seconds. If you feel discomfort or pain while performing any of the stretches, you should stop immediately and then ease back into the stretch until you feel a slight pull without any pain.

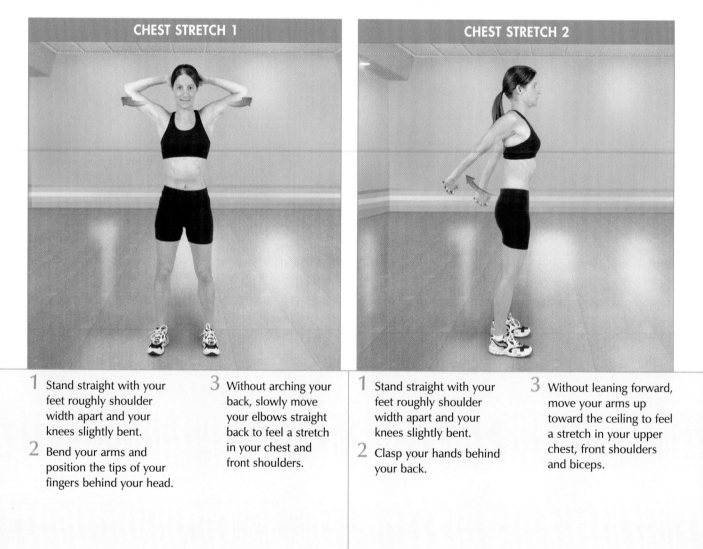

CHEST STRETCH 1

1 Stand straight with your feet roughly shoulder width apart and your knees slightly bent.

2 Bend your arms and position the tips of your fingers behind your head.

3 Without arching your back, slowly move your elbows straight back to feel a stretch in your chest and front shoulders.

CHEST STRETCH 2

1 Stand straight with your feet roughly shoulder width apart and your knees slightly bent.

2 Clasp your hands behind your back.

3 Without leaning forward, move your arms up toward the ceiling to feel a stretch in your upper chest, front shoulders and biceps.

Are there assisted chest stretches I can perform?

Yes. When performing Chest Stretch 1 shown on page 256, a partner can stand behind you and place his or her palms on the front of your elbows to gently apply pressure and give you a better stretch. When performing Chest Stretch 2 shown on page 256, place your arms straight behind you, instead of clasped. Then have your partner stand behind you, grab your wrists with his or her palms facing up and pull up toward the ceiling.

How can I stretch my chest and front shoulders at the same time?

To stretch your chest and front shoulders at the same time, lie on a bench and stretch your arms out to your sides, keeping your arms at shoulder level. Then slowly drop your arms, allowing gravity to pull them down.

CHEST STRETCH 3

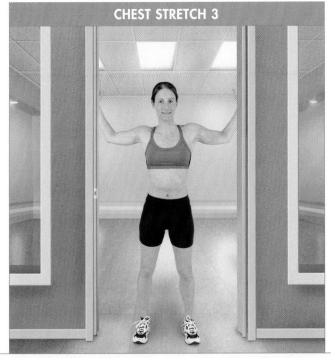

1 Stand straight in front of a doorway with your feet roughly shoulder width apart and your knees slightly bent.

2 Bend your arms at 90-degree angles and position each palm on the edges of the doorway.

3 Lean your body forward to feel a stretch in your chest and front shoulders.

CHEST STRETCH 4

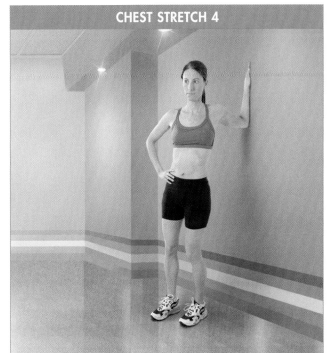

1 Stand with your left side to a wall with your feet roughly shoulder width apart and your knees slightly bent. Position your right hand on your hip.

2 Bend your left arm and place your forearm and palm on the wall. Your elbow should be at shoulder height.

3 Take several small steps to twist your body to the right to feel a stretch in your chest and front shoulder.

4 Repeat the exercise with your right side.

back stretches

Back stretches help to keep your spine healthy. Performing back stretches also helps to keep your vertebrae loose and mobile so that when you bend over to pick up an object, you avoid injuring yourself.

You can perform back stretches after each set of a back exercise and at the end of your workout. You can also perform back stretches every morning if you have time. If you work at a desk all day, you may want to perform the Upper Back Stretch while seated.

As with other stretching exercises, you should try to hold each stretch for 15 to 30 seconds.

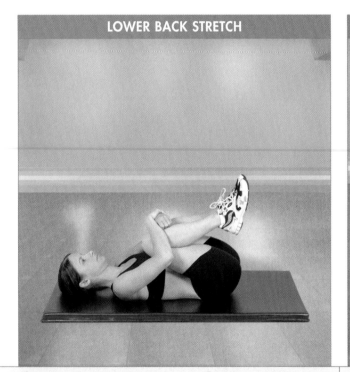

LOWER BACK STRETCH

1 Lie on your back on a mat with your legs together and your knees bent. Lift your feet off the floor.

2 Wrap your arms around both legs in front of your knees.

3 Slowly bring your knees toward your chest to feel a stretch in your lower back. Make sure you keep your head on the mat.

UPPER BACK STRETCH

1 Stand with your feet roughly shoulder width apart and your knees slightly bent.

2 Bend your right arm and place your right hand on top of your head.

3 Bend your left arm and place your left hand on your lower back with your palm facing back.

4 Slowly tilt your head to the right to feel a stretch in your upper back and neck.

5 Repeat the exercise, switching the positions of your arms and tilting your head to the left.

When stretching my lower back, can I focus on stretching one side at a time?

Yes. To focus on stretching one side of your lower back at a time, perform the Lower Back Stretch as shown on page 258, except with your arms wrapped around only one leg and your other leg straight on the floor. You may feel the stretch easier when you have your arms wrapped around one leg rather than both legs.

If I do not have an object to grasp for the Middle Back Stretch, is there an alternative stretch?

Yes. While standing, place your arms straight in front of you at shoulder height and put your hands together with your fingers interlocked. Turn your palms outward as you stretch your arms forward. Pretend you are pushing an object away from you. In addition to stretching your middle back, you should also feel a stretch in your shoulders, arms, hands, fingers and wrists.

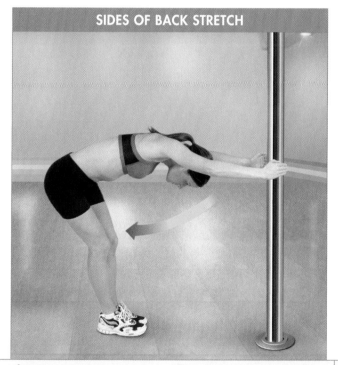

SIDES OF BACK STRETCH

1 Stand with your legs together and knees slightly bent in front of an object you can grasp, such as a piece of gym equipment or a post or column at home.

2 Grasp the object with both hands at waist level with your palms facing each other.

3 Bend forward at the hips until your upper body is parallel to the floor.

4 Slowly bend your knees and pull your body slightly back and to the left to feel a stretch in the right side of your back.

5 Repeat the exercise, leaning your body to the right.

MIDDLE BACK STRETCH

1 Stand with your legs together and knees slightly bent in front of an object you can grasp, such as a piece of gym equipment or a post or column at home.

2 Grasp the object with both hands at chest height with your palms facing each other.

3 Bend slightly forward at the hips and round your back.

4 Slowly bend your knees and pull your body slightly back to feel a stretch in your middle back.

shoulder stretches

Stretching your shoulders helps to loosen and lengthen your shoulder muscles so your shoulders look leaner. Shoulders stretches also make you less prone to common injuries such as tendonitis and bursitis. For more information on stretching, see page 254.

You may want to perform shoulder stretches after each set of a shoulder exercise and at the end of your workout. If you have time, you can stretch your shoulders every morning.

When you stretch, hold each stretch for 15 to 30 seconds. Remember to keep your breathing even and regular. As with any exercise, you should not continue a shoulder stretch if you feel pain in your shoulders.

SHOULDER STRETCH 1

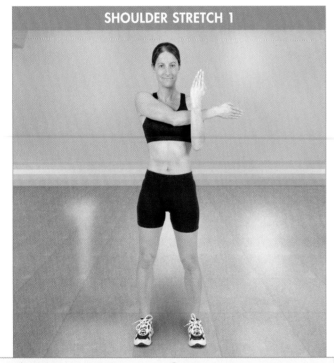

1 Stand with your feet roughly shoulder width apart, knees slightly bent.

2 Place your right arm across your chest with your palm facing back.

3 Place your left forearm on the front of your right forearm with your fingers pointing up and your palm facing back.

4 Slowly push your left forearm back to feel a stretch in your right shoulder and tricep.

5 Repeat the exercise to stretch your left shoulder.

SHOULDER STRETCH 2

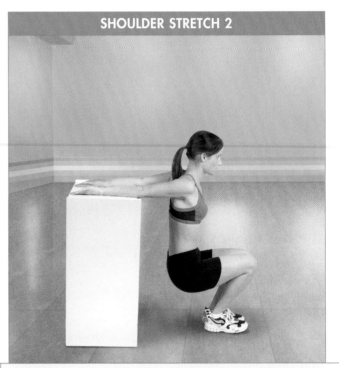

1 Stand with your back to a table or ledge and your feet together.

2 Position your arms straight behind you and place your palms facing up on the table or ledge with your fingers pointing back.

3 Keeping your back straight and elbows slightly bent, slowly lower your body by bending your knees to feel a stretch in the front of your shoulders.

How can I warm up my upper body before stretching?

You can perform arm circles to warm up your upper body. Stand with your feet shoulder width apart and your arms extended straight out to the sides at shoulder level. Start by moving your arms in small circles and then gradually move to larger circles. After completing the largest circle you can make, repeat this exercise in the opposite direction. This is a good exercise for warming up your shoulders, neck and chest before stretching or weight training exercises.

Is there another exercise I can perform to warm up my shoulder joints before stretching?

Yes. Stand with your left side facing a bench or chair. Position your feet shoulder width apart and then bend forward at the hips and place your left hand on the bench or chair for support. Your upper and lower body should form a 90-degree angle. Let your right arm hang down so your fingers point to the floor and then move your arm in small circles, gradually increasing to larger circles. After completing a set, perform the exercise with your left arm.

SHOULDER STRETCH 3

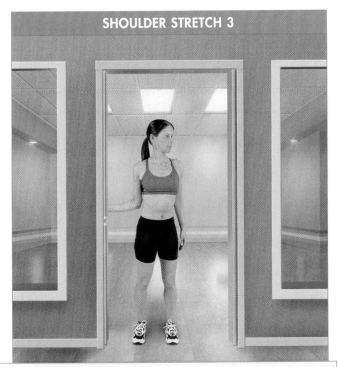

1 Stand in a doorway or beside the edge of a wall with your feet slightly apart and your knees slightly bent.

2 Position your palm and part of your right forearm at waist level on the edge of the doorway or wall.

3 Keeping your elbow close to your body and your wrist straight, slowly turn your body to the left to feel a stretch in your right shoulder.

4 Repeat the exercise with your left arm.

SHOULDER STRETCH 4

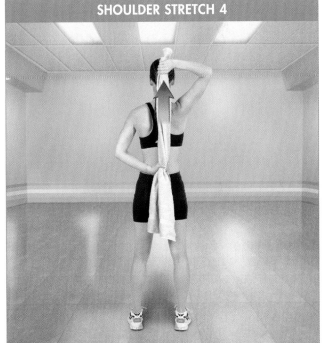

1 Stand with your feet roughly shoulder width apart and your knees slightly bent.

2 Grasp one end of a towel with your right hand. Position your right hand behind your head, palm facing forward.

3 Grasp the towel behind your lower back with your left hand, palm facing backward.

4 Slowly pull the towel up with your right hand to feel a stretch in your left shoulder.

5 Repeat the exercise to stretch your right shoulder.

bicep and tricep stretches

Stretching your bicep and tricep muscles helps to lengthen your muscles and increase the flexibility in your arms. You use your triceps and biceps when you carry objects. Since your biceps are attached to your shoulders, where you tend to slouch, stretching your biceps can help improve your posture. Your triceps are larger muscles than your biceps and should be stretched more often. For more information on stretching, see page 254.

You may want to perform the stretches described below after each set of a bicep or tricep exercise and at the end of your workout. When you perform the exercises, try to hold each stretch for 15 to 30 seconds before releasing.

If you have a recent shoulder injury, you should be careful when performing bicep and tricep stretches. Remember that stretches should not be painful, so do not continue a stretch if you experience any pain in the area you are stretching.

BICEP STRETCH 1

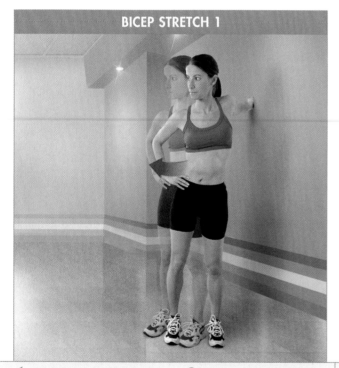

1 Stand with your left side beside a wall, your feet slightly apart and knees slightly bent. Position your right arm on your hip.

2 Position your left palm on the wall at shoulder level with your arm straight and your fingers pointing back.

3 Take several small steps to slowly turn your body to the right to feel a stretch in your left bicep, forearm and the front of your shoulder.

4 Repeat the exercise to stretch your right arm.

BICEPS STRETCH 2

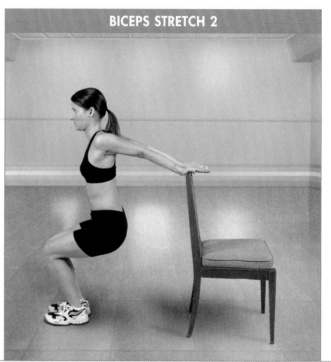

1 Stand with your back to the back of a chair with your feet slightly apart.

2 Position your arms straight behind you at roughly waist height and place your palms on the chair with your fingers pointing back.

3 Keeping your back straight and elbows slightly bent, slowly lower your body by bending your knees to feel a stretch in your biceps and the front of your shoulders.

What other tricep stretches can I perform?

Stand with your right side facing a wall, your feet slightly apart and your knees slightly bent. Place your left hand on your hip. Position your right elbow on the wall with your elbow pointing to the ceiling and your right hand behind your head. Lean your body into the wall to stretch your right tricep. Then switch sides and repeat the exercise to stretch your left tricep. This is a good exercise if you are not very flexible.

TRICEP STRETCH 1

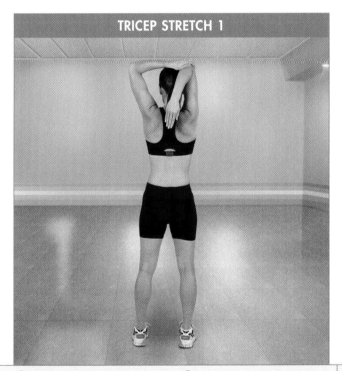

1 Stand with your feet slightly apart and knees slightly bent.

2 Bend your right arm and point your elbow to the ceiling with your palm facing your back.

3 Position your left hand on your right elbow.

4 Use your left hand to slowly push your right elbow back and slightly to the left to feel a stretch in your right tricep.

5 Repeat the exercise to stretch your left tricep.

TRICEP STRETCH 2

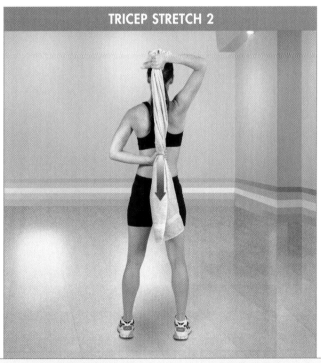

1 Stand with your feet slightly apart and your knees slightly bent.

2 Grasp one end of a towel with your right hand. Position your right hand behind your head, palm facing forward.

3 Grasp the towel behind your middle back with your left hand, palm facing back.

4 Slowly pull the towel down to feel a stretch in your right tricep.

5 Repeat the exercise to stretch your left tricep.

forearm stretches

Stretching your forearms increases the flexibility and relieves the tension in your wrists, which is important for people who constantly work with their hands or fingers, such as individuals who work for long periods of time on a computer.

Your forearm muscles tend to get tight very fast, so you should stretch these muscles frequently. If your job requires constant wrist or finger movements, you should perform the forearm stretches shown below at

least every hour. You can also perform the stretches after each set of a forearm exercise and at the end of your entire workout.

When you perform forearm stretches, try to hold each stretch for 15 to 30 seconds. Remember to stretch only to the point where you feel a slight tension in your forearms, not to the point of pain. For more information on stretching, see page 254.

FOREARM STRETCH 1

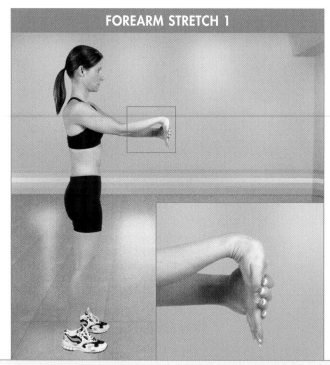

1 Stand with your feet apart, knees slightly bent.

2 Position your right arm in front of your body, elbow slightly bent, palm facing up.

3 Place your left hand on your right hand, palm facing down.

4 Use your left hand to slowly push your right hand down to bend your right wrist. You should feel a stretch in your right forearm and wrist.

5 Repeat the exercise to stretch your left forearm.

FOREARM STRETCH 2

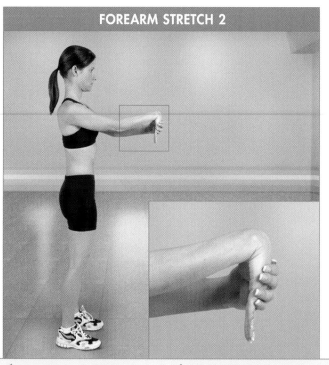

1 Stand with your feet apart, knees slightly bent.

2 Position your right arm in front of your body, elbow slightly bent, palm facing down.

3 Place your left hand on your right hand, palm facing down.

4 Use your left hand to slowly push your right hand down to bend your right wrist. You should feel a stretch in your right forearm and wrist.

5 Repeat the exercise to stretch your left forearm.

neck stretches

Stretching your neck muscles is a good way to relieve stress, since your neck tends to store a lot of the tension your body accumulates during the day.

To keep your neck muscles flexible, you should stretch regularly. You can perform neck stretches at the end of your workout. If you work for long periods at a desk, you should stretch your neck every hour or so. The stretches shown below can be done while sitting or standing. When you perform the stretches,

hold each stretch for 15 to 30 seconds.

If you have a stiff neck, you can start with a less intense stretch and then gradually progress to the stretches shown below. For a basic stretch, perform the steps for Neck Stretch 1 below, except do not move your chin towards your shoulder in step 2.

You should avoid neck stretches that bend your head backward, as these stretches compress the vertebrae in your spine.

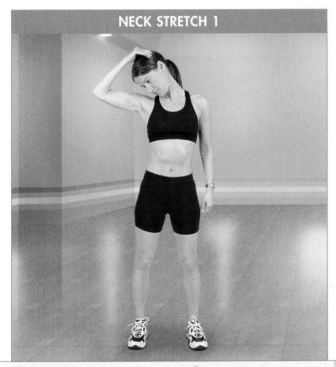

NECK STRETCH 1

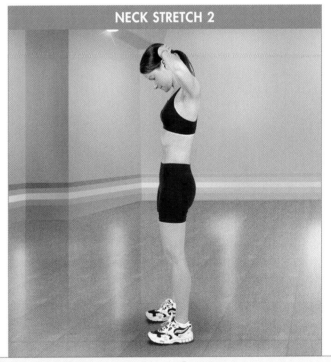

NECK STRETCH 2

1 Stand with your feet slightly apart and your knees slightly bent.

2 Slowly tilt your right ear towards your right shoulder and then move your chin slightly towards your right shoulder to feel a stretch in the left side of your neck.

3 Place your right hand on top of your head to add slight pressure. Do not pull your head with your hand.

4 Repeat the exercise to stretch the right side of your neck.

1 Stand with your feet slightly apart and your knees slightly bent.

2 Slowly lower your chin towards your chest to feel a stretch in the back of your neck.

3 Place both hands on top of your head to add slight pressure. Do not pull your head forward with your hands.

quadricep stretches

Quadricep stretches focus on muscles used in everyday activities, such as walking and climbing stairs. These stretches are very important to perform if you plan to do lower body workouts or cardiovascular exercise. You can perform quadricep stretches after each set of a quadricep exercise and at the end of a workout.

If you are not very flexible, Quadricep Stretch 1 would be easier to perform. In the seated position, you can easily grab your foot and get into the stretch. Quadricep Stretch 2 is a more relaxing type of stretch that is easy to do if

you are already on the floor performing other stretches. Quadricep Stretch 3 and 4 are more advanced stretches for people who are flexible and have good balance.

When performing quadricep stretches, pushing your hips forward is important since one of the quadricep muscles attaches to the pelvis and this movement allows you to fully stretch the entire muscle group so you do not create imbalances.

Be careful performing quadricep stretches if you have knee problems.

QUADRICEP STRETCH 1

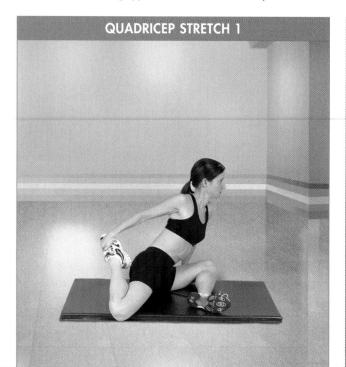

1 Sit and place your left foot in front, knee pointing sideways.

2 Place your right foot behind, knee pointing to the side.

3 Place your left hand beside you for support. Grasp your right foot with your right hand.

4 Pushing your hips forward, use your right hand to slightly pull your foot toward your buttocks to feel a stretch in your right quadricep and hip flexor.

5 Repeat the exercise with your left leg.

QUADRICEP STRETCH 2

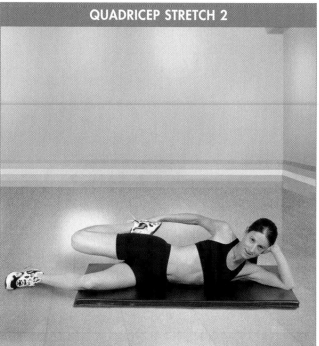

1 Lie on your left side and rest your head in your left hand. Bend your left leg for support.

2 Bend your right leg and grasp the top of your right foot with your right hand behind you.

3 Pushing your hips forward, use your right hand to slightly pull your foot toward your head to feel a stretch in your right quadricep and hip flexor.

4 Repeat the exercise with your left leg.

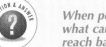

QUESTION & ANSWER

When performing Quadricep Stretch 2 and 3, what can I do if I am not flexible enough to reach back and grasp my foot with my hand?

If you are not flexible enough to reach back and grasp your foot, you can loop a rope or towel around your foot and hold on to the rope or towel with your hand.

How can I get a better stretch when performing Quadricep Stretch 3?

If you have good balance and flexibility, you can remove your hand from the wall and get a better stretch by placing both hands around your foot.

I am very flexible. Is there a more advanced quadricep stretch I can perform?

Yes. For a more advanced quadricep stretch, sit on your heels with the front of your lower legs on the floor and your toes pointing back. Place your hands on the floor behind you and lean back as far as you can to get a stretch in your quadriceps and hip flexors.

QUADRICEP STRETCH 3

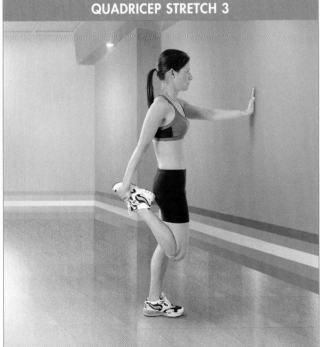

1 Stand facing a wall and position your left hand on the wall for support.

2 Bend your right knee and grasp the top of your right foot with your right hand behind you. Slightly bend your left knee.

3 Pushing your hips forward, use your right hand to slightly pull your foot up to feel a stretch in your right quadricep and hip flexor.

4 Repeat the exercise with your left leg.

QUADRICEP STRETCH 4

1 Stand with your back to a weight machine or table with your hands on your hips.

2 Bend your right leg and position the top of your toes on the weight machine or table.

3 Pushing your hips forward, slowly bend your left leg to lower your body to feel a stretch in your right quadricep and hip flexor.

4 Repeat the exercise with your left leg.

hamstring stretches

The hamstrings are typically tight muscles for the majority of people. Hamstring stretches can loosen up the muscles and make daily activities, such as walking and climbing stairs, easier. Stretching your hamstrings also helps prevent back injury and lower back pain.

You can perform the stretches shown below after each set of a hamstring exercise and at the end of your workout. If you have time, you can stretch your hamstrings every morning or night. Try to hold each stretch for 15 to 30 seconds.

The stretches below are shown in order of their level of difficulty, starting with the easiest. When performing each stretch, remember to keep your back and neck in a straight line. If you have trouble performing Hamstring Stretch 1 or 2, wrap a towel or rope around your thigh or foot and gently pull on the ends to feel the stretch.

If you have lower back problems, do not perform Stretch 4 and be careful performing Stretches 2 and 3.

HAMSTRING STRETCH 1

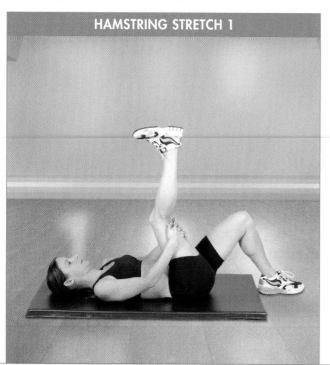

1 Lie on your back on a mat with your left foot flat on the floor.

2 Straighten your right leg with your knee slightly bent and pull your toes toward your shin.

3 Keeping your back and buttocks on the mat, raise your right leg.

4 Grasp your right leg with both hands.

5 Use your hands to slowly pull your right leg toward your head to feel a stretch in your right hamstring.

6 Repeat the exercise with your left leg.

HAMSTRING STRETCH 2

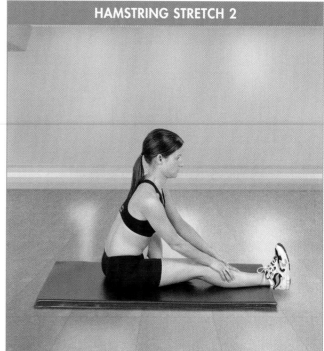

1 Sit on a mat with your right leg straight and your toes pulled toward your shin.

2 Place the bottom of your left foot against the inside of your right thigh. Place your hands on your right leg.

3 Keeping your back straight, slowly bend forward at your hips toward your right leg to feel a stretch in your right hamstring and lower back.

4 Repeat the exercise with your left leg straight.

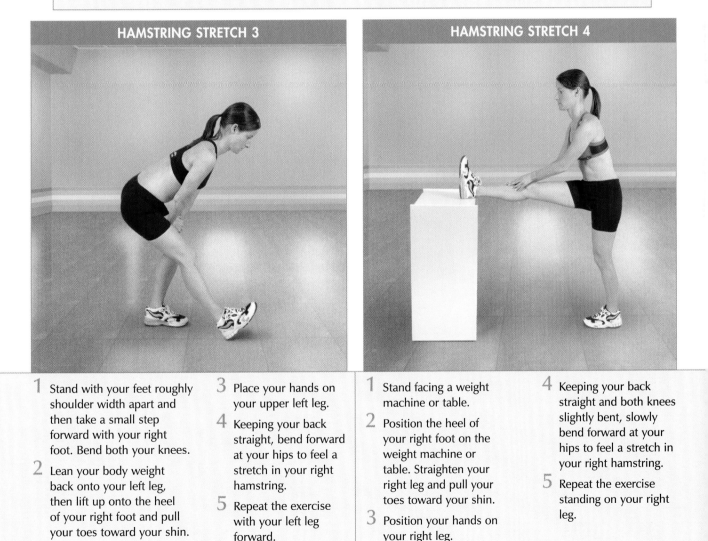

Can I use a wall to stretch my hamstrings?

Yes. Lie on a mat facing the edge of a wall or doorway. Bend your left leg and place your foot flat on the floor. Position your right heel against the edge of the wall or doorway with the toes on your right foot pointed toward your shin. With your hands beside you, slide your body forward to move your right leg closer to the wall or doorway. Repeat the exercise with your left leg. This variation is useful when you do not have a rope or towel handy to help you stretch.

Can I use another person to help stretch my hamstrings?

If you are not flexible, a partner can help stretch your hamstrings more effectively. Lie on a mat with both legs straight, knees slightly bent and the toes on your right foot pointed toward your shin. Have your partner kneel in front of you, lift your right leg and position your calf on his or her left shoulder. Your partner can place his or her left hand on your right upper thigh and then move forward until you feel a stretch in your right hamstring. Repeat the exercise with your left leg.

HAMSTRING STRETCH 3

1 Stand with your feet roughly shoulder width apart and then take a small step forward with your right foot. Bend both your knees.

2 Lean your body weight back onto your left leg, then lift up onto the heel of your right foot and pull your toes toward your shin.

3 Place your hands on your upper left leg.

4 Keeping your back straight, bend forward at your hips to feel a stretch in your right hamstring.

5 Repeat the exercise with your left leg forward.

HAMSTRING STRETCH 4

1 Stand facing a weight machine or table.

2 Position the heel of your right foot on the weight machine or table. Straighten your right leg and pull your toes toward your shin.

3 Position your hands on your right leg.

4 Keeping your back straight and both knees slightly bent, slowly bend forward at your hips to feel a stretch in your right hamstring.

5 Repeat the exercise standing on your right leg.

inner thigh stretches

Stretching your inner thighs maintains flexibility in the muscles and helps prevent injury. If you perform weight training exercises to strengthen your inner thighs or are involved in sports that require sudden stops and starts, such as squash or soccer, it is important to stretch your inner thighs frequently.

You can perform the stretches shown below after each set of an inner thigh strength training exercise and at the end of your entire workout. For more

information on stretching, see page 254.

When you perform the exercise, try to hold each stretch for 15 to 30 seconds before releasing. Concentrate on keeping your breathing even and regular as you stretch.

You should be careful performing inner thigh stretches if you have knee problems. Remember to stretch only to the point where you feel tension in your inner thighs. You should not continue stretching if you experience pain.

INNER THIGH STRETCH 1

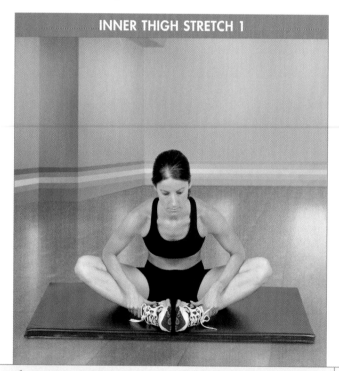

1 Sit on a mat with your knees bent and the bottom of your feet together in front of you. Position your feet as close to your body as you can.

2 Grasp an ankle with each hand and rest your elbows on your thighs.

3 Slowly bend at your hips to move your upper body forward and use your elbows to apply a gentle downward pressure to your thighs. You should feel a stretch in your inner thighs and lower back.

INNER THIGH STRETCH 2

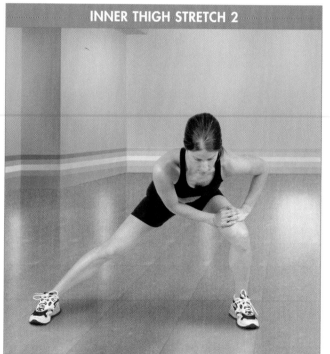

1 Stand with your feet roughly triple shoulder width apart and your toes pointing forward. Bend your left leg and straighten your right leg without locking your right knee.

2 Bend forward at your hips and place your palms on your left thigh.

3 Keeping your back straight, slowly move your body to the left to feel a stretch in your right inner thigh.

4 Repeat the exercise to stretch your left inner thigh.

hip flexor stretches

Your hip flexor muscles, located at the front of your hips, are used in daily activities such as walking, running and climbing stairs. Stretching these muscles not only makes it easier to perform everyday activities, but can also improve your posture and prevent lower back pain.

You can perform hip flexor stretches after each set of a hip flexor exercise and at the end of your workout. Try to hold each stretch for 15 to 30 seconds.

If you have trouble maintaining your balance when performing Hip Flexor Stretch 1 shown below, you can perform the exercise with your side facing a wall and place one hand on the wall for support.

Depending on your flexibility, you can place either your hand or your elbow on the mat behind you when performing Hip Flexor Stretch 2 shown below. You should be careful when performing this stretch if you have knee problems.

HIP FLEXOR STRETCH 1

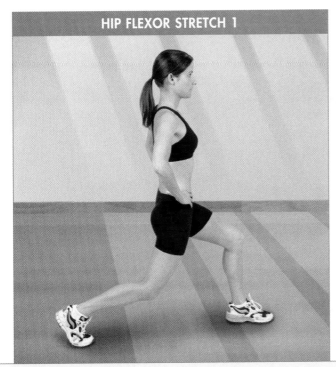

1 Stand with your feet roughly shoulder width apart and then take a large step forward with your left foot. Slightly bend both of your knees.

2 Position your left foot flat on the floor and your right foot on the ball of your foot.

3 Place your hands on your hips.

4 Tilt your pelvis forward and then bend your knees to feel a stretch in your right hip flexor and quadricep.

5 Repeat the exercise with your right foot forward.

HIP FLEXOR STRETCH 2

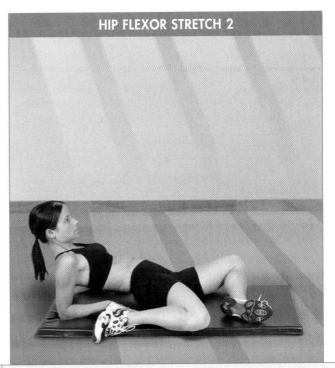

1 Sit on a mat and place your left foot in front of you with your knee pointing sideways.

2 Place your right foot behind you with your knee pointing forward.

3 Slowly lean back and place your elbows or hands on the mat behind you to feel a stretch in your right hip flexor and quadricep.

4 Repeat the exercise with your right foot in front of you.

buttocks and
outer hip stretches

You can perform buttocks and outer hip stretches to help relax the muscles in these areas, which can feel stiff due to activities such as walking, running and cycling. In addition to keeping your back healthy and flexible, performing buttock stretches is a good way of balancing out your hip flexors, which are opposing muscles to your buttocks.

You should keep the following things in mind when performing these stretches. Although Buttocks Stretch 1 is easier on your back, you should be careful performing

this stretch if you have knee problems. You should also keep your head and shoulders on the mat when performing Buttocks Stretch 1. Be careful performing Buttocks Stretch 2 if you have lower back problems. With Buttocks Stretch 3, you should be careful if you have knee, lower back or hip problems. When performing the Outer Hip Stretch, do not lean forward or back as you move your hip toward the wall.

As with other stretching exercises, try to hold each stretch for 15 to 30 seconds.

BUTTOCKS STRETCH 1	BUTTOCKS STRETCH 2
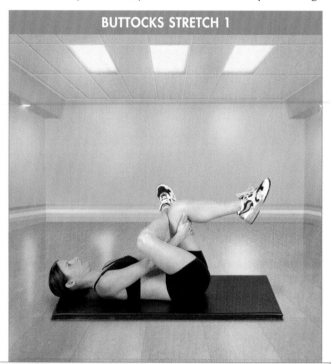	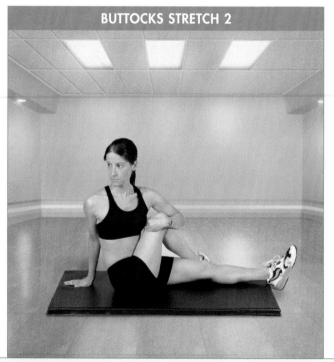

BUTTOCKS STRETCH 1

1 Lie on your back on a mat with your knees bent and feet flat on the floor.

2 Place your right ankle on the top of your left thigh.

3 Lift both legs off the floor and interlace your fingers behind your left thigh.

4 Use your hands to slowly pull your left thigh toward your chest to feel a stretch in your right buttock and lower back.

5 Repeat the exercise to stretch your left buttock.

BUTTOCKS STRETCH 2

1 Sit on a mat with your left leg straight.

2 Cross your right leg over your left leg and place your right foot flat on the floor beside your left knee.

3 Rest your left arm on the outside of your right knee.

4 Slowly turn to the right and place your right hand on the mat behind you to feel a stretch in your right buttock, outer hip and lower back.

5 Repeat the exercise with your left side.

QUESTION & ANSWER

What can I do if I am not flexible enough to properly perform Buttocks Stretch 1?

If you are not flexible enough to properly perform Buttocks Stretch 1, you can wrap a towel or rope behind your thigh and hold on to the ends with both hands to help pull your thigh toward your chest.

Can I stretch my outer hips without using a wall?

Yes. When pushing your right hip to the side, you can extend your right arm straight over your head instead of placing your right hand on the wall.

How can I get a better stretch when performing Buttocks Stretch 3?

If you are flexible, try placing your front foot closer to your front thigh and extending your back leg straight behind you. You will be able to lean forward more and get a better stretch. In addition to feeling a stretch in your buttocks, you will also feel a stretch in your hip flexors.

BUTTOCKS STRETCH 3

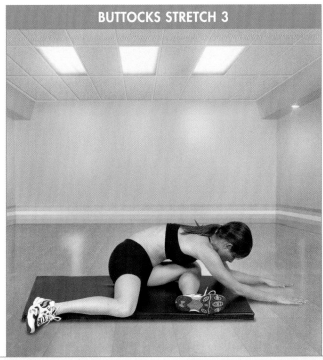

OUTER HIP STRETCH

1 Sit on a mat. Place your left foot in front, knee pointing to the left.

2 Place your right foot behind, knee pointing forward.

3 Bend both knees at a 90-degree angle.

4 Bend forward at your hips and reach forward with your hands to feel a stretch in your left buttock.

5 Repeat the exercise with your right foot in front of you.

1 Stand next to a wall and position your left hand on the wall, elbow slightly bent.

2 Cross your right foot over your left foot. Straighten your left leg and slightly bend your right leg.

3 Slowly lean your left hip toward the wall to feel a stretch in your left outer hip.

4 Repeat the exercise with your right outer hip.

calf and shin stretches

It is important to stretch your calf and shin muscles to keep them flexible, since many essential daily activities utilize these muscles. For example, calf and shin muscles are used in everyday activities such as walking and climbing stairs. If you run for cardiovascular exercise, it is important to stretch these muscles to prevent injury. For more information on stretching, see page 254.

You can perform the stretches described below after each set of a calf or shin exercise and at the end of your workout. If you have time, it is a good idea to perform these stretches every morning or evening.

When you perform the exercises, try to hold each stretch for 15 to 30 seconds before releasing. Remember that stretches should not be painful, so do not continue a stretch if you experience any pain in the area you are stretching.

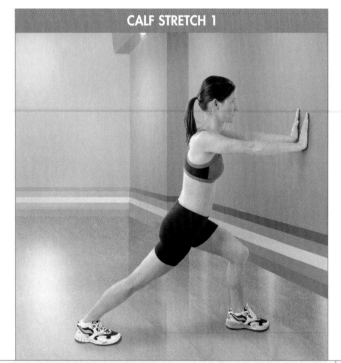

CALF STRETCH 1

1 Stand facing a wall and position your feet roughly shoulder width apart. Take a large step back with your right foot.

2 Position both palms on the wall at shoulder level, fingers pointing up.

3 Keeping your feet flat on the floor and your toes pointing forward, bend your left knee to move your body forward to feel a stretch in your right calf.

4 Repeat the exercise with your right foot forward.

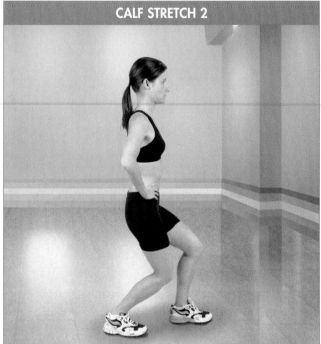

CALF STRETCH 2

1 Position your feet roughly shoulder width apart and take a step forward with your left foot. Place your hands on your hips.

2 Keeping your feet flat on the floor and your toes pointed forward, slowly bend your legs to feel a stretch in your right calf.

3 Repeat the exercise with your right foot forward.

The calf stretches below don't seem to stretch my calves enough. Is there a more intense calf stretch?

Yes. Stand facing a wall and then step back with your left foot, placing the foot flat on the floor. Place your palms on the wall at shoulder level and then position the toes of your right foot against the wall so only your right heel is touching the floor. Push forward off the heel of your left foot to feel a stretch in your right calf.

I have trouble balancing when performing the shin stretch shown below. Is there an easier shin stretch?

Yes. You can stretch your shins while sitting. Kneel on the floor and then sit back on your heels so your lower legs are on the floor and your toes are pointing straight back. Place your hands on top of your thighs and lean back slightly to get a stretch in your shins and a slight stretch in your quadriceps. If you have knee problems, be careful when performing this stretch.

CALF STRETCH 3

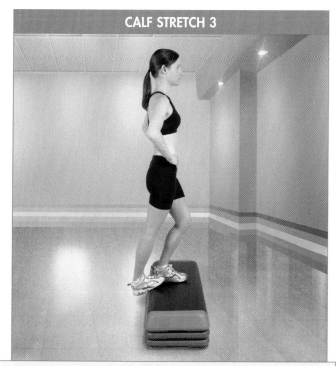

SHIN STRETCH

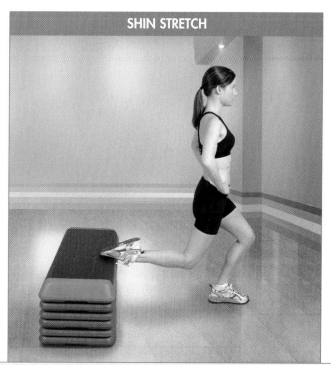

1 Stand on a step with your left foot flat and your right heel hanging over the edge. Slightly bend your left knee, making sure your weight is mainly on your left leg.

2 Position your hands on your hips or grasp a stable object for support, if available.

3 Slowly lower your right heel toward the floor to feel a stretch in your right calf.

4 Repeat the exercise with your left calf.

1 Stand with your back to a step, bench or chair with your hands on your hips.

2 Bend your right leg and position your toes on the step, bench or chair behind you.

3 Slowly bend your left leg to lower your body to feel a stretch in your right shin.

4 Repeat the exercise standing on your right leg.

abdominal stretches

Abdominal stretches are important for improving flexibility in your midsection, which can make performing everyday activities and sports easier.

Some abdominal stretches can also open your diaphragm to help you breathe easier, which can increase your energy, improve your blood circulation and overall health. For more information on the benefits of stretching, see page 254.

You may want to perform abdominal stretches in the morning or after you finish your weight training workout. When you perform the exercises, hold each stretch for 15 to 30 seconds.

While the abdominal stretches described below are relatively gentle exercises that will help your body relax, you should take care when performing these stretches if you have back or neck problems. If you feel discomfort or pain during any of the exercises, you should stop immediately.

FRONT ABDOMINAL STRETCH 1

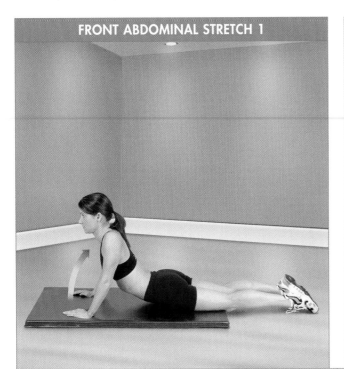

1 Lie on your stomach on a mat with your legs together and straight.

2 Place your palms on the mat under your shoulders.

3 Pushing your hips into the floor, slowly straighten your arms to lift your upper body. You should feel a stretch in your front abdominal muscles.

• Do not shrug your shoulders, lock your elbows or bend your neck back.

FRONT ABDOMINAL STRETCH 2

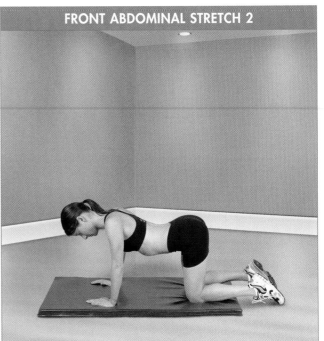

1 Position yourself on your hands and knees on a mat. Make sure your hands and knees are roughly shoulder width apart and your elbows are slightly bent.

2 Position your hands directly under your shoulders and your knees directly under your buttocks.

3 Slowly lower your stomach toward the floor. You should feel a stretch in your front abdominal muscles.

Is there an abdominal stretch that will also stretch my entire body?

Yes. You can perform a full body stretch to stretch your abdominal muscles as well as your upper and lower body. Lie on your back on a mat with your legs together and straight. Point your toes as you stretch your arms above your head. This is a good stretch to help ease the stress of sitting for long periods. To perform the stretch while standing, rise up onto your toes as you stretch your arms above your head.

After I stretch my abdominal muscles, how can I further relax?

You can practice diaphragm breathing. Diaphragm breathing is a more efficient way of breathing than chest breathing, allowing you to take deeper, more calming breaths. To practice diaphragm breathing, place two fingers on your diaphragm, just below your breast bone. Your fingers should rise as you inhale and move downward, rather than inward, as you exhale. As you inhale and exhale, you should notice a rise and fall in your abdominal area rather than your chest.

SIDE ABDOMINAL STRETCH 1

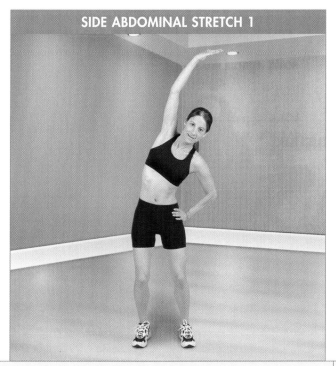

SIDE ABDOMINAL STRETCH 2

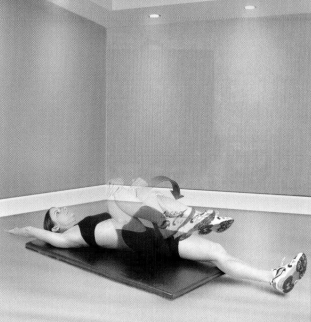

1 Stand with your feet roughly shoulder width apart and your knees slightly bent.

2 Place your left hand on your hip for support.

3 Slowly extend your right hand over your head as you bend to the left at your waist. You should feel a stretch in your side abdominal muscles.

4 Repeat the exercise with your left side.

1 Lie on your back on a mat with your right leg bent, your left leg straight and your right arm straight above your head.

2 Keeping both shoulders on the mat, slowly bring your right knee over your left thigh toward the floor.

3 Place your left hand on the outside of your right knee for support. You should feel a stretch in your side abdominal muscles, buttocks and chest.

4 Repeat the exercise with your left side.

Section 7

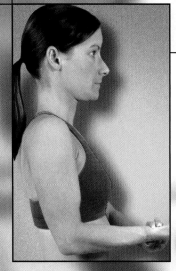

In addition to weight training, you need to perform cardiovascular exercise and maintain a proper diet to achieve overall physical health and fitness. Regular cardiovascular exercise and a balanced diet help improve the health of your heart, increase endurance and energy levels and reduce body fat. Section 7 covers essential information about cardiovascular exercise and nutrition. You can use this information to develop an effective cardiovascular routine and a nutrition plan that can help you become stronger and healthier.

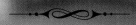

Cardiovascular Training and Nutrition

In this Section...

Cardiovascular Training

Cardiovascular Training Basics

Common Cardiovascular Machines

Take Your Pulse

Determine Your Target Heart Rate

Nutrition

Nutrition Basics

Nutritional Supplements

The Food Guide Pyramid

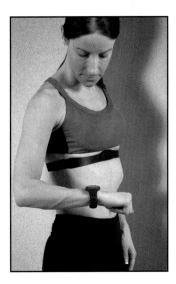

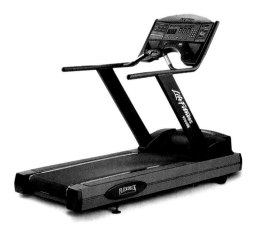

cardiovascular training basics

Cardiovascular exercise is an important complement to your weight training program. In addition to getting your heart pumping and your blood circulating, cardiovascular exercise can help you burn a lot of calories in a short period of time and burn fat to make your muscles appear more defined. You may have difficulty seeing your weight training results due to the layers of fat that hide your muscles. The best cardiovascular exercises are the ones that work large muscle groups, such as your legs.

Benefits of Cardiovascular Exercise

Cardiovascular exercise improves the health of your heart, lowers blood pressure, increases endurance and energy levels, reduces body fat, improves mood and can make you less susceptible to fatigue and illness. By making cardiovascular exercise part of your regular workout routine, you also reduce the risk of developing heart disease, diabetes and other serious medical conditions.

Clothing and Shoes

With cardiovascular exercise, you should wear light, comfortable clothing that allows you to move freely. It is a good idea to wear multiple layers of clothing so you can remove a layer when you get hot. You should also wear athletic shoes with good ankle support and sufficient cushioning. When shopping for a new pair of shoes, you should run in the shoes for a few minutes, try on a few different pairs to compare and ensure you have a good fit.

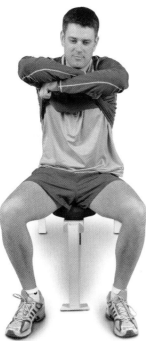

Frequency and Duration

If you are a beginner, you can participate in cardiovascular exercise 2 to 3 times a week, for about 15 minutes each time. As you become more comfortable, you can first increase each session by a few minutes each time and then increase the number of days you work out, up to 4 to 5 times a week. Your goal should be to exercise 3 to 5 times a week, for about 20 to 30 minutes each time.

MAY 2003

Sun	Mon	Tue	Wed	Thu	Fri	Sat
				1	2 *Swim*	3
4	5 *Bike*	6	7 *Run*	8	9 *Swim*	10
11	12 *Bike*	13	14 *Run*	15	16 *Swim*	17
18	19 *Bike*	20	21 *Run*	22	23 *Swim*	24
25	26 *Bike*	27	28 *Run*	29	30 *Swim*	31

Warm Up and Cool Down

For the first 5 minutes of cardiovascular exercise, you should work out gradually to slowly increase your heart rate. This is safer for your heart and is important for preventing injury. If you start out too fast, you will quickly experience fatigue. For the last 5 minutes, you should cool down to slowly decrease your heart rate.

Fitness Classes

Many gyms offer different types of fitness classes to suit the wide range of individual tastes. You can choose to participate in low-impact aerobic classes, which are suited for beginners, or high-impact aerobic classes, which are more intense and can be harder on your joints. You can also join kickboxing, step aerobic, indoor cycling and toning classes. The group dynamics and high-energy music in many fitness classes can help keep you motivated. For a fun way of varying your workout routine, you can try participating in more than one type of fitness class.

Common Cardiovascular Activities

There are numerous cardiovascular activities you can choose from. You can run, swim, bike, hike or cross-country ski. If you enjoy participating in any of these activities, you can incorporate them into your routine to make your workouts more fun.

Keep Motivated

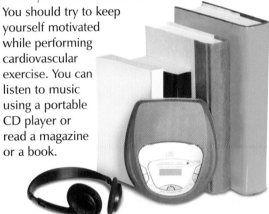

You should try to keep yourself motivated while performing cardiovascular exercise. You can listen to music using a portable CD player or read a magazine or a book.

Many gyms have TVs hanging from their ceilings so you can watch a show while working out. You can also keep yourself motivated by working out with a friend.

Weight Train Before or After Cardiovascular Exercise

You can weight train before or after cardiovascular exercise. Although it usually does not make a difference which you perform first, cardiovascular exercise is recommended after weight training if you plan to lift very heavy weights. When lifting heavy weights, you want to ensure your muscles are fresh and energized.

common cardiovascular machines

Gyms offer a wide variety of cardiovascular machines. When determining the best cardiovascular machine for you, you should select a machine you will enjoy using on a regular basis. Most cardiovascular machines simulate common activities, such as running, climbing stairs and biking. When using a cardiovascular machine for the first time, you should begin slowly to get a good feel for the machine and then gradually increase the intensity. You can start by using the machine 2 to 3 times a week, for about 15 to 20 minutes each time. As you become more comfortable, you can increase the time of each session by a few minutes and then increase the number of days you use the machine, up to 4 to 5 times a week.

Treadmill

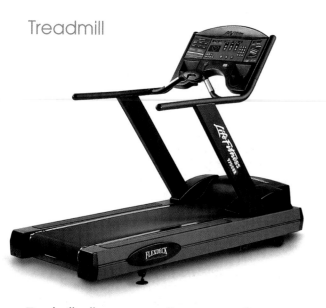

Treadmills allow you to walk or run on a flat or inclined, moving platform. This machine is easy to start off with since walking and running are activities familiar to everyone. As such, treadmills are one of the most heavily used cardiovascular machines in gyms. Be careful not to increase the speed too much to avoid falling off the treadmill. If a treadmill has a safety switch, you should attach the clip to your clothing so the machine will automatically stop if you lose your footing. If you suffer from lower back problems, you should be careful using a treadmill and walk instead of run.

Stationary Bike

A stationary bike suits a wide range of fitness levels, from the advanced cyclist to the absolute beginner. Stationary bikes are also ideal for individuals recovering from an injury. Using a stationary bike is just like riding a regular, outdoor bike. There are two types of stationary bikes—upright, which is similar to a regular bike, and recumbant, which features back support. The recumbant bike provides better support for people with back problems, but may be more difficult to use due to the angle in which you have to pedal. You should adjust the seat height so your bottom leg is slightly bent at the bottom of the movement. Unfortunately, people who are very tall or very short may find it difficult to find a proper seat height adjustment. Some stationary bikes have panels that light up as soon as you start pedaling. You should be careful using stationary bikes if you have knee problems.

Rowing Machine

Using a rowing machine is similar to rowing a boat. Rowing machines allow you to work both the upper and lower parts of your body. This machine works many muscles at once so you can burn a lot of calories. A rowing machine involves non-impact movements, which is great for people with hip, knee and ankle problems. You should start off slowly and gradually increase the intensity as you become more comfortable with the machine. Avoid locking your knees or leaning back at the end of the movement. You should be careful using a rowing machine if you have lower back problems.

Elliptical Machine

Elliptical machines simulate the motion of running. When using this machine, your feet stay on pedals, which move and guide your feet in an elliptical pattern. Since your feet stay on the pedals, there is no impact, which is beneficial for people with knee, hip or lower back problems. Some elliptical machines have moving handlebars that allow your arms to move forward and back, while some allow you to incline, which simulates running up a hill. To use this machine properly, you should avoid bouncing through the movement. An elliptical machine requires good coordination and is not easy to learn how to use, so it is best for beginners to skip this machine.

Stair Climber

Stair climbers mimic the motion of climbing stairs. This machine provides an intense cardiovascular workout and can work your lower body muscles more than other exercises. To avoid an elbow injury or placing unnecessary stress on your knees and lower back, do not put weight on your arms or lean forward at your hips. Make sure you keep your back straight at all times. You should also avoid locking your knees and taking small steps. It is best to take big, full steps. If you are a beginner or have hip, knee or lower back problems, you should not use a stair climber.

Common Features of Cardiovascular Machines

Most cardiovascular machines have preset programs that can guide you through different workout programs. You can generally find an intensity that will meet your needs. Many machines also allow you to set the amount of resistance, the length of time you plan to exercise and the speed at which the machine moves. Most new machines can measure your heart rate when you place your hand on a sensor and they can also measure the amount of calories burned. Just keep in mind that these measurements are not always precise. More sophisticated cardiovascular machines can more accurately measure your heart rate by reading a heart rate monitor that straps around your chest. For more information on heart rate monitors, see page 284.

take your
pulse

You should regularly check your heart rate to ensure you are exercising safely and effectively. Your heart rate, which is often referred to as your pulse, indicates how many times your heart beats per minute.

How to Take Your Pulse

The simplest way of taking your pulse is to place your middle and index fingers on your wrist, just under the base of your thumb. Make sure not to use your thumb. Feel for a pulse and count how many times your heart beats in 15 seconds. Multiply that number by 4 to determine your pulse.

When taking your pulse, you should count the first beat you feel as zero and then start counting from that point. You can also take your pulse by placing your middle and index fingers on either side of your neck, just underneath your jaw. When taking your pulse on your neck or wrist, be careful not to press too hard to avoid cutting off your pulse.

Heart Rate Monitor

For a more accurate way of taking your pulse, you can use a heart rate monitor. Position the heart rate monitor around your chest. The device will transmit your pulse readings to a wristwatch that acts as a receiver. There are also several cardiovascular machines, such as treadmills and stair climbers, that can read your pulse directly from your heart rate monitor.

Cardiovascular Machine

Some cardiovascular machines can measure your heart rate by placing your hand on a sensor. However, these measurements are not always accurate. Sensors on cardiovascular machines should be used as an estimate as they typically display results that are higher than your actual heart rate. Inaccurate readings can be caused by your hand being too sweaty, your hand not having direct contact with the sensor or the machine being improperly calibrated.

determine
your target heart rate

Your target heart rate indicates the range at which your heart should be beating while exercising. You should always try to train within this range to receive the full benefit of your workouts.

Calculate Your Target Heart Rate

To calculate your target heart rate, first determine your maximum heart rate by subtracting your age from 220. You will then need to calculate the top and bottom ends of your target heart rate.

To do so, multiply your maximum heart rate by percentages corresponding to your skill level. You can use the chart below to help you.

Your Maximum Heart Rate	SKILL LEVEL			Your Target Heart Rate
	Beginner	Intermediate	Advanced	
220 – your age = [ ]	x 0.65	x 0.80	x 0.90	= [ ] Top End
220 – your age = [ ]	x 0.50	x 0.65	x 0.70	= [ ] Bottom End

For example, if you are 30 years old and a beginner:

Maximum heart rate:	220 – 30 = 190
Top end of target heart rate:	190 x 0.65 = 124
Bottom end of target heart rate:	190 x 0.50 = 95

The next time you work out, check to see if your heart rate falls between the top and bottom ends of your target heart rate. If your heart rate is lower than the bottom end, you are not exercising hard enough. If your heart rate is higher than the top end, you are exercising too hard. If you are more fit, this calculation may not be as accurate. You should consult with a fitness professional, who can help determine a more accurate heart rate.

The "Talk" Test

The "talk" test is a very simple way of determining how hard you are exercising. If you are able to talk while exercising, you are training at the ideal intensity. However, if you have difficulty saying even a few words, you are exercising too hard.

Rate of Perceived Exertion (RPE)

Another way of gauging how hard you are exercising is to use the modified rate of perceived exertion (RPE) scale. The RPE is a simple, personal assessment that is measured on a scale of 1 to 10, where 1 indicates no effect and 10 indicates you are exhausted. The ideal RPE is from 4 to 8. Beginners should aim for an RPE of 3 to 4.

1	Nothing
2	Very Easy
3	Easy
4	Comfortable
5	Somewhat Difficult
6	Difficult
7	Hard
8	Very hard
9	Extremely hard
10	Exhausted

nutrition basics

Combining proper nutrition with exercise is the best way to maintain good health and stay in shape. Healthy eating does not have to be expensive, time consuming or painful. Eating properly is about moderation, balance and making the right choices. You can continue to eat the foods you love, but in moderation.

Essential Nutrients

Food is composed of five essential nutrients:
CARBOHYDRATES, PROTEIN, FAT, VITAMINS AND MINERALS.

CARBOHYDRATES

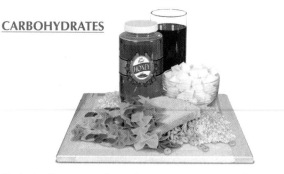

Carbohydrates are the primary energy source for your body and they come in two forms—simple and complex. Simple carbohydrates are easily converted into energy. They are found in foods rich in sugar, such as honey and fruit juice. Complex carbohydrates supply a slower and steadier release of energy into your body and are generally lower in calories than simple carbohydrates. Foods rich in complex carbohydrates include bread, cereals and pasta.

PROTEIN

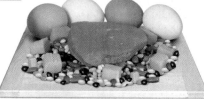

Protein is a main structural component of all muscle tissues and is needed for muscle growth and repair. Foods rich in protein include meat, fish, eggs, dairy products and legumes.

FAT

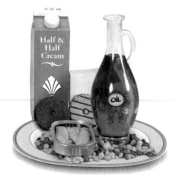

Your body needs a certain amount of fat to help maintain tissues and absorb vitamins A, D, E and K. However, avoid consuming foods with too much fat to prevent obesity and heart disease. The amount of fat in your diet should not amount to more than 30 percent of your total calories.

There are two types of fat—saturated and unsaturated. Consuming foods containing saturated fat can raise your blood cholesterol and increase your risk of heart disease. Foods that contain an abundance of saturated fat include meats, dairy products and coconut oil. Unsaturated fat is better for your body and is found in some fish, nuts and olive oil. You should also avoid hydrogenated fats, such as butter and shortening, which are commonly-used ingredients in cookies, crackers and other baked goods.

VITAMINS AND MINERALS

Vitamins and minerals are important for the everyday functions of your body and are needed to maintain good health. A varied, well-balanced diet that includes fruits, vegetables, grains and dairy products can provide most of the vitamins and minerals your body needs.

Water

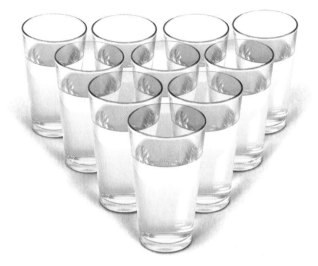

When you consider that approximately two-thirds of your body is composed of water, you can better understand why water is such an important part of a healthy diet. Drinking enough water every day can help you lose weight, help with digestion and help cleanse toxins from your body. The average person needs to drink at least 8 to 10 glasses of water each day. You may need to drink more water if you work out often or consume large quantities of coffee or alcohol, which can contribute to dehydration.

During exercise, water helps control your body's temperature and prevent overheating. You need to constantly replenish the water that your body loses through sweating when you exercise. To keep hydrated, you should drink plenty of water 20 to 30 minutes before, throughout and after your workouts.

Calories

A calorie is a unit of energy and is commonly used to measure the energy value of foods. These days, most food products have labels that indicate how many calories a serving of the food contains. The amount of calories that a person needs on a daily basis depends on the person's gender, age and level of activity. Older adults and sedentary women usually need about 1,600 calories a day. Active women, sedentary men, teenage girls and most children usually require about 2,200 calories a day. Active men, very active women and teenage boys usually need about 2,800 calories a day. When trying to lose weight, you should eat fewer fatty foods and consume fewer calories than what is normally recommended. However, to maintain your weight, you should consume as many calories as you burn during the day.

Salt and Sodium

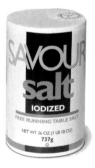

Your diet can include a moderate amount of salt and sodium, but should not exceed approximately 2,400 milligrams, which is equivalent to slightly more than one teaspoon of salt, each day. Eating foods that are high in sodium, such as soy sauce, fast food and canned soups and vegetables, can lead to high blood pressure. You should try to find low salt or no salt alternatives for these types of foods. When shopping for food, keep in mind that the more a food is processed, the more sodium it is likely to have. For example, a fresh pork loin has trace amounts of sodium, but ham or bacon is very high in sodium. A large portion of the sodium people consume comes from the salt they add to their food when cooking. When adding flavor to your food, you should consider using herbs and spices instead of salt.

nutrition basics

Cholesterol

Cholesterol is a substance similar to fat that is naturally produced in your body and stored in your liver. It is also found in meats, milk, poultry, egg yolks and fish. Eating too much of these types of foods can raise the cholesterol in your system and increase your risk of developing heart disease. To help limit the amount of cholesterol in your body, you should try to eat more foods that are low in saturated fat and cholesterol.

Sugar

You should avoid consuming foods rich in sugar as much as possible, since too much sugar can lead to obesity and tooth decay. Sweet foods, such as jams, cakes, canned fruits, chocolates, candies and soft drinks tend to have a lot of calories, but offer little else nutritionally. This is why calories from these sweet foods are sometimes referred to as empty calories.

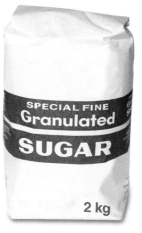

In addition to avoiding sweets, you should watch out for foods that have added sugars. Many common foods have sugar added in the form of white or brown sugar, molasses, honey or corn syrup. When reading food labels, try to look for foods that do not include these ingredients or that list these ingredients toward the end of the list, since ingredients are listed in order of quantity.

Caffeine

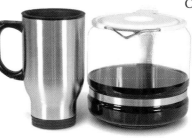

Caffeine is a stimulant that can temporarily boost energy levels, raise metabolism, elevate heart rate and blood pressure and increase mental alertness. You can find caffeine in chocolate and in various drinks, such as tea, coffee and soft drinks. It is important to take caffeine in moderation. The average diet should not contain more than 300 milligrams of caffeine, or the equivalent of 3 cups of coffee, per day. Too much caffeine can make you feel shaky and can cause sleeping problems. Instead of using caffeine to give you a boost, try other methods of increasing your energy levels, such as taking a brisk walk or getting a good night's sleep.

Alcohol

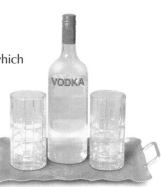

Alcohol is a depressant which slows down your body's ability to metabolize fats. Excessive consumption of alcohol can result in heart or liver disease, high blood pressure and some forms of cancer. Calories from alcohol are considered empty calories because they have little or no nutritional value. You should try to limit your intake of alcohol to 1 to 2 servings of alcohol per day. Twelve ounces of beer, 5 ounces of wine or a cocktail with 1 1/2 ounces of 80-proof spirits are all considered a standard serving of alcohol.

Fad Diets

You should always be wary of fad diets that offer quick-fix solutions and make unrealistic weight loss promises. Fad diets that restrict the consumption of certain foods may actually adversely affect your health by depriving your body of important vitamins and minerals. Some diets that require you to eat food with more protein and no carbohydrates may help you lose weight in the short term, but can be harmful to your body over time. When you go back to your normal diet, you end up gaining the weight back. Remember that to properly lose weight, you must exercise and eat a healthy, sensible diet.

Weight Training and Healthy Eating

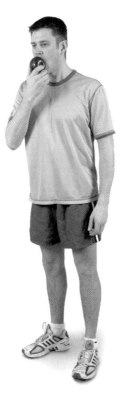

You should always try to eat enough food to give you the most energy for your workouts. However, do not eat too much food, as this can slow you down and cause stomachaches and cramps. It is best to wait about 2 hours after a meal before beginning your workout. You should also avoid going to the gym on an empty stomach. If you are hungry, you can eat a light snack, such as an energy bar or a banana, half an hour before working out.

Tips for Healthy Eating

* To help get all the vitamins and nutrients your body needs, you should eat a wide variety of food on a daily basis.

* You should eat slowly, chew your food thoroughly and stop eating as soon as you are full.

* Instead of having 3 large meals, try eating 5 or 6 small meals or snacks throughout the day.

* Keep healthy snacks, such as apples, bananas and carrot sticks, with you at all times so you will not be tempted to eat foods high in fat, sugar and calories.

* Learn to differentiate between hunger and cravings. If you are craving junk food, try eating a healthy alternative or satisfy your craving with a small portion of the food you desire.

* You should eat more fresh foods and avoid processed foods, which tend to be rich in fat, salt and calories.

* Do not go to the grocery store on an empty stomach. Also, remember to make a list of things you have to buy to avoid making unnecessary food purchases.

* When cooking or at the table, add fats, condiments and flavorings, such as butter, salad dressing, salt and sugar, in moderation.

* Avoid frying food. It is healthier to grill or broil food.

* Make a habit of reading food labels to learn more about the nutrition and ingredients of the foods you eat.

nutritional supplements

Although nutritional supplements can be useful to hard-core weight lifters and professional athletes, the average person would not benefit from taking nutritional supplements to build muscle mass and lose weight. If you decide to take nutritional supplements, make sure you carefully read the labels and research the products.

Some supplements, even those labeled "all-natural," may actually cause more harm than good, especially when taken in excessive amounts. Also, be aware of companies that make outrageous claims about their supplements. You can purchase nutritional supplements from gyms, health food stores and muscle magazines.

Creatine

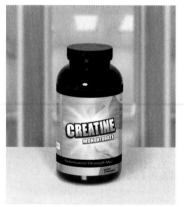

Creatine is used to enhance performance in activities which require explosive movements, such as hockey and power lifting. Creatine itself does not increase muscle mass, but helps you push harder. The extra weight gained when taking creatine comes mostly from water retention. When working out, creatine can give you that extra burst of energy to help you complete a few extra repetitions. The risks and benefits of creatine have not been fully proven.

Protein Supplements

Protein supplements can help repair muscles and increase their size. People who are training heavily to build muscle mass use protein supplements. Just be aware that taking too much can put stress on your kidneys. Instead of taking protein supplements, you should eat food rich in HBV (high biological value) protein, such as lean cuts of meat, chicken, fish and eggs.

Ephedra

People take ephedra to boost their metabolism and increase their heart rate. Ephedra is an unsafe supplement due to its harmful effects on the heart. It has been known to cause seizures and heart attacks and has been linked to several deaths. Many weight loss products contain ephedra, so read the labels carefully before taking any of these products.

Energy Bars

Energy bars are convenient snacks that contain a combination of carbohydrates, proteins and fats. Bars are a great source of energy when exercising for long periods of time or when you want a snack before going to the gym. If you are trying to lose weight, avoid eating energy bars on a regular basis since they are usually rich in calories.

Multivitamins

Multivitamins can provide you with the vitamins and minerals you may be missing from your regular diet. You do not need to take multivitamins if you are eating healthy, well-balanced meals.

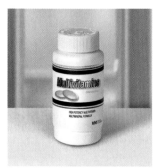

the food guide pyramid

The Food Guide Pyramid is a guideline of what you should eat each day to maintain good health. You can use the Pyramid as a guide to plan a healthy diet.

To obtain all the nutrients your body needs, you should eat at least the lowest number of servings for each of the major food groups. A serving size is not suggested for the Fats, Oils and Sweets Group, but you should make sure you eat these foods sparingly.

The serving suggestions for each group are a rough guide, since the ideal number of servings for each person may vary.

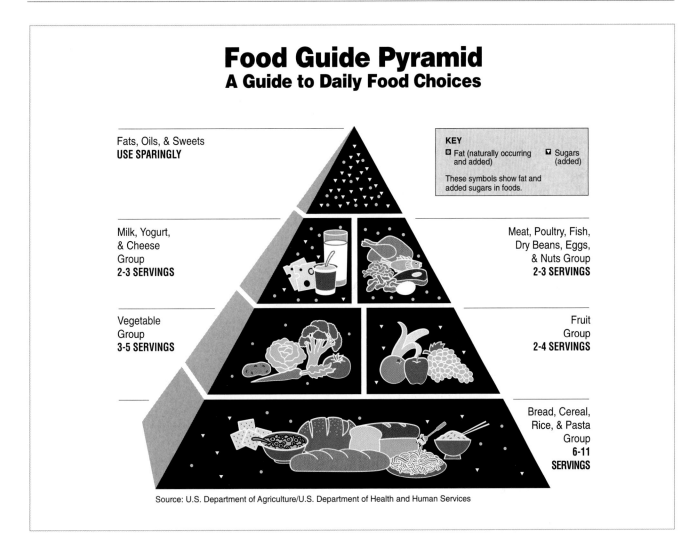

Food Guide Pyramid
A Guide to Daily Food Choices

Fats, Oils, & Sweets
USE SPARINGLY

KEY
▫ Fat (naturally occurring and added)   ✓ Sugars (added)

These symbols show fat and added sugars in foods.

Milk, Yogurt, & Cheese Group
2-3 SERVINGS

Meat, Poultry, Fish, Dry Beans, Eggs, & Nuts Group
2-3 SERVINGS

Vegetable Group
3-5 SERVINGS

Fruit Group
2-4 SERVINGS

Bread, Cereal, Rice, & Pasta Group
6-11 SERVINGS

Source: U.S. Department of Agriculture/U.S. Department of Health and Human Services

the food guide pyramid

Fats, Oils & Sweets

The Pyramid does not specify serving quantities for the Fats, Oils and Sweets Group, since you should consume these foods sparingly. Foods from this group include butter, margarine, cream, salad dressing, sugar, candy and desserts. These foods generally contain little or no nutrients and are high in calories.

Milk, Yogurt & Cheese Group
(2-3 servings)

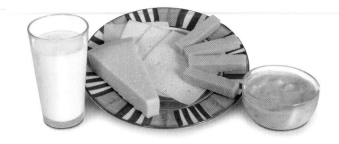

EXAMPLES
  1 cup of milk or yogurt
  1 1/2 ounces of natural cheese
  2 ounces of processed cheese

In addition to contributing protein, vitamins and minerals to your diet, this food group provides the best source of calcium. The nutrients you obtain from this group are essential to maintaining strong, healthy bones.

To avoid adding a lot of fat to your diet, you should choose milk products that are low in fat, such as skim milk, non-fat or low-fat yogurt and low-fat cheese.

Meat, Poultry, Fish, Dry Beans, Eggs & Nuts Group (2-3 servings)

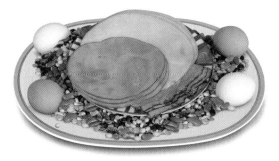

EXAMPLES
  2-3 ounces of cooked lean meat, poultry or fish (example: a hamburger or 1/2 a chicken breast)
  1/2 cup of cooked dry beans (about 1/3 serving)
  1 egg (about 1/3 serving)
  1/3 cup of nuts (about 1/3 serving)

The foods in this group provide a wealth of essential vitamins and minerals. Meat, poultry and fish contain protein, B vitamins, zinc and iron. Eggs, dry beans and nuts also contain protein and many vitamins and minerals.

Whenever possible, choose lower fat items such as lean meat, fish and dry beans and peas. Avoid processed foods, such as sausage, bacon, hot dogs and pepperoni, which are usually high in fat and sodium. Try to reduce the fat in cooked meat by trimming all visible fat before preparing. When preparing meat, you should roast, boil or broil instead of frying.

You can cut the fat in eggs and retain the nutrients by using only the egg whites and discarding the yolk, which contains most of the fat.

Vegetable Group (3-5 servings)

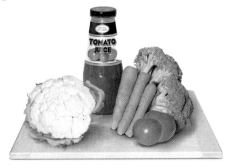

EXAMPLES

1 cup of raw leafy vegetables

1/2 cup of other vegetables, cooked or chopped raw

3/4 cup of vegetable juice

Vegetables supply vitamins, minerals and fiber and are naturally low in fat. Dark green and orange vegetables are especially rich in vitamins A and C. Fresh or frozen vegetables are better than canned vegetables. To preserve the nutrients, vegetables are best when not overcooked.

Fruit Group (2-4 servings)

EXAMPLES

1 medium apple, banana or orange

1/2 cup of chopped, cooked or canned fruit

3/4 cup of fruit juice

Fruit and fruit juices are important sources of vitamins A and C and potassium. Since different fruits contain different nutrients, you should eat a variety of fruits to maximize the nutrients you consume.

Although fruit and fruit juices are both low in fat and sodium, fruit contains more fiber and fewer calories than fruit juices.

Whenever possible, choose fresh, frozen or dried fruit. When choosing fruit juice, keep in mind that only 100 percent fruit juice counts as fruit.

Bread, Cereal, Rice & Pasta Group (6-11 servings)

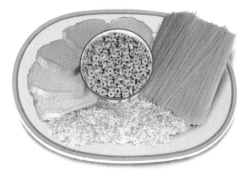

EXAMPLES

1 slice of bread

1 ounce of ready-to-eat cereal

1/2 cup of cooked cereal, rice or pasta

The foods in this group supply complex carbohydrates or starches, as well as vitamins, minerals and fiber, to your diet. Carbohydrates are a key energy source.

The majority of the calories in these foods often come from extra fats and sugars that are added during preparation, such as sauces, seasonings, spreads and toppings. Choose foods that are made without high-calorie additives, such as bread, rice and pasta and use toppings or high-fat seasonings in moderation.

Whole grain and enriched high-fiber products, such as whole grain bread, are best. The extra fiber they contain will not only keep you feeling satisfied longer, but has also been shown to help decrease blood cholesterol, promote regularity and prevent certain cancers. Baked goods such as cookies, cakes and pastries have a high sugar and fat content and should be eaten sparingly.

index

index

index

index

negative phase, of lowering weight, 236
negatives, weight training technique, 236
non-assisted
    chin-ups, 71
    dips, 39
nutrients, essential, 286
nutrition, overview, 286-289
nutritional supplements, 290

O

obliques
    external, location on body, 6, 7
    internal, location on body, 6
Olympic barbells
    for home gym, 11
    overview, 14
one-arm dumbbell row, 64-65
opposing muscle super sets, 242
osteoporosis, prevent though weight training, 4
outer hip
    exercises
        on cable machine, hip abduction, 155
        on exercise mat, side-lying leg lift, 152-153
        with exercise tubing, lying leg abduction, 208-209
        on multi-hip machine, hip abduction, 155
        using machines, hip abduction, 154-155
    stretches, 272-273
outer hips, location on body, 6
overhead press, 46-47
overuse injuries, overview, 246

P

pec
    deck machine, 43
    fly
        with exercise ball, 179
        on pec fly machine, 42-43
    fly/rear deltoid machine, 54-55
pectoralis
    major, location on body, 6
    minor, location on body, 6
pelvic tilt, 113
    with exercise ball, 195
personal trainers, choosing, 22-23
plank, 118-119
    side, 120-121
plate loaded machines, overview, 15
positive phase, of lifting weight, 236
power cage
    exercises for legs, barbell squat, 128
    overview 16

preacher
    curl, 98-99
        benches, overview, 16
progress, track for weight training, 244
Proprioceptive Neuromuscular Facilitation (PNF), 255
protein
    overview, 286
    supplements, overview, 290
pull split, 241
pull-ups, versus chin-ups, 71
pulse, 284
push split, 241
pushdown
    reverse-grip, 82-83
    triceps, 82-83
push-ups, 36-37
    with exercise ball, 181
    with exercise tubing, 212-213
    modified, 37
        with exercise tubing, 213
    to target triceps, 85
    wall, 37
pyramids, weight training technique, 237

Q

quadricep
    exercises
        with exercise ball
            lunges, 172-173
            wall squats, 170-171
        with exercise tubing, squats, 200-201
        lunges, 138-139
        step-ups, 140-141
        using free weights
            barbell squat, 128-129
            dumbbell squat, 126-127
        using machines
            hack squat, 130-131
            leg extension, 134-135
            leg press, 132-133
    stretches, 266-267
quadriceps, location on body, 6

R

rate of perceived exertion (RPE), 285
rear
    deltoid fly machine, 54-55
    shoulder exercises
        on cable machine, bent over lateral raise, 51
        with exercise ball, bent over lateral raise, 182-183
        with exercise tubing, bent over lateral raise, 215

index

Teach Yourself VISUALLY
WEIGHT TRAINING

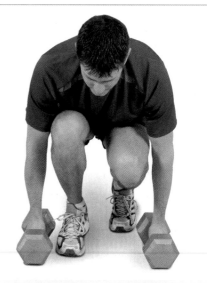

Teach Yourself VISUALLY Weight Training is an information-packed guide that covers all the basics of weight training, as well as more advanced techniques and exercises.

Teach Yourself VISUALLY Weight Training contains more than 500 full-color photographs of exercises for every major muscle group, along with clear, step-by-step instructions for performing the exercises. Useful tips provide additional information and advice to help enhance your weight training experience.

Teach Yourself VISUALLY Weight Training provides all the information you need to start weight training or to refresh your technique if you have been weight training for some time.

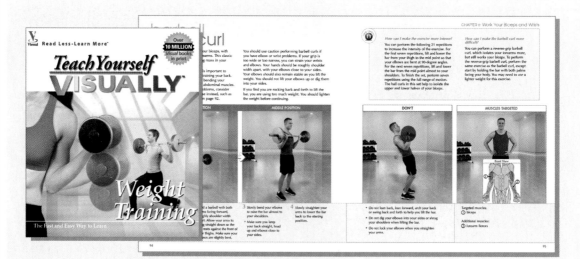

ISBN: 0-7645-2582-4
Price: $24.99 US; $36.99 CDN; $14.99 UK
Page count: 320

Teach Yourself VISUALLY
GUITAR

Teach Yourself VISUALLY Guitar is an excellent resource for people who want to learn to play the guitar, as well as for current musicians who want to fine tune their technique. This full-color guide includes over 500 photographs, accompanied by step-by-step instructions that teach you the basics of playing the guitar and reading music, as well as advanced guitar techniques. You will also learn what to look for when purchasing a guitar or accessories, how to maintain and repair your guitar, and much more.

Whether you want to learn to strum your favorite tunes or play professionally, Teach Yourself VISUALLY Guitar provides all the information you need to become a proficient guitarist.

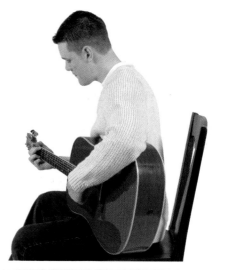

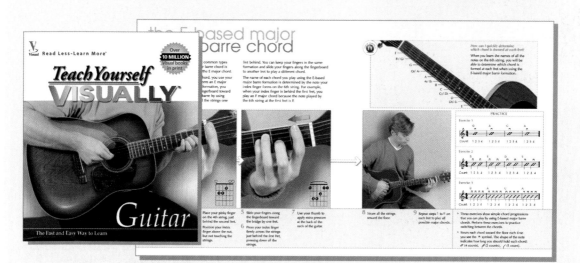

ISBN: 0-7645-2581-6
Price: $24.99 US; $36.99 CDN; $14.99 UK
Page count: 320

Teach Yourself VISUALLY
YOGA

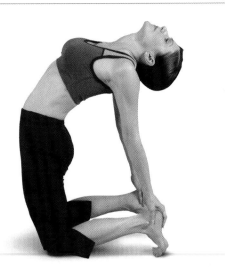

Teach Yourself VISUALLY Yoga provides a wealth of simplified, easy-to-follow information about the increasingly popular practice of Yoga. This easy-to-use visual guide is a must for visual learners who prefer to see and do without having to read lengthy explanations.

Using clear, step-by-step instructions accompanied by over 500 full-color photographs, this book includes all the information you need to get started with yoga or to enhance your technique if you have already made yoga a part of your life. Teach Yourself VISUALLY Yoga shows you how to safely and effectively perform a variety of yoga poses at various skill levels, how to breathe more efficiently, how to customize your yoga practice to meet your needs, and much more.

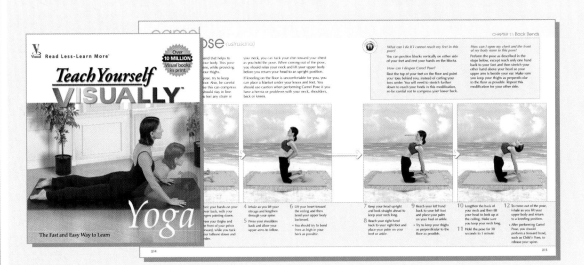

ISBN: 0-7645-2580-8

Price: $24.99 US; $36.99 CDN; $14.99 UK

Page count: 320